LIGAND ASSAY

Analysis of International Developments on Isotopic and Nonisotopic Immunoassay

Ligand Assay

Analysis of International Developments on Isotopic and Nonisotopic Immunoassay

edited by

John Langan, Ph.D.
President, Princeton Medical Services
Princeton, New Jersey

and

Jeremy J. Clapp, Ph.D.
Division of Clinical Biochemistry
Mount Sinai Hospital
Toronto, Ontario, Canada

MASSON Publishing USA, Inc.
New York • Paris • Barcelona • Milan • Mexico City • Rio de Janeiro

Library of Congress Cataloging in Publication Data
Main entry under title:

Ligand assay.

Bibliography: p.
Includes index.
1. Radioimmunoassay. 2. Immunoassay.
3. Immunodiagnosis. 4. Biological chemistry—
Technique I. Langan, John, 1932-
II. Clapp, Jeremy J.
OP519.9.R3L52 616.07'57 80-39663
ISBN 0-89352-094-2

ISBN 0-89352-094-2

Library of Congress Catalog Card Number: 80-39663

Printed in the United States of America

Contributors

F. R. Bishai, PhD
Laboratory Services Branch
Ontario Ministry of Health
Box 9000
Toronto, Ontario, Canada

R. C. Boguslaski, MD
Ames Research Laboratory
Ames Division
Miles Laboratories, Inc.
P.O. Box 70
Elkhart, IN

E. S. Bos, PhD
Organon Scientific Development Group
Oss, The Netherlands

A. Broughton, MD
Vice President
Nichols Institute
1300 S. Beacon St.
San Pedro, CA

R. J. Carrico, MD
Ames Research Laboratory
Ames Division
Miles Laboratories, Inc.
P.O. Box 70
Elkhart, IN

R. D. Falb, MD
Ames Research Laboratory
Ames Division
Miles Laboratories, Inc.
P.O. Box 70
Elkhart, IN

T. C. J. Gribnau, MD
Organon Scientific Development Group
Oss, The Netherlands

J. Landon
Professor, Department of Clinical Pathology
The Medical College of St. Bartholomew's Hospital
London, England

A. L. Nichols, MD
Nichols Institute
1300 S. Beacon St.
San Pedro, CA

P. Rathnam, MD
Cornell University Medical College
Department of Medicine
Division of Endocrinology
1300 York Ave.
New York, NY

D. Rodbard, MD
Biophysical Endocrinology Section
Endocrinology and Reproduction Research Branch
National Institute of Child Health and Human Development
National Institutes of Health
Bethesda, MD

E. Rosemberg, MD
The Medical Research Institute of Worcester, Inc.
The Worcester City Hospital
University of Massachusetts Medical School
Worcester, MA

J. Savory, PhD
Departments of Pathology and Biochemistry
University of Virginia Medical Center
Charlottesville, VA

B. B. Saxena, MD
Cornell University Medical College
Department of Medicine
Division of Endocrinology
1300 York Ave.
New York, NY

R. S. Schneider, PhD
Syva Research Institute
3181 Porter Drive
Palo Alto, CA

H. R. Schroeder, MD
Ames Research Laboratory
Ames Division
Miles Laboratories Inc.
P.O. Box 70
Elkhart, IN

A. H. W. M. Schuurs, PhD
Organon Scientific Development Group
Oss, The Netherlands

E. F. Ullman, MD
Syva Research Institute
3181 Porter Drive
Palo Alto, CA

B. Van Weeman, PhD
Organon Scientific Development Group
Oss, The Netherlands

K.-K. Yeung, MD
Ames Research Laboratory
Ames Division
Miles Laboratories Inc.
P.O. Box 70
Elkhart, IN

M. Young, MD
Department of Biochemistry and Molecular Biology
University of Florida
College of Medicine
Gainesville, FL

Contents

Chapter 1

Introduction to Nonisotopic Ligand Immunoassays

J. LANDON

INTRODUCTION

As the name implies, an immunoassay is an analytical procedure based on the use of an antibody, while the term nonisotopic immunoassay (NIIA) denotes that none of the reactants are labeled with a radioisotope. This chapter will classify the place of immunoassays with regard to other analytical techniques, suggest an appropriate terminology, briefly discuss some of the existing NIIA procedures, and consider their general advantages and disadvantages as compared with radioimmunoassay (RIA). Finally, a personal view will be given as to the present role of NIIA.

Analytical procedures can be classified into three broad categories,[28] namely, biological techniques (also termed bioassays), those based on physical and/or chemical methods, and others that depend upon the noncovalent binding of one reactant by another (Table 1). The term binding assay is employed to cover the latter, which comprise a variety of methods that depend upon the specific reaction between a ligand and a binding protein and which obey the Law of Mass Action:

$$\underset{\text{(free fraction)}}{L + BP} \underset{k_2}{\overset{k_1}{\rightleftharpoons}} \underset{\text{(bound fraction)}}{L:BP}$$

Department of Chemical Pathology, The Medical College of St. Bartholomew's Hospital, London EC1A 7BE, U.K.

Table 1. A General Classification of Analytical Techniques with Especial Reference to Binding Assays

Analytical techniques

- Bioassays
- Binding assays
  - For binding protein
  - For ligand
    - (i) Employing antibodies as binding protein (immunoassay)
    - (ii) Employing receptor proteins
    - (iii) Employing natural circulating binding proteins
- Physical/chemical assays

← Assess Function → ← Assess Structure →

where L represents the ligand, BP the binding protein, and L:BP the bound complex. At equilibrium, some of the free reactants will be combining with a rate constant k_1 to form more of the complex, while some of the complex will be dissociating, with a rate constant k_2, to give free ligand and binding protein. Such assays can be subdivided into immunoassays (in which the binding protein is a specific antibody and the ligand an antigen), receptor binding protein assays (in which the receptor protein is usually extracted from the target organ of a hormone or drug), and circulating binding protein assays, employing a naturally occurring plasma protein, for example, thyroxine binding globulin (TBG) for the assay of thyroxine (T_4) and transcortin for the assay of cortisol or progesterone.

Immunoassays are by far the most common form of binding assay,[30] because antibodies can be raised against an immense range of compounds; they display marked structural specificity; the high affinity with which antibodies bind their appropriate antigen enables great sensitivity to be achieved and, indeed, sets the ultimate sensitivity that can be attained; and, finally, they can be employed to determine the concentration of an antigen or, as discussed briefly in the next section, to detect the presence of antibodies.

It should be noted that estimates of concentration based on biological activity or *function* may differ significantly from estimates using an immunoassay. This is because the latter are *structural* assays which, indeed, assess only part of the antigen's structure — termed the antigenic determinant. In the case of a peptide or protein, the antigenic determinant (that part of the molecule bound by the antibody) comprises only some four to six amino acids and, for example, most

RIAs will determine any circulating prohormone, the hormone itself, and any fragments of the hormone which contain the antigenic determinant. In contrast, bioassays will usually determine only the hormone itself. An elegant example of bioassay, immunoassay dissociation follows cleavage of the S–S ring of oxytocin or arginine vasopressin, which causes a complete loss of biological activity but does not effect most RIA results.

It follows from the above that values obtained by bioassay may be lower than those determined by RIA. Furthermore, the cytochemical group of bioassays, introduced by Chayen and his colleagues,[24] are more sensitive than RIA and can, for example, detect plasma levels of adrenocorticotrophin as low as 20 fg (1 fg = 10^{-15} g) per ml and be applied to heelprick samples from neonates.[36] Physical and chemical methods (like immunoassays) depend upon the structure of the compound to be determined, such as the need for a hydroxyl group in the 11 position of the steroid nucleus in the fluorimetric assay for cortisol described by Mattingly.[55] Some of the techniques, including gas chromatography/mass spectroscopy, are both more specific and sensitive than RIA. For example, one such method can routinely measure 50 fg of prostaglandin $F_{2\alpha}$ with a precision of $\pm 10\%$.[80] However, none of these assays approach the practicality and wide application of RIA and related analytical techniques.

GENERAL CLASSIFICATION OF IMMUNOASSAY PROCEDURES

Immunoassays are commonly considered as techniques for the detection and quantitation of antigens. However, as stated earlier, they can be used to determine the presence of antibodies. Indeed, Berson and his colleagues' pioneer work in RIA followed their use of ^{131}I-labeled insulin to demonstrate circulating antibodies in patients treated with insulin.[11] A similar approach was later adopted to show that the failure of several dwarfed children to maintain their response to early preparations of relatively impure human growth hormone (HGH) was due to antibody production, and such assays are also being employed to enable the rapid detection of antibodies against other hormones, including porcine and salmon calcitonin, arginine vasopressin and adrenocorticotrophin,[44] and against other proteins of interest to endocrinologists, such as human antibodies to thyroglobulin.[62] For reasons of space, they will not be discussed further.

Immunoassays for the detection and quantitation of antigen can be categorized into those in which no labeled reactant is required, those employing labeled antigen, and others in which specific antibodies are labeled (Table 2).

Table 2. A General Classification of Immunoassays

A. For the detection of antibodies
B. For the quantitation of antigens
   1. Employing no labeled reactant
   2. Employing labeled antigen (including radioimmunoassay)
      With a separation step
      With no separation step
   3. Employing labeled antibodies (including immunoradiometric assays)
      Single site
      Two site sandwich techniques

Nonlabeled Immunoassays

Several immunoassay techniques do not require the use of a labeled reactant. One group depends on the precipitin line that forms in a gel support when a protein antigen comes into contact with its specific antibody, such as immunoelectrophoresis and radial immunodiffusion. For example, the rocket system described by Laurell has been employed to assay serum TBG levels, and several hundred samples can be run in a working week, with a coefficient of variation less than 5%.[13] A second group comprise manual and automated assays for many of the plasma proteins in which the formation of antigen:antibody complexes is detected by the increase in light scattering produced. Recent developments in this general area include a kinetic approach and the use of a laser beam as the light source; the application of such nephelometric techniques is discussed in a later chapter by J. Savory.

Despite their relative simplicity, nonlabeled immunoassays have several limitations because of the need to form very large antigen:antibody complexes for these to be detectable. Thus they are applicable only to the assay of proteins (since hapten:antibody complexes do not form a precipitin line or scatter light), and high concentrations of such proteins must be present, which limits their sensitivity to the micromole per liter (μmol/liter) or upper nanomole per liter (nmol/liter) range. These nonlabeled immunoassays also employ relatively high concentrations of monospecific antisera. They are not, unless a kinetic endpoint or "blank" measurement is made, suitable for very turbid or hemolyzed samples. Finally, they may give spurious results in the presence of antigen excess, due to the prozone phenomenon.

Immunoassays Employing Labeled Antigen

The development of the first RIA, for insulin, by Yalow and Berson[82] in 1960 has proved to be an important milestone, because use of antigen labeled with an isotope has enabled the assay of haptens (such as drugs and the steroid and thyroid hormones) as well as proteins; resulted in a millionfold increase in sensitivity; removed the need for monospecific antisera and markedly reduced the concentration of antisera required; overcome the problem of antigen excess and enabled the assay of hemolyzed and turbid samples by both manual and automated procedures. In the same year Ekins had recognized the wider implications of binding assays, and developed techniques for both serum T_4[29] and vitamin B_{12},[7] employing circulating carrier proteins. His use of the general term "saturation analysis" and, more recently, "limited reagent methods" was to indicate that the concentration of binding protein must be insufficient to bind all the ligand.[30] The labeled antigen is employed as a tracer to enable determination of the distribution of total antigen between the antibody bound and unbound (free) fractions. If the amounts of labeled reactant and of antiserum are kept constant, then the percentage of the counts present in the bound fraction will be inversely related to the initial amount of unlabeled ligand in the standards or samples being assayed.

The dominant reactant in all immunoassays for antigens is the antibody, since it is this which, in large part, determines both the specificity and ultimate sensitivity that can be achieved; the latter, as mentioned earlier, depending on the affinity with which the antibody binds the antigen. The labeled antigen is employed only as a tracer, and any label is suitable provided (1) its determination is relatively simple and sufficiently sensitive for the purpose to which the assay will be applied, (2) there are no significant problems with other materials present in the sample, (3) means are available to link the label to the antigen, and (4) the antibody does not distinguish significantly between labeled and unlabeled antigen.[43]

Immunoassays Employing Labeled Antibody

In 1968 Miles and Hales introduced a new type of immunoassay, which they termed immunoradiometric analysis (IRMA), based on the use of isotopically labeled specific antibodies. Such antibodies were prepared by affinity chromatography on columns containing the antigen covalently linked to a support, radioiodinated on the column (to prevent introduction of isotope into their binding sites), and then eluted for use. In an assay, standards or unknown samples are incubated with an excess of labeled antibody and, after equilibrium has been attained, the unused labeled antibody is removed by affinity chromatography and the bound fraction counted. They employed the technique successfully for both the assay of insulin and human growth hormone.[56-58]

IRMA differs markedly from RIA as an analytical technique (Table 3). In the standard procedure only two, not three, reactants are required and, of course, antibody as opposed to antigen is labeled. Since excessive

Table 3. Differences Between Radioimmunoassay and Immunoradiometric Analysis

IRMA	RIA
Ag + Ab* ⇌ Ag:Ab*	Ag + Ag* + Ab ⇌ Ag:Ab:Ag*
Two reactants	Three reactants
Employs labeled antibody	Employs labeled antigen
Separate bound and free antibodies	Separate bound and free antigens
Counts in bound fraction *directly* related to initial concentration of antigen	Counts in bound fraction *inversely* related to initial concentration of antigen
Reagent excess technique, therefore: 1. Rapid 2. Pipetting accuracy not critical	Limited reagent technique, therefore: 1. Slow 2. Pipetting accuracy critical
No problems in labeling antibodies	May have problems in labeling some antigens
Labeled antibodies have long shelf life	Some labeled antigens have short shelf life
Can employ only high affinity antibodies with improved sensitivity	Employ both high and low affinity antibodies

amounts of labeled antibody are added to ensure that all the hormone is bound, IRMA can be defined as a "reagent excess" procedure as distinct from the "limited reagent" techniques described above. It is necessary to separate the antibody (as opposed to the antigen) in the bound form from that in the free fraction and, finally, the counts in the bound fraction are related *directly* to the total amount of antigen present, in contrast to the *inverse* relationship characteristic of RIA. These differences offer several advantages in favor of IRMA. The labeled antibodies are, in general, more stable than labeled antigens and are relatively easy to prepare, whereas difficulties may arise in iodinating haptens, fragile antigens, or peptides lacking tyrosine or histidine residues.[67] Use of a reagent excess shortens the time necessary to reach equilibrium (which depends on the concentrations of the various reactants) and, since it is possible to employ only the high affinity antibodies in an antiserum, there is a potential (though seldom realized) gain in sensitivity. However, considerable expertise is required to prepare the immunoadsorbants and labeled antibodies, and IRMA is more wasteful of antisera than RIA.

In addition to conventional IRMA, "sandwich" techniques have been developed for the assay of large molecules with more than one antigenic determinant, an approach pioneered by Wide and his colleagues,[79] and shown to be suitable for the assay of such hormones as human growth hormone[1] and follicle stimulating hormone.[65] The standard or sample is first incubated with an excess of an antibody covalently linked to an insoluble support and directed against one antigenic determinant. After careful washing, excess of a second, isotopically labeled antibody directed against another part of the molecule is added (Fig. 1a) and, after further washes, the counts present in the bound fraction can be determined and will be related *directly* to the amount of antigen added. Such "sandwich" techniques have the advantage of improved specificity, since fragments of an antigen containing only one of the antigenic determinants will not affect the result. Subsequently, Beck and Hales[9] further modified "sandwich" assays for HGH, insulin, glucagon, and parathyroid hormone (PTH) by adding an excess of an isotopically labeled second antibody. This has the merit that, for example, labeled goat antirabbit gamma globulin sera can be used for all assays based on a rabbit first antibody (Fig. 1b).

TYPES OF NONISOTROPIC IMMUNOASSAY

The number of different materials that have been employed to label the antigen or antibody for immunoassay procedures is increasing rapidly and includes gamma and beta emitting isotopes; free radicals;

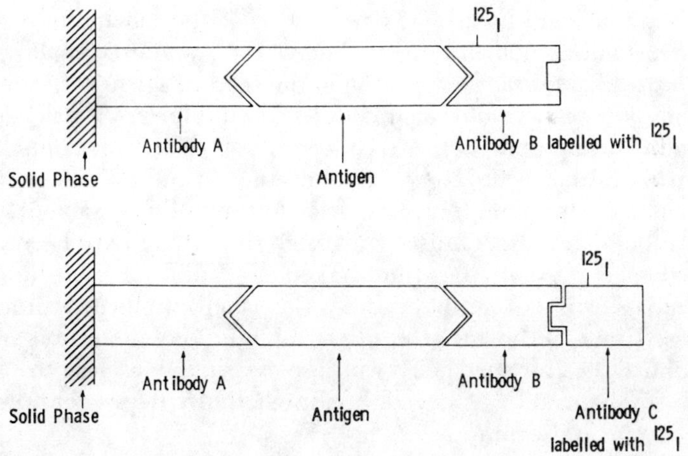

Fig. 1a. Representation of a "sandwich" immunoradiometric assay for an antigen with two antigenic determinants. Antibody A, attached to a solid phase, is directed against one determinant, and antibody B, which is labeled with ^{125}I, is directed against the other.

Fig. 1b. The principle of "sandwich" immunoradiometric assays employing a common label, similar to Fig. 1a, except that antibody A, in addition to being directed against a different antigenic determinant than antibody B, is from a different species. For example, antibody A may be raised in a sheep and antibody B in a rabbit, in which case a third antibody (c), labeled with ^{125}I would be added, which is directed against rabbit immunoglobulins.

enzymes; coenzymes and enzyme inhibitors; viruses; proteins; fluorescent, bioluminescent, and chemiluminescent molecules; red blood cells; and latex and other particles. Considerable confusion is inevitable unless a terminology is employed that, for example, clearly distinguishes whether what is being referred to is an RIA for an enzyme or an immunoassay employing an enzyme as the label.

Any terminology should give regard to the names suggested by the originators, to the suitability of any likely acronym and, in particular, to the principles involved. Thus the term radioimmunoassay and its acronym RIA is excellent in that it signifies that a radioisotope is employed and that the assay is based on an immunological reaction. It is suggested that NIIA, in which the antigen is labeled other than isotopically, should follow this convention; for example, enzymoimmunoassay (EIA), fluoroimmunoassay (FIA), and viroimmunoassay (VIA). The term immunoradiometric analysis and its acronym IRMA is also well known and well suited for immunoassays employing specific antibodies labeled with an isotope. Thus it would seem correct to employ similar terms for NIIA, such as immunoenzymometric assays (IEMA) and immunofluorometric assays (IFMA), involving the use of specific antibodies labeled with enzymes and with fluorogenic molecules, respectively.

All manual immunoassays, irrespective of the label employed, have much in common, including the need for standards, quality control samples, and antisera; the addition of the reactants in a set order, usually in μl amounts; a period of incubation until equilibrium is reached, which depends, in large part, on the concentration of the reactants and may vary from minutes (for compounds present in the μmol/liter range) to several days (for compounds in the low pmol/liter range); and the calculation of results. It must be stressed, since there have been claims to the contrary,[46] that the time taken to attain equilibrium in an immunoassay is not influenced by the label employed (although, as discussed below, the time required for endpoint detection may vary substantially). The specificity will also be similar as will the ultimate sensitivity that can be achieved, because both are dependent predominantly on the antiserum used.

Employing Labeled Antigen and a Separation Step

All immunoassays employing labeled antigen involve the series of steps listed in Table 4. Of these only two, the separation step and the method of endpoint detection, may vary, depending on the label. The term "homogeneous" has been suggested for those immunoassays that do not require separation of the antibody-bound and free fractions prior to endpoint detection, and "heterogeneous" for those, including RIA, in which a separation step is essential. These terms have other connotations

Table 4. Essential Steps in Immunoassays Employing Labeled Antigen

1. Addition of sample (or standard) labeled antigen and appropriate dilution of antiserum
2. Incubation until equilibrium is achieved (other than with some automated systems)
3. Separation of antibody-bound and free antigen[a]
4. Endpoint detection of the label in the antibody-bound and/or free fraction[a]
5. Calculation of results

[a]The only steps that may vary dependent on the label employed.

to some immunoassayists, and it would seem preferable, therefore, to classify NIIA employing labeled antigen into a separation and nonseparation group (Table 5).

For those assays requiring separation of the bound and free fractions, this step can serve a second important function, namely, to separate the exogenous compound being employed as the label from any endogenous compounds in the sample that have similar effects or from any other constituents in the sample, such as enzyme inhibitors, which could affect the signal. Indeed, only if such background influences are removed can the sensitivity of present-day EIA, based on the amplification that is inherent in all enzyme substrate reactions, approach that of RIA.

Such assays have a specificity similar to RIA, which is inherent in all analytical techniques involving use of an antibody. Furthermore, some separation NIIAs, including EIA, are able to determine serum levels of compounds such as thyroid stimulating hormone (TSH), which lie in the low pmol/liter range, which shows that the same sensitivity can be

Table 5. Classification of Immunoassays Employing Labeled Antigen

A. Requiring a separation step, such as RIA and ELISA
B. Not requiring a separation step
   1. Due to antibody binding changing the nature of the signal (such as FRAT)
   2. Due to antibody binding decreasing the signal
      - Direct quenching (some examples of EMIT)
      - Excitation transfer[a]
      - Release immunoassays
   3. Due to antibody binding increasing the signal
      - Enhancement
      - Indirect quenching
      - Polarization fluorescence[a]

[a]Applicable only to FIA.

attained as by RIA. It is important to appreciate that no NIIA can achieve a *greater* sensitivity than RIA. Thus the sensitivity of any immunoassay is ultimately set by the affinity with which the antibody binds the antigen. Use of gamma-emitting isotope to label an antigen, or antibody, enables this sensitivity to be obtained.

Employing Labeled Antigen and No Separation Step

It is perhaps surprising that the first nonseparation NIIA was described in 1953, several years before the introduction of RIA (Stavitsky and Arquilla, 1953). Thus Stavitsky and Arquilla[72] employed insulin labeled with erythrocytes to detect the presence of antibodies in diabetics treated with insulin and to assay nanogram (ng) amounts of insulin in buffer. Following incubation, complement (in the form of guinea pig serum) was added and caused lysis of erythrocytes in the bound, but not in the free, fraction; the resultant release of hemoglobin into the supernatant was then quantitated spectrophotometrically. The assay was not sufficiently sensitive to detect insulin in biological fluids, and little further attention was given to nonseparation NIIA until the development of a spin immunoassay procedure by Leute and his colleagues in 1972.[45] They employed morphine labeled with a free radical and determined the change in electron spin resonance that followed antibody binding for the detection of morphine in urine, which they termed the *free radical assay technique* (FRAT).

Nonseparation NIIAs depend on antibody binding either changing the nature of the signal (as with free radical labeling), decreasing the signal, or increasing the signal. No other possibilities exist, and if one of these three changes does not result, then a separation step is essential.

DIRECT QUENCHING

Figure 2 represents a direct quenching EIA of the type first introduced by the Syva Corporation. The antibody in the bound fraction can be considered (probably naively) to sterically hinder the reaction between the substrate and the active site of the enzyme, so that only the free fraction retains full enzymatic activity. Several examples of FIA and VIA of this type have also been described with, in the former, antibody binding either impairing the excitation of, or emission from, the fluorogenic molecule and, in the latter, impeding the fixation of the virus to the bacteria.

ENHANCEMENT

In direct contrast to quenching EIA, other assays exist of the "enhancement" type, in which antibody binding potentiates the activity of the enzyme employed to label the antigen (Fig. 3). In one example, the tracer is a thyroxine derivative covalently linked to malate dehydrogenase, of beef or pork heart origin, such that the enzyme has little activity. However, there is a marked increase in enzymatic activity following addition of antibodies raised against T_4, enabling the assay of T_4 employing only 50 μl of serum, with results that correlate well with those of RIA. An enhancement FIA for T_4 has also been described,[70] in which fluorescein-labeled T_4 was found to give an abnormally low fluorescence yield, probably due to intramolecular quenching of the fluorophore by the iodine-containing thyroxine moiety. A fourfold increase in fluorescence was caused by antibody binding (presumably by inhibiting the quenching effect) and served as the basis of an FIA.

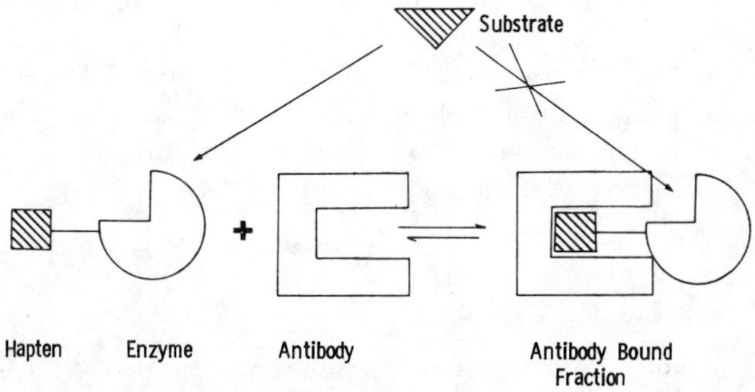

Fig. 2. Representation of a direct quenching enzymoimmunoassay, in which the enzyme activity in the bound fraction is impaired due to the antibody sterically hindering the reaction between the enzyme and its substrate.

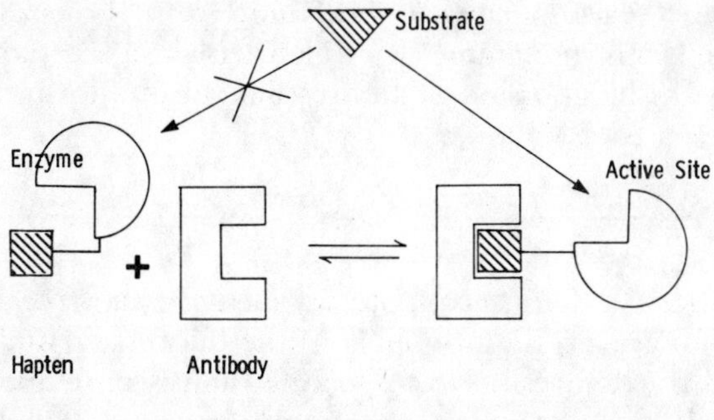

Fig. 3. Representation of an enhancement enzymoimmunoassay, in which the enzyme activity in the bound fraction is enhanced following antibody binding.

Indirect Quenching

The techniques described above are applicable only to the assay of haptens since, for example, antibody binding of a protein labeled with a fluorophore rarely results in any significant change in fluorescence intensity,[25] probably because of the distance between the antigenic determinant and the site of label attachment (Fig. 4b). Nonetheless, it has proved possible to develop nonseparation FIA for proteins based on an indirect approach, which makes use of the fact that binding of fluorescein-labeled compounds[47,78] by antifluorescein sera causes virtually complete quenching of fluorescence.

Sample (or standard), labeled antigen and antibody are incubated and, after equilibrium has been attained, an excess of the antifluorescein sera is added. This immediately binds to, and quenches, the fluorescence of the free fraction but, because of steric hindrance by the first antibody, is unable to bind the fluorescein label in the bound fraction (Fig. 4c), which continues to fluoresce. Indirect quenching FIAs have been developed for human albumin,[59] immunoglobulin G and placental lactogen.[60] This indirect quenching approach should also be applicable to other labels. Thus, for example, enzymes are excellent immunogens,[44] and the resultant antibodies often inhibit enzyme activity.

Polarization Fluorescence

This technique was described independently by two groups[26,71] and will not be discussed further at this point since it is the subject of a separate chapter by R. Spencer.

Excitation Transfer

This novel approach, introduced by the Syva Corporation,[76] involves the use of one reactant labeled with fluorescein (F) as donor, and a second labeled with rhodamine (R), which acts as an acceptor because of its overlap with the emission of fluorescein. In one form, the reaction can be represented as follows:

$$\mathrm{Ag-F+AB-R} \quad \rightleftharpoons \quad \mathrm{Ag-F:Ab-R}$$

Upon excitation at the appropriate wavelength, the free fraction will give a signal; however, the proximity of the fluorescein and rhodamine in the bound fraction results in up to 70% fluorescence quenching, due to energy transfer to the acceptor molecule by a dipole-dipole resonance mechanism.

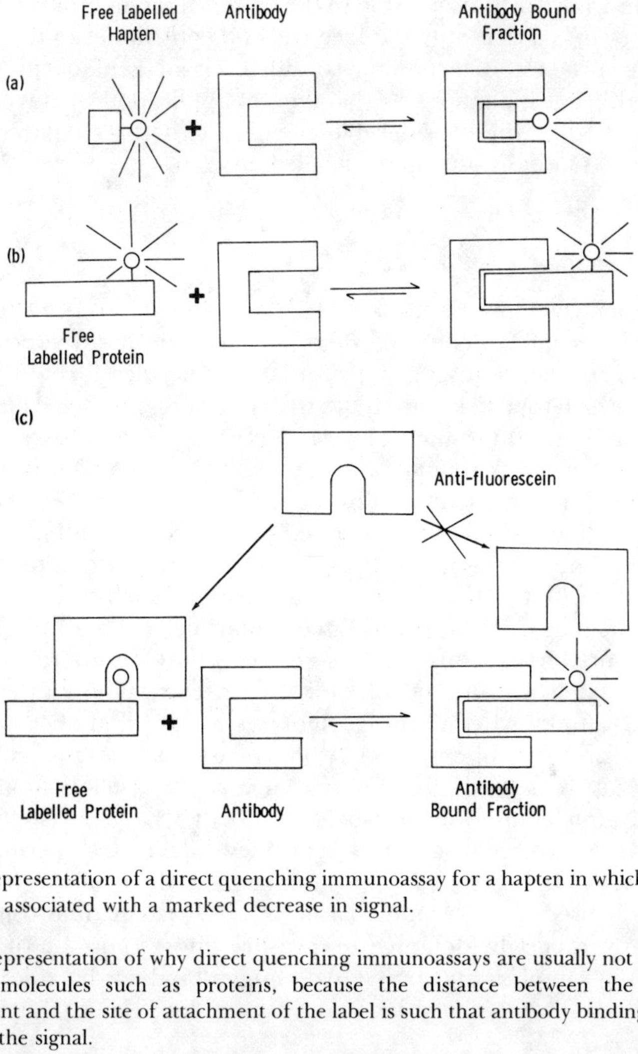

Fig. 4a. Representation of a direct quenching immunoassay for a hapten in which antibody binding is associated with a marked decrease in signal.

Fig. 4b. Representation of why direct quenching immunoassays are usually not applicable to large molecules such as proteins, because the distance between the antigenic determinant and the site of attachment of the label is such that antibody binding does not influence the signal.

Fig. 4c. Representation of an indirect quenching immunoassay in which an antiserum to the label is added to Fig. 4b. This binds to and completely quenches the signal in the free fraction, but does not bind to the label in the bound fraction because of steric hindrance by the first antibody.

Release Immunoassays

Another type of nonseparation NIIA, introduced by Burd and colleagues,[15] involves the use of a nonfluorescent labeled antigen that releases a fluorophore when split by an appropriate hydrolytic enzyme.

Steric hindrance by the antibody in the bound fraction inhibits the action of the enzyme so that only the free fraction contributes to the signal. A practical assay for determining serum levels of gentamicin has been described,[16] but limitations to the general application of this approach may prove to be the considerable chemical expertise required for the design and synthesis of suitable labeled antigens.

Employing Labeled Antibodies

Immunoenzymometric assays (IEMA), similar to two-site IRMA except with regard to endpoint detection, have been developed,[8,51,77] as have assays of the "sandwich" type for large molecules, including rat and human alpha fetoprotein with more than one antigenic determinant.[10,52]

Early immunofluorometric assays (IFMA) were based on the precipitin reaction and separation of the bound complex from excess unreacted labeled antibody by centrifugation[35,73] or filtration.[61] Techniques have also been developed in which the binding of labeled antibodies onto antigens attached to the surface of paper disks is assessed by a fluorimeter designed to measure surface fluorescence[74] and in which agarose beads and microfluorimetry are employed.[21,28,39] Most recent work has involved use of the sandwich approach. Excess antibody attached to a solid phase is first used to bind all the antigen from the sample. After washing, fluorescent-labeled antibody is added in excess, and that bound to the solid phase, via the antigen, gives a direct measurement of the amount of antigen. Quantitation can be achieved after elution of the labeled antibodies from the solid phase.[2] Alternatively, techniques have been developed that permit direct fluorimetry of fluorescent antibody on the solid phase, of which the most extensively used is the commercial FIAX/StiQ system. This comprises a fluorimeter especially designed to measure fluorescence on the surface of the StiQ samplers and individual antigen-binding disks designed to facilitate the several incubation and washing steps required in assays of this type.

All the labeled antibody techniques so far described in this chapter have required a separation step. However, Ullman and his colleagues[76] have successfully developed a nonseparation IFMA based on fluorescent excitation transfer for large antigens, such as proteins with more than one antigenic determinant. Thus one population of highly specific antibodies directed against human IgG was labeled with fluorescein (F) and another population with rhodamine (R). When an excess of both were added to the sample,

$$\mathrm{Ag + Ab - R + Ab - F \quad \rightleftharpoons \quad Ab - R : Ag : Ab - F}$$

Only the free fractions fluoresced fully, quenching in the bound fraction resulting from energy transfer from the donor (F) to the acceptor (R). This differs from the excitation transfer FIA described earlier in that only labeled antibodies are employed, with no labeled antigen.

As with IRMA, the expertise necessary to first isolate and then label specific antibodies, together with the relatively large amounts of antiserum needed, explains the limited number of publications relating to the nonisotopic labeling of antibodies as compared with antigens.

TYPES OF NONISOTOPIC LABEL EMPLOYED

Most work relating to NIIA has been based on the use of enzymes, fluorescent molecules, and bacteriophages for labeling. These together with bioluminescent immunoassay systems are considered later in this volume and will only be discussed briefly. Some attention will also be given to a few other labels.

Enzymes

A later chapter by A. Bosch and B. Van Weeman deals with the coupling of enzymes to proteins, and another chapter by F. Bishai deals with EIA requiring a separation step and termed *enzyme labeled immunosorbent assays* (ELISA). These are similar to RIA, other than that a different endpoint detection system is required. An enzyme also differs from a radioisotope in terms of its size, so that there is less difference between the bound and free fractions with regard to molecular weight and charge.[41] In general, this lack of difference limits the separation procedures that can be applied to those based on addition of a second antibody, or to solid phase systems in which the first antibody is absorbed onto, or covalently bound to, an insoluble matrix or to a combination of the two, such as the *double antibody solid phase* (DASP) system.

The subject of nonseparation EIA of the direct quenching and enhancement types, termed the *enzyme multiplied immunoassay technique* (EMIT) will be reviewed in a later chapter by R. Schneider.

Fluorogenic Molecules

The general subject of FIA is considered later in this volume by R. Schneider, and the basis of some nonseparation techniques has already been discussed. This is the area of NIIA with which our group has had the most experience, and more than 15 assays have been developed. Several are of the direct or indirect quenching type. However, for antigen circulating in the nmol/liter range (such as cortisol and thyroxine), it is necessary to employ a separation step, while for those in the pmol/liter range (such as estradiol 17β and dihydrotestosterone) a polylabel is also required.

Bacteriophages

The term bacteriophage is applied to a virus that has bacteria as its host. Initial independent studies on the use of such viruses as labels in immunoassay were performed by Haimovich and Sela[34] and by Mäkelä.[53] This subject will be discussed in a later chapter by M. Young and A.L. Nichols.

Proteins

The limitations of nonlabeled immunoassays have been outlined earlier. Thus, for example, only large antigen:antibody aggregates form a precipitin line or scatter light, and such aggregates are found only when the antigen is a protein (with several antigenic determinants) and is present in high concentration. However, such techniques can be applied to the assay of haptens provided hapten conjugated to protein is employed as label. Thus Cambiaso and his colleagues[18,19] described automated immunoprecipitation techniques for the assay of DNP-lysine (with a sensitivity of l ng/ml) and of progesterone (with a sensitivity of 10 ng/ml), although difficulties were experienced in applying such a procedure to serum when, for example, the presence of rheumatoid factor or Clq may influence the results obtained.

Metals

Recently, metalloimmunoassays have been described[17] employing metal atoms, in the form of their organometallic or coordination complexes, for labeling haptens and larger antigens. After separation of the antibody-bound and free fractions, the amount of metal present in one or the other is determined by suitable methods such as emission, absorption, fluorescence spectrometry, or neutron inactivation. Among the haptens studied were estrone, estradiol-17β, estriol, cannabis, and barbiturate, while bovine serum albumin was employed as a protein model. It does not seem likely that such assays will have wide relevance in clinical practice in the near future, because of their lack of sensitivity (2–50 ng/ml) and the complexity of available endpoint detection systems.

Chemiluminescence and Bioluminescence

Chemiluminescence is associated with certain chemical reactions that result in the emission of photons of light. One of the best known and efficient reactions of this type is the oxidation of luminol (5-amino-2,3′-

dihydrophthalazine-1, 4-dione) by, for example, H_2O_2 in the presence of a catalyst. Bioluminescence refers to chemiluminescent reactions that involve a biological reactant. The best known of these, the luciferin-luciferase system, was discovered nearly a century ago by Dubois. Such assays are discussed in a later chapter by R.D. Falb and coworkers.

Cofactors

The use of cofactors would seem an attractive alternative to enzyme labeling, especially since it would be anticipated that the antibody in the bound fraction would be more likely to sterically hinder the approach of both substrate and enzyme than, as in most EIAs, of the substrate alone. Schroeder and his colleagues[69] successfully labeled biotin and dinitrofluorobenzene with an NAD analogue and developed a nonseparation assay employing a bioluminescent endpoint. This group[22] were also successful in preparing ATP-labeled antigens as the basis of a homogeneous assay.

We have also successfully coupled NAD to various ligands; however, it is a formidable chemical task that significantly decreases cofactor activity. Of more importance, cofactors are present in all biological fluids, and even in distilled water (probably as a result of prior bacterial contamination), which makes nonseparation assays of a sensitivity appropriate for hormone measurement impractical. As separation procedures, such techniques would not appear to offer any advantages over EIA and, in all probability, would have some additional disadvantages.

Particles

Reference has already been made to early work by Arquilla and Stavitsky.[4] Many other examples of immunoassays employing RBC as the label exist, including, for example, a hemagglutination-inhibition assay for the detection of morphine.[4] Large numbers of tests have also been developed in which antigens or antibodies are labeled with latex particles with the endpoint being visual determination of latex agglutination. Among the most common are pregnancy tests employing particles coated with antisera to HCG, which agglutinate in the presence of HCG in a urinary sample. Kits of this type are available commercially for a wide range of antibodies (including antithyroglobulin and antimicrosomal) and antigens (such as fibrin degradation products, several plasma proteins, and some viral and bacterial antigens). Indeed, the number of samples currently assayed by this means may well approach that by RIA.

Such techniques are usually qualitative rather than quantitative. However, the availability of instruments to count platelets and other blood cells has made possible the recent introduction of sensitive, quantitative *particle counting immunoassays* (PACIA), based on the reduction of the total number of particles when they are agglutinated. In its simplest form, for the assay of large molecules with several antigenic determinants, latex particles of some 0.8-μm size are coated with antiserum and, after incubation, the number of single particles remaining will be inversely proportional to the amount of antigen present in the sample.

For the assay of haptens with only a single antigenic determinant, the technique must be modified slightly. For example, in the assay of T_4, macromolecules of destran to which several T_4 molecules have been linked (the T_4 conjugate) are incubated with the antibody-coated latex particles and the sample (or standard). In the absence of T_4 several of the latex particles will become bound to the T_4 conjugate, and the number of single particles will be small. In the presence of increasing levels of T_4, which will block binding sites on the antibody-coated latex particles so that they no longer agglutinate with the T_4 conjugate, the number of single particles will increase proportionally.

Sensitivities of about 1 nM were achieved for both HPL and alpha-fetoprotein by the first procedure and of about 10 n*M* for T_4 by the inhibition technique. Coefficients of variation ranged from 2 to 10%, and both manual and automated assays were developed.[20] Specialized and hence expensive equipment is necessary, and problems were encountered initially with some samples due to latex particle agglutination by rheumatoid factor or Clq. However, these are being successfully overcome by prior treatment of the samples and a modification of the procedures using the $F(ab')_2$ fragments.[48] Furthermore, new approaches to PACIA are enabling even greater sensitivity to be achieved.

COMPARISON OF THE ADVANTAGES AND DISADVANTAGES OF ISOTOPIC AND NONISOTOPIC LABELING IN IMMUNOASSAY

The future of NIIAs will depend upon their advantages and disadvantages as compared with RIA and IRMA. Thus any alternative should be equally rapid and practical, employ as simple and efficient a detection system as possible, and enable a specificity, sensitivity, and precision to be achieved appropriate to the compound being assayed. The relative merits of some alternative labels are discussed below.

Preparation and Stability of Labeled Reactant

Much of the early success of RIA can be attributed to the development by Greenwood and his colleagues,[33] of an efficient and simple means for radioiodinating peptides and proteins containing tryosine and/or histidine residues. Many other procedures have since been introduced for labeling steroids, thyroid hormones, and other haptens as well as alternative techniques for labeling protein and glycoprotein hormones. Reactants labeled with gamma-emitting isotopes, in particular ^{125}I, are being employed increasingly for clinical purposes in preference to those labeled with a beta-emitting isotope, such as ^{3}H or ^{14}C. This is because of the much shorter counting times required, the avoidance of the need for a liquid scintillant, and for applying corrections for quenching or chemiluminescence.

Excellent methods exist for the labeling of haptens and proteins with enzymes and with fluorescent molecules, in part because of the prior use of such labeled products in histopathology and other fields. However, there are two types of alternative label, namely, phages and some chemiluminescent molecules, where the actual labeling may pose difficulties. Thus there are problems in retaining the viability of bacteriophages during the labeling procedure, while chemiluminescent molecules, such as luminol, may fail to react after the conjugation to other molecules.

Considerable concern is often expressed about the radiation hazards associated with RIA and IRMA. Thus isotopes can be absorbed through the skin while volatile ^{125}I can be released into the atmosphere and inhaled.[12] It is essential to distinguish clearly between the risk of performing a radioiodination and of carrying out an actual RIA or IRMA. In the former, 1 or 2 mCi of ^{125}I are commonly employed, with the need for proper facilities and precautions. However, performing an RIA involves the use of less than 0.1 μCi of ^{125}I, and there are no risks provided simple rules are obeyed, such as not using a mouth pipette or eating or smoking in the laboratory. The Radiochemical Centre, Amersham, has demonstrated that the rate of release of volatile ^{125}I during the course of any assay is less than 1% and that it is impossible for a laboratory worker, irrespective of the number of RIA performed, to inhale more than a miniscule percentage of the maximum permitted dose.

The prolonged shelf life, measured in years, is a major advantage of reactants labeled with enzymes, fluorescent molecules, and various other alternatives as compared to those labeled with gamma-emitting isotope. The latter have a relatively limited shelf life due to the short halflife of such isotopes (about 60 days in the case of ^{125}I) and the rapid degradation of some labeled antigens. The use of new and gentler radioiodination procedures together with the availability of purer and more stable antigens and antibodies is helping to improve the situation. Thus isotopically labeled antigens can now normally be used for at least 12 weeks, while radioiodinated antibodies can be employed for up to 6 months. Nonetheless, the short shelf life of antigens labeled with a gamma-emitting isotope poses considerable problems for commercial kit producers, since it necessitates frequent radioiodinations and markedly increases the cost of production, quality assurance, and distribution.

Legislation

Most countries base their legislation concerning RIA and IRMA on the use and disposal of radioisotopes as recommended by the International Commission on Radiation Protection. However, wide differences exist in the interpretation of these regulations. The aim should be to enable maximum use of clinically valuable *in vitro* procedures while safeguarding the health of laboratory staff and the general public. Since, as discussed earlier, there is no significant hazard involved in performing such assays, it might be expected that no significant legislative problems would exist.

Such is the fortunate situation that exists in the United Kingdom and United States, while in West Germany and despite very detailed regulations, the only problems concern the disposal of solid radioactive waste and the requirement to keep extremely careful records. However, in some countries (including France), legislation has been so framed as to prohibit all but a few centers from performing RIA, with consequent difficulties in the practice of some clinical disciplines such as endocrinology. It might also be expected that in other countries, especially Japan, there may be emotive problems in employing radioisotopes.

No such problems exist with the majority of nonisotopic labels (although it is possible that difficulties might arise if viruses were to be employed extensively for labeling). Thus it is certain that in countries with very restrictive legislation or a strong emotive bias against the use of isotopes, increasing use will be made of some forms of NIIA irrespective of their merits and demerits as compared with RIA.

Influence of Biological Samples

A major advantage of employing a gamma-emitting isotope as a label is that there is virtually never any radioactivity in the biological fluids to be assayed and nothing present in the sample either decreases or increases the number of counts recorded. Thus lipemic, jaundiced, or hemolyzed specimens can be assayed, and it is not necessary to make "blank" corrections. Unfortunately, many types of NIIA may be markedly affected by endogenous compounds, especially with non-separation procedures and when low levels of the antigen to be determined necessitate that a large volume of the biological fluid is assayed and a prolonged incubation period is required.

Examples of interference with a NIIA by endogenous compounds include the presence of enzymes with similar biological effects to those of an enzyme employed as the label; the presence of enzyme inhibitors or other factors that influence endpoint detection in an EIA; high levels of bilirubin, which has an excitation and emission spectrum that overlaps with those of the fluorescein usually employed as the label in an FIA; inner filter effects with turbid samples; and fluorescence quenching due to nonspecific binding of the label to albumin.

These problems do not arise in assays for haptens, such as drugs, which circulate in the μmol/liter range, because the sample volume can be limited to a few μl and a large amount of labeled reactant can be employed. They can also usually be overcome during the separation step, as discussed earlier, or by the late addition of the label. Thus, as an example of the latter, sample and antiserum linked to magnetizable particles are incubated till equilibrium has been attained, the serum is aspirated, and the solid phase washed with buffer; only then is the labeled antigen added.

Need for Separation Step

The separation step essential in all RIA and IRMA is one of the main sources of imprecision. It requires considerable work and technical expertise; it adds to the time taken to complete an assay if centrifugation and multiple washes are necessary; and, finally, it has posed problems in the development of fully automated RIA systems.

It is not surprising, therefore, that those NIIAs that do not require a separation step are simpler, take less time to perform, and are potentially more precise *provided* endpoint detection is also simple, quick, sensitive, and precise. Unfortunately, when sensitivity is required, as it often is in the measurement of hormone levels and the detection of tumor associated products, nonseparation EIA, FIA, and VIA may be affected significantly by endogenous materials present as discussed above. Indeed, under such circumstances, it may be necessary to reintroduce a separation step to remove such interfering factors. Furthermore, such a step appears to be a requisite of virtually all assays employing labeled antibodies, irrespective of the label used, since the act of binding seldom influences the signal.

Endpoint Detection

It would seem logical first to consider the criteria on which the ideal endpoint detection system should be based and then assess how these criteria are met with various labels. Some suggested criteria are given in Table 6.

The use of detection systems for reactants labeled with gamma-emitting isotopes offers many advantages. Relatively inexpensive manual and automated gamma counters are widely available and becoming increasingly so, and such counters are very efficient (greater than 70% efficiency when ^{125}I is being counted). It is difficult to envisage a simpler method of endpoint detection than the introduction of the sample into the well of a sodium iodide crystal. Further, counting precision obeys known physical laws such that, when 10,000 counts are collected, the coefficient of variation is only 1% for repeated counts on the same sample. Finally, the time taken to generate 10,000 counts is short (usually 10–120 sec) with the high specific activity ^{125}I-labeled reactants commonly employed. Of particular importance in many fields, the use of isotopically labeled reactants enables attainment of the maximum sensitivity set by the affinity of the antibody.

Some NIIAs, such as VIA and metalloimmunoassay, have such complex, insensitive, or prolonged endpoint detection systems that it is difficult to envisage them playing a major role. Instruments for determining enzyme activity are the most widely available of all and no hazards are involved. However, the additional step of determining enzyme activity prolongs the assay, and makes it more complex, and increases imprecision. The amplification made possible by use of an enzyme to attain sensitivity will also magnify an error. Finally, it is difficult to check a value, and a change in temperature of less than 1°C greatly influences enzymatic activity.

Endpoint detection systems for FIA offer a surprising number of advantages. Manual and flow-through fluorimeters are efficient and relatively inexpensive, introduction of the sample is easy, and the result

Table 6. Some Criteria for Choosing an Endpoint Detection System for an Immunoassay

1. Cost, speed, and simplicity of detection technique
2. Cost and availability of appropriate instrumentation
3. Precision, accuracy, and sensitivity of endpoint detection: dependent on signal-to-background ratio
4. No influence of biological samples on endpoint detection
5. Ability to check
6. Nonhazardous
7. Suitable for automation

is available within seconds. Precision of measurement is excellent (with coefficients of variation less than 0.2%). The results are not significantly affected by normal changes in ambient temperature, there are no hazards, and rechecking poses no problem. However, fluorimeters are not widely available and, at their present stage of development, FIAs are relatively insensitive, covering only the μmol/liter and nmol/liter range, in part due to other compounds present in samples (such as bilirubin), which cause a variable background.

Automation

There are several factors that suggest the need for fully automated immunoassay systems[41] and indicate that their introduction may have the same profound impact as did the Auto Analyzer in clinical chemistry. These include the rapidly increasing demand for existing assays, the application of immunoassay to a rapidly increasing range of compounds in several diverse fields; and the need to improve precision and reduce costs (by such means as reducing reagent volumes and removing the need for running duplicates). Such systems may also significantly shorten assay time. Thus in a manual immunoassay it is essential to attain equilibrium because of the impossibility of keeping the time between reagent addition and the separation step constant. In automated systems, particularly those of the continuous-flow type, accurate timing is simple and disequilibrium assays can be employed.

Much recent work has related to the automating of RIA, and developments have reflected closely those seen previously in routine clinical chemistry. Thus, following the introduction of partially automated equipment, fully automated procedures are being introduced, which can be divided into discrete and continuous-flow systems (Table 7). The main problem concerned the separation step. However, this has been overcome in a number of ingenious ways, including the use of antibodies covalently linked to magnetizable particles and a magnetic field[31] and of magnetizable charcoal.[27]

Similar approaches are certain to come with those NIIAs which require a separation step. Indeed, a generation of fully automated immunoassay systems can be envisaged in which several different endpoint detectors are employed, depending on the particular label. However, the development of fully automated equipment is particularly easy for those immunoassays that do not require separation of the bound and free fractions. Thus automated immunoprecipitation procedures have been introduced, by Technicon, for large numbers of specific plasma proteins and references have been made, during the course of this chapter, to automated FIA and EIA. Developments in the field of automated particle counting immunoassays (PACIA) are of especial

Table 7. Some Available Automated Radioimmunoassay Systems

Name	Separation procedure	References
Continuous Flow		
	Second antibody/filtration	Pollard and Waldron[64]
	Second antibody/filtration	Bagshawe et al.[5]
	Second antibody/sedimentation	Johnson et al.[38]
	Antibodies attached to RBC/sedimentation	Lunar[50]
Gammaflow (Squibb)	Column of Dowex and charcoal	Brooker et al.[14]
ARIA II (Becton Dickinson)	Reusable immobilized antibodies	Reese and Johnson[66]
Star (Technicon)	Antibodies linked to magnetizable particles	Forrest[31]
Southmead System	Immobilized antibodies/filtration	Ismail et al.[37]
Discrete		
Centria (Union Carbide)	Centrifugation through Sephadex G25 columns	Lo and Ertingshausen[49]
Concept 4 (Micro Medic)	Antibody coated tubes	Painter and Hasler[63]
Pace 4 (Picker)	Second antibody/filtration	Bagshawe[6]
Ismatec	Second antibody/filtration	Marschner et al.[54]

interest in endocrinology because of their potential sensitivity and precision.

Nonetheless, in the immediate future, it seems certain that most automated immunoassay systems will employ an isotopically labeled reactant, since many large commercial companies are making a major investment in this area. This fact more than any other may determine the relative use made of RIA and NIIA.

CONCLUSIONS AS TO THE ROLE OF NONISOTROPIC IMMUNOASSAYS IN ENDOCRINOLOGY

The immense impact that RIA has had reflects its specificity, sensitivity, precision, practicality, and wide applicability. It is possible that the availability of fully automated RIA will have a further impact by decreasing individual sample assay costs and enabling virtually unlimited sample numbers to be handled. Current NIIAs share this specifity (which is a function of the antibody), wide applicability (which reflects the ease of raising antibodies against a vast range of molecular species), and ability to automate. However, problems may arise with regard to sensitivity, precision, and practicality.

To date, of the commonly employed NIIA, only the separation EIA can attain a sensitivity equivalent to that of RIA. Nonseparation EIA and most forms of FIA are currently limited to the assay of compounds that circulate at concentrations in the μmol/liter or nmol/liter range and, even then, difficulties may be encountered at low nmol/liter levels. As shown in Table 8, most hormones circulate in the low pmol/liter range, well below their present sensitivity. It is of interest that the majority of hormones lying in the nmol/liter range are either those associated with pregnancy (estriol and HPL), or others that circulate largely bound to carrier proteins (such as T_4 and T_3), and whose free levels lie in the pmol/liter range.

These low levels are in sharp contrast to those of drugs. Thus alcohol at twice the permitted driving level has the third highest blood concentration of any compound, at about 40 mmol/liter, while therapeutic levels of lithium and salicylates are also in the mmol/liter range. The majority of drugs for which nonseparation EIA and FIA have been developed circulate in the μmol/liter range, about one million times higher than many hormones. Digoxin is an exception in this respect, since its therapeutic levels lie in the low nmol/liter range.

Despite its potential sensitivity, separation EIA must remain technically more complex and less precise than RIA for the reasons considered above relating to endpoint detection. Even the manual nonseparation EIA for T_4 is more complex and takes longer to perform than many of

Table 8. Approximate Circulating Levels, in Molar Terms, of a Variety of Natural Compounds

Natural compound	(mmol/liter)	Natural compound	(μmol/liter)
Sodium	140	Albumin	600
Chloride	105	Urate	250
Bicarbonate	30	Phenylalanine	125
Glucose	5	Immunoglobulin G	90
Urea	4	Ammonia	30
Cholesterol	4	Iron	20
Calcium	2.5	Bilirubin (total)	10
Triglycerides (fasting)	1	Immunoglobulin M	1
Natural compound	**(nmol/liter)**	**Natural compound**	**(pmol/liter)**
Estriol (late pregnancy)	600	Aldosterone	180
Thyroxine binding globulin	500	Insulin	120
Cortisol	400	Parathyroid hormone	100
Placental lactogen	300	Growth hormone	50
Thyroxine (total)	125	Luteinizing hormone	10
Corticosterone	20	Triiodothyronine (free)	10
Triiodothyronine	2	Adrenocorticotrophin	10
Prolactin	1	Thyroid stimulating hormone	5
Estradiol 17β (women)	1	Angiotensin 11	4
Progesterone	1	Oxytocin	1
		Arginine vasopressin	1

its RIA counterparts unless appropriate automated instrumentation is used. Nonetheless, NIIA has undoubted value in many areas of clinical practice.

First, NIIA is playing an increasingly important role in detecting the presence of antibodies against a wide range of parasites, bacteria, viruses, and other organisms. Examples include the screening of pregnant women for the presence of IgM and IgG antibodies to rubella and the use of EIA with a simple visual endpoint in the developing world. Similar procedures would be of value in endocrinology for the detection of, for example, circulating antibodies to the thyroglobulin or thyroid microsomal antigens; but this is a relatively limited requirement.

Second, NIIA has an extensive and valuable role in detecting the presence of antigens such as Australian antigen.[81] There are many medical situations of the plus/minus type for which precision is unimportant. The detection of human chorionic gonadotrophin or its β subunit provides such an example, and NIIAs (with antibodies covalently bound to erythrocytes or latex particles) are already used extensively. However, it is usually important to quantitate hormone levels in endocrinology, as opposed to merely detecting their presence.

Third, NIIA has a much less important role in the exact quantitation of antigens, and especially hormones and tumor associated products. Indeed, in the latter context, the role of NIIAs in their present stage of development may well be limited to the following:

1. The developing world, which does not have easy access to gamma counters and where the relative instability of reactants labeled with a gamma emitting isotope may cause problems.
2. Countries with severe legal restrictions on the use of isotopes or an emotive bias against their use. Under such circumstances laboratory staff will be willing to perform technically more complex, time consuming, and imprecise analytical procedures.
3. Detecting antigens that circulate in the μmol/liter and high nmol/liter range and for which nonseparation techniques exist. Immunoassays not employing labeled reactants are sufficiently sensitive for most plasma proteins. Nonseparation EIAs and FIAs have proved suitable for the assay of serum levels of most drugs and of total T_4, and assays for estriol and cortisol should not pose a problem. However, it is not yet certain if the practicality and precision of such assays will be such that they will replace conventional RIA.

Thus I conclude (and, hopefully, my experience with both RIA and NIIA prevents bias) that the use of isotopically labeled reagents will continue to dominate in endocrinology and in some other areas, such as the assay of tumor associated antigens, during the next decade, and that RIA and NIIA will have complementary rather than exclusive roles. I believe that NIIA will prove of immense value in many other medical fields, for example, therapeutic drug monitoring and microbiology. I would also conclude (but would admit bias) that FIA will prove more practical than EIA for quantitative situations. Finally, it is too early to forecast the impact of other alternative labels, but the use of particle counting immunoassay and chemiluminescent labeling may prove to be of special interest.

REFERENCES

1. G.M. Addison and C.N. Hales, *Horm Metab Res* **3**:59, 1971.
2. R.C. Aalberse, *Clin Chim Acta* **48**:109, 1973.
3. F.L. Adler and C.T. Lau, *J Immunol* **106**:1684, 1971.
4. E.R. Arquilla and A.B. Stavitsky, *J Clin Invest* **35**:458, 1956.
5. K.D. Bagshawe, F.W. Harris, and A.H. Orr, *In Automation in Analytical Chemistry*, Vol. 2, Technicon Symposia, Mediad, Inc., New York, p. 53.
6. K.D. Bagshawe, *Lab Pract* **24**:573, 1975.
7. R.M. Barakat and R.P. Ekins, *Lancet* **ii**:25, 1961.
8. H.M. Barbour, *J Immun Methods* **11**:15, 1976.
9. P. Beck and C.N. Hales, *Biochem J* **145**:607, 1975.
10. L. Belanger, C. Sylvestre, and D. Dufour, *Clin Chim Acta* **48**:15, 1973.
11. S.A. Berson, R.S. Yalow, A. Baumann, M.A. Rothschild, and K. Newerly, *J Clin Invest* **35**:170, 1956.
12. E.M. Bogdanove and A.M. Strash, *Nature* **257**:426, 1975.
13. A.R. Bradwell, D. Burnett, D.B. Ramsden, W.A. Burr, H.P. Prince, and R. Hoffenberg, *Clin Chim Acta* **71**:501, 1976.
14. G. Brooker, W.L. Terasaki, and M.G. Price, *Science* **194**:270, 1976.
15. J.F. Burd, R.J. Carrico, M.C. Fetter, R.T. Buckler, R.D. Johnson, R.C. Boguslaski, and J.E. Christner, *Anal Biochem* **77**:56, 1977.
16. J.F. Burd, R.C. Wong, J.E. Feeney, R.J. Carrico, and R.C. Boguslaski, *Clin Chem* **23**:1402, 1977.
17. M. Cais, S. Dani, Y. Edden, O. Gandolfi, M. Horn, E.E. Issacs, Y. Josephy, Y. Saar, E. Slovin, and L. Snarsky, *Nature* **270**:534, 1977.
18. C.L. Cambiaso, P.L. Masson, and J.F. Heremans, *J Immunol Methods* **5**:153, 1974.
19. C.L. Cambiaso, H.A. Riccomi, P.L. Masson, and J.F. Heremans, *J Immunol Methods* **5**:293, 1974.
20. C.L. Cambiaso, A.E. Leck, F. de Steenwinkel, J. Billen, and P.L. Masson, *J Immunol Methods* **18**:33, 1977.
21. P.J.A. Capel, *J Immunol Methods* **5**:295, 1974.
22. J.R. Carrico, K.K. Yeung, H.R. Schroeder, R.C. Boguslaski, T.R. Buckler, and J.E. Christner, *Anal Biochem* **76**:95, 1976.
23. T. Chard, *In An Introduction to Radioimmunoassay and Related Techniques*, T.S. Work, and E. Work (eds.), Elsevier/North-Holland Biomedical Press, New York, 1978.

24. J. Chayen, N. Loveridge, and J.R. Daly, *Clin Edocrinol* **1**:219, 1972.

25. W.B. Dandliker and V.A. de Saussure, *Immunochemistry* **7**:799, 1970.

26. W.B. Dandliker, R.J. Kelly, J. Dandliker, J. Farquhar, and J. Levin, *Immunochemistry* **10**:219, 1973.

27. C. Dawes and J. Gardner, *Clin Chim Acta* **86**:353, 1978.

28. A.M. Deelder and J.S. Ploem, *J Immunol Methods* **4**:239, 1974.

29. R.P. Ekins, *Clin Chim Acta* **5**:453, 1960.

30. R.P. Ekins, *In Hormone Assays and Their Clinical Application,* J.A. Loraine, and E.T. Bell (eds.), Churchill Livingstone, New York, p. 1.

31. G.C. Forrest, *Ann Clin Biochem* **14**:1, 1977.

32. R.S. Galen, and D. Forman, *Clin Chem* **23**:119, 1977.

33. F.C. Greenwood, W.M. Hunter, and J.S. Glover, *Biochem J* **89**:114, 1963.

34. J. Haimovich and M. Sela, *J Immunol* **97**:338, 1966.

35. W.F. Head, *J Pharm Sci* **51**:662, 1962.

36. I.M. Holdaway, L.H. Rees, and J. Landon, *Lancet* **ii**:1170, 1973.

37. A.A.A. Ismail, P.M. West, and D.J. Goldie, *Clin Chem* **24**:571, 1978.

38. H.K Johnson, B.E. Brann, R.F. Ritchie, and J. Graves, *In Automation in Analytical Chemistry,* Vol. 2, Technicon Symposia, Mediad, Inc., New York, p. 69.

39. W. Knapp and J.S. Ploem, *J Immunol Methods* **5**:259, 1974.

40. J. Landon, M. Friedman, and F.C. Greenwood, *Lancet* **i**:652, 1967.

41. J. Landon, L. Rees, and L. Nye, *Br J Hosp Equip* **1**:29, 1975.

42. J. Landon, J. Crookall, and A. McGregor, *In Steroid Immunoassay*, E.H.D. Cammeron, S.G. Hiller and K. Griffiths, (eds.), Alpha-Omega, Cardiff, U.K.

43. J. Landon, *Nature* **268**:483, 1977.

44. J. Landon, J. Carney, and D. Langley, *Ann Clin Biochem* **14**:90, 1977.

45. R.K. Leute, E.F. Ullman, A. Goldstein, and L.A. Herzenberg, *Nature New Biol* **236**:93, 1972.

46. R.K. Leute, E.F. Ullman, and A. Goldstein, *JAMA* **221**:1231, 1972.

47. S.A. Levison, F. Kierszenbaum, and W.B. Dandliker, *Biochemistry* **9**:322, 1970.

48. J.N. Limet, C.H. Moussebois, C.L. Cambiaso, J.P. Vaerman, and P.L. Masson (to be published).

49. D.H. Lo and G. Ertingshausen, *Clin Chem* **22**:1165, 1976.

50. S.J. Lunar, *Anal Biochem* **65**:355, 1975.

51. R. Maiolini, B. Ferrua, and R. Masseyeff, *J Immunol Methods* **6**:355, 1975.

52. R. Maiolini and R. Masseyeff, *J Immunol Methods* **8**:223, 1975.

53. O. Mäkelä, *Immunology* **10**:81, 1966.

54. I. Marschner, F. Erhardt, J. Henner, and P.C. Scriba, *Z Klin Chem Klin Biochem* **13**:481, 1975.

55. D. Mattingly, *J Clin Pathol* **15**:374, 1962.

56. L.E.M. Miles and C.N. Hales, *Nature (London)* **219**:186, 1968.

57. L.E.M. Miles and C.N. Hales, *Biochem J* **108**:611, 1968.

58. L.E.M. Miles and C.N. Hales, *Lancet* **ii**:492, 1968.

59. R.D. Nargessi, J. Landon, and D.S. Smith, *Clin Chim Acta,* in press.

60. R.D. Nargessi, J. Landon, and D.A. Smith, *J Immunol,* in press.

61. A.R. Neurath, *Z Naturforsch* **206**:974, 1965.

62. L. Nye, M.J. Anderson, C. Dawes, J. Landon, and G.C. Forrest, *Clin Chim Acta* **87**:307, 1978.

63. K. Painter and M.J. Hasler, *Clin Chem* **22**:1164, 1976.

64. A. Pollard and C.B. Waldron, *In Automation in Analytical Chemistry,* Vol. 1, Technicon Symposia, Mediad, Inc., New York, p. 49.

65. C. Readhead, G.M. Addison, C.N. Hales, and H. Lehmann, *J Endocrinol* **39**:313, 1973.

66. M.G. Reese and L.R. Johnson, *Clin Chem* **24**:342, 1978.

67. D. Rodbard and G.H. Weiss, *Anal Biochem* **52**:10, 1973.

68. R.S. Schneider, P. Lindquist, E.T. Wong, K.E. Rubenstein, and E.F. Ullman, *Clin Chem* **19**:821, 1973.

69. H.R. Schroeder, R.J. Carrico, R.C. Boguslaski, and J.E. Christner, *Anal Biochem* **72**:283, 1976.

70. D.S. Smith, *FEBS Lett* **77**:25, 1977.

71. R.D. Spencer, F.B. Toledo, B.T. Williams, and N.L. Yoss, *Clin Chem* **19**:838, 1973.

72. A.B. Stavitsky and E.R. Arquilla, *Fed Proc* **12**:461, 1953.

73. R.P. Tengerdy, *Anal Chem* **35**:1084, 1963.

74. A.J. Toussaint and R.I. Anderson, *Appl Microbiol* **33**:552, 1965.

75. E.F. Ullman, J. Blackmore, R.K. Leute, W. Eimstad, and A. Jaklitsch, *Clin Chem* **21**:1011, 1975.

76. E.F. Ullman, M. Schwarzberg, and K.E. Rubenstein, *J Biol Chem* **251**:4172, 1976.

77. B.K. Van Weeman and A.H.W.M. Schuurs, *FEBS Lett* **43**:215, 1974.

78. E.W., Voss, W. Eschenfeldt, and R.T. Root, *Immunochemistry* **13**:447, 1976.

79. L. Wide, H. Bennich, and S.G.O. Johansson, *Lancet* **ii**:1105, 1967.

80. B.W. Wilson, W. Snedden, and R.B. Parker, *Adv Mass Spec Biochem Med* **11**:487, 1976.

81. G. Wolters, L. Kuijpers, J. Kacaki, and A. Schuurs, *J Clin Pathol* **29**:873, 1976.

82. R.S. Yalow and S.A. Berson, *J Clin Invest* **39**:1157, 1960.

Chapter 2

Selection of Standards for the Measurement of Pituitary Hormones: Problems of Standardization

EUGENIA ROSEMBERG, M.D.

This chapter is intended to review the purpose of standardization in comparative assay systems and the problems related to standardization. Criteria will be considered for selection of appropriate substances that should serve as standards and reference preparations in various types of assay systems. Further, we will consider expression of assay results, describe the quality control procedures to be used in order to achieve standardization, and provide information concerning the official agencies responsible for the distribution of these materials.

STANDARDIZATION, PURPOSE AND PROBLEMS: CRITERIA FOR SELECTION OF SUITABLE STANDARDS AND REFERENCE PREPARATIONS

A standard is not, and seldom can be, an example of the "perfect" preparation of a substance. This common point of reference is simply a sample of a material considered to be suitable in the light of knowledge and of the preparations available at the time it is set up. Common reference materials are essential to provide results which, in accordance

The Medical Research Institute of Worcester, Inc., The Worcester City Hospital, and The University of Massachusetts, Medical School, Worcester, Mass.

This work was supported, in part, by Grant AM-07564, USPHS, NIH, Bethesda, Maryland.

with biometric principles, should be quantitatively consistent, and could be reliably related from one laboratory to another, from time to time in the same laboratory, and from time to time to its replacement.[1-4]

Establishing the suitability of a reference preparation for dose interpolation in any assay system either biologic, immunologic, or chemical, depends upon its fulfilling the criteria for similarity to the substance being measured in samples where the concentration of these substances is not known. Suitability is defined operationally when dilutions of the unknown are indistinguishable from dilutions of the reference preparation. However, demonstration of similarity in the response of unknown and reference preparations is not to be interpreted as proof that the two substances have a "common effective constituent." Using a reference preparation, results are truly valid when relative potencies obtained for given unknown samples are independent of the method used for testing. In biologic assays, the hallmark of similarity is parallelism of linearized dose-response curves such that relative potencies of substances remain the same irrespective of dose level at which the determination is made. Moreover, a standard or reference should serve the purpose for which the measurement is intended.

Ideally, individual standards should be available for each substance to be measured. These materials should be as alike as possible as the material being assayed. The alikeness means biological, chemical, physical, and immunological alikeness. Because of the inherent difficulties in attaining this goal, the problem of setting up suitable standards and reference preparations presents a real dilemma, and compromise has been inevitable.

We should have assays that recognize specifically the hormone under study. Where two hormone molecules have a common physiological effect, it is too readily assumed that a bioassay which reflects that specific effect is not influenced by differences in the molecule other than the active site. In bioassays, the extent to which nonidentity of standard and unknown may cause trouble depends upon the specificity and precision of the bioassay systems employed. In the case of radioimmunoassay, similarity between the unknown and standard or reference material implies that the antigen binding sites involved in binding radioactive trace antigen to antibody react identically with both substances.

It is clear from evolving research that hormones differ at the molecular level with respect to species, source (gland, plasma, or urine), methods of extraction, and possibly in the occurrence of isomeric forms. Likewise, precursors and metabolic products of a hormone may also react in immunoassay systems. The very fact that a variety of chemically related and frequently biologically inactive molecular species may react in immunoassay systems has yielded much information about precursors and metabolic products of hormones. However, all these various forms may interfere with the conditions for comparison of identical materials so that invalid estimates are obtained.

A full discussion of the various assay systems is beyond the scope of this chapter. However, some salient points will have to be made to provide some basis for rational use of standards and reference preparations. It is best to observe the conditions of similarity by assaying unknown preparations against standards or reference materials that are qualitatively as similar as possible with respect to species, tissue or fluid of origin, and extent of purification. Examples of the importance of this principle in the bioassay (BIOA) field is illustrated in the assay of ovine pituitary FSH and LH (NIH-FSH-S1 and NIH-LH-S1) by the ventral prostate (VPW) and ascorbic acid depletion (OAAD) assays, using a reference preparation of human urinary origin, i.e., 2nd IRP-HMG. When unknown preparations of human urinary LH were assayed by these two methods, using ovine NIH-LH-S1 as the reference preparation, it was found that the urinary materials contained 12 times more LH activity by the VPW than by the OAAD method. The discrepancy was understandable on the basis that it was attributable to physical and chemical characteristics and possible metabolic differences in the standard used (NIH-LH-S1, an ovine pituitary LH), and the materials (human urinary LH) tested.[1,5,6,] Also, discrepancies in relative potency obtained using these two bioassay systems have been related to the concept that the OAAD represents "an acute biochemical response," and the VPW represents a "chronic growth response."[5] In any case, the discrepancy disappeared when a urinary standard was used for the BIOA of urinary LH. Similarly, the use of a material of human urinary origin, such as the 2nd IRP-HMG as a reference preparation in radioimmunoassay (RIA), ia associated with overestimation of the FSH and LH content of human pituitary tissue extracts. Conversely, a pituitary tissue extract such as the National Pituitary Agency (NPA) preparation LER 907, is satisfactory, or almost so, as reference material in the RIA of FSH and LH in pituitary tissue extracts.[7]

In general, by modification of structure, the biologic activity of glyprotein hormones is more readily destroyed than immunological reactivity. These modifications could be the result of loss of sialic acid groups, deamination, oxidation, aggregation, radioiodination, photo-oxidation, etc. Some of the altered products, however, retain certain *in vitro* biologic activities, that is, they may bind to receptors, promote steroidogenesis, stimulate follicular growth in organ culture, etc. Consequently, *in vivo* and *in vitro* BIOAs and various types of RIAs may yield significantly different results. It should be noted that in BIOAs, when substances are compared using fundamentally the same techniques and the same assay animals, variability within and between laboratories can be minimized and, therefore, conversion factors have been utilized. However, the indiscriminate use of conversion factors can be hazardous and is applicable only if it is demonstrated that bioassay conditions in different laboratories are basically the same.

Assay of individual hormones, or for a group of structurally related derivatives representing "the hormone" in a test sample, requires that the assay system be specific for that hormone or for that particular group of compounds. In BIOAs, the specificity resides in the structure of the active compounds, and in their reaction with the specific receptor present in the target tissue of the animal used. In RIAs, the specificity resides in the structure of the immunoreactive compounds, and in their reaction with the antibodies available in the antiserum used, as well as in the interaction of these with the other reagents comprising the assay system. It should be noted that the use of a pure or homogeneous standard does not confer specificity to RIAs.

In contrast to BIOAs, RIAs are specific for a hormone from a limited number of species only. Moreover, RIAs are performed with a unique set of reagents: antisera, antigens used for labeling, etc. Therefore, the problems confronting the assayist performing these assays are extremely complex. As in BIOAs, the validity of RIAs depends on the assumption that the substances compared are identical or so similar that the test sample behaves in the system as a dilution of the standard. Most test samples (pituitary extract, plasma, or urine), contain variable quantities of structurally related hormones, subunits, structurally related derivatives such as precursors and metabolites, and large amounts of unrelated materials. As there is evidence that immunochemical differences exist between a hormone material extracted from the gland of origin and similar material found in blood and urine, it is important when performing RIAs to employ standards or reference materials that are comparable to the samples being examined.

There is a need for agreement in the criteria to be used in assessing specificity of RIAs. Ultimately, specificity of an RIA system is defined by the list of compounds and their potency which, if present in the test sample, are known to contribute to assay results. However, RIAs have hardly ever been assessed in these general terms. Traditionally, studies of RIA systems have always been based on the degree of agreement of RIAs with BIOAs.[8-10] Correlative studies between RIAs and BIOAs are complex to interpret when discrepancies arise. For example, it is known that removal of sialic acid from hCG, LH, and FSH differentially affects bio and immunoreactivities. *In vivo* biologic potency is impaired.[11] Binding to and activation of hormone-specific receptors *in vitro* is unaffected,[12] and the loss of *in vivo* biologic activity is related to an increased rate of disappearance of the hormone from the circulation.[13] However, immunological potency is unimpaired by removal of sialic acid. Since, as a result of extraction procedures, different preparations of these compounds may contain different amounts of sialic acid, it can be appreciated that disparities in relative potency estimates develop between BIOAs and RIAs.

Theoretically, the essential attributes of a standard or reference preparation are that one sample should be identical to another. The sample should be free from substances that interfere in assays, and if it is to be widely used, it should be tested in a variety of assay systems. However, from the preceding discussion, it can be visualized that the selection of materials to be used in various assay systems presents difficulties.

When prepared, standards and reference preparations should be available for distribution to provide these materials to many laboratories for long periods of time. They should not be altered while being isolated or handled. Ideally, the ampouled standard or reference preparation should be characterized as far as possible by chemical and physical means. The reactivity of the material as well as that of other related substances that may be contained in the ampoules should be examined using ligand assays and BIOAs, if applicable. The stability of the materials should also be tested by studying the rate by which the activity in unopened ampoules of the dry preparation is lost when stored for several months at elevated temperatures.

The collected information about the standard of reference preparation, the source, its preparation, the identity and homogeneity of the material, its distribution into ampoules, the results of biochemical, physical, and stability tests, including an analysis and interpretation of assay results, should be made available to users of these materials.

The nature of the material used as a reference preparation and the type and degree of its characterization are greatly influenced by the type of the assay (bio, immuno, or cytochemical) in which they are to be used. Moreover, its suitability for use in a particular assay must be determined not only by the basic principles of comparison of like with like, but in reference to the particular question to which the answer is sought.

UNITAGE

It does not seem possible at present to suggest a rational and generally acceptable solution to the problem of unitage of standards and reference preparations and, therefore, to the problem of expression of results in the various assay systems where these materials are utilized. Currently, there are two ways of expressing estimates of the relative potencies of unknowns in terms of standards or reference preparations. One is in terms of *mass,* the other in terms of *units.**

In 1968, the Expert Committee on Biological Standardization of the World Health Organization (WHO) recommended that, where a standard or reference preparation exists to which a unitage has been assigned, the relative potencies should be expressed in units, with the proviso that the standard or reference preparation and the method of assay used, whether chemical, BIOA, RIA, or other receptor assays, be specified.[14,15] For many substances now being measured by immunoassay, a biologic unit has already been assigned. Thus, the *imm* (unit of immunological reactivity of antigen), and the *bion* (unit of biological activity) for any substance (nomenclature suggested by Borth[16]), should refer to the same quantity at least for a first standard or reference preparation. In other words, the number of units assigned to a WHO standard for immunoassay (imms) will be made equal to the number of units it contains by bioassay (bions).

Each possibility, that is, the application of the mass or the unit system, has its shortcomings. The unit notation system in use in biologic assays allows for direct transfer of estimates of activity (units) from one preparation to another without reference to conversion factors. However, this system makes it difficult to compare the relative amounts of different materials in terms of either mass or molecular concentration. In the past, units for bioassay were usually assigned on an arbitrary basis to a standard or reference preparation before there was real knowledge of the molecular structure of "pure" hormone or substance being assayed. Moreover, the amount of substance present in the ampoule being distributed, to which a unitage has been assigned, might be merely an intelligent guess as to the mass of pure substance that it contains; it might be based on the unitage of a previously existing standard, it might be defined on an arbitrary basis, or perhaps is related to the fraction of the gram molecule of the active substance present. The official WHO position is that standards or reference preparations are the materials as they exist in the ampoules. Thus the material includes the active ingredients together with the other constituents, such as moisture, and carrier or buffer salts. The potency should be taken as the number of units per ampoule stated on the labels, and no attempt should be made to weigh out portions of the freeze-dried plugs.

For substances for which RIA methods have been or are being developed, work on isolation, molecular weight, characterization, and general structure is quite advanced. Because ligand assays do not

*NIAMDD, Research materials available to qualified investigators, *J Clin Endocrinol Metab* **46:** 179, 1978 (Announcement).

necessarily estimate the same characteristics of a molecule that are responsible for biologic activity, there is a need for an unambiguous distinct unit notation system for the expression of ligand assay estimates.[17] As stated previously, in practice, results of RIAs are expressed in terms of existing standards and reference preparations, which had been set up for use in BIOAs. These preparations are impure; they vary in the degree of homogeneity, nature, and amount of contaminants, and in physicochemical properties. A great majority of RIAs measure more than one molecular form, and the estimates differ when different antisera are used leading to a marked discontinuity of estimates. In order to diminish the degree of discontinuity, RIA standards and reference preparations might be set up with essentially pure hormone peptides in their intact native form. However, judging from the present "state of the art," this possibility may not be forthcoming.

The use in RIAs of standards and reference preparations set up for use in BIOAs has created a considerable amount of confusion. This practice, however regrettable, may continue until appropriate materials can be developed, indeed if this is possible.

QUALITY CONTROL: CALIBRATION AND REPLACEMENT OF STANDARDS

The reproducibility of test results within a laboratory is usually effectively monitored by employing quality control procedures, which involve the repeated estimation of hormone concentrations in control samples of appropriate test materials, e.g., serum pools, and of the available reference materials.[18] Such sera are generally selected to contain different concentrations of the substance being assayed. These samples should be distributed in portions, each appropriate for a single assay and kept "deep frozen." Whereas standardization of procedure is necessary for precision within an assay, standardization of test animals and reagents is essential to provide comparability between assays, a fact that is extremely important in RIAs, where differences between antisera exist, and their specificity is dependent on the particular combination of antiserum and labeled antigen. Also, in RIAs, a certain degree of discontinuity of results occurs following change from one batch of reagents to another. In order to diminish the frequency and extent of discontinuity, it is preferable to use one large pool of antisera as a source of antibodies. Similarly, antigens can be prepared in large batches of identical samples in a form that is stable and appropriate for labeling. Care should also be taken to ensure that all test samples are kept under suitable and similar conditions. RIAs are particularly amenable to the application of automated and computerized quality control techniques, and for the automated calculation of results, thus providing better analyses of data and of quality control procedures.[19-21]

If every assay system were entirely specific, or if we were concerned only with a series of assays with identical specificities, calibration of working standards or the transfer of units from estimates made in one assay system to another would not present problems. This situation does not exist at present. Therefore, there is an urgent need for availability of well-characterized reference materials necessary for testing assay specificity. Some suitable preparations are available and can be obtained from official agencies.

Once standards or reference preparations are in widespread use, the problem of replacing them with a like preparation will be inevitable. Theoretically, it could be done. However, in practice, the preparations in use may contain various amounts of denatured, damaged, or isomeric forms, and it may be difficult to replace such preparations with others having essentially identical immunological properties. In other situations, a hormone may be found that shows closely comparable immunological activity to that of the original preparation. In this situation, replacement should prove to be relatively easy. In any case, replacement of standards or reference preparations may involve difficult decisions concerning continuity of unitage.

OFFICIAL AGENCIES THAT PROVIDE STANDARDS OR REFERENCE PREPARATIONS

The time, work, and financial resources necessary for the preparation, testing, and distribution of substances designed to serve as standards and reference preparations for use by the scientific and medical community on worldwide basis can only be accomplished by an official body such as the World Health Organization (WHO), long recognized for its important role in this area of activity.

For many years, WHO has provided materials for the biologic estimation of pituitary hormones. These materials are of various categories: international standards, international reference preparations and reference reagents, working standards, and research standards.

The *international standard* is a preparation to which an *international unit* (IU) is assigned on the basis of an extensive international collaborative study. The IU is defined as the specific biological activity contained in a defined weight of the current international standard. The standard is the material as it exits in the ampoules; the "material" thus includes the active ingredients together with all the other constituents such as moisture, and in some instances carrier and buffer salts. The potency of the international standard should be taken as the number of IUs stated on the label, although the unit is still formally defined in terms of weight.

International reference preparations may serve a function similar to that of the international standard, but are established without the full international study that precedes the establishment of an international standard or, when a collaborative study has shown that the preparation is, for some reason, not entirely suitable to serve as an international standard. In some instances, an international unit is assigned to an international reference preparation, especially when an early definition of such a unit is desirable to prevent the emergence of a multiplicity of systems for designating potencies.

International biological reference reagents are used for specific laboratory tests for the identification of microorganisms. They are highly specific for the organism concerned, and since they are used mainly for the purpose of qualitative identification, unitage is not usually assigned to them.

Working standards are not normally provided by WHO. An international working standard may be made available however, from the Division of Biological Standards, WHO, in a special case when the benefit of having one is exceptional. The assumption is made that the ampoules of the working standard are equivalent to those of the international standard itself. Assays are carried out on each batch to verify its potency, but it is for individual national control authorities to decide whether to adopt the working standard as an official national standard.

Research standards do not have the official status of standards, reference preparations, or reference reagents, but they are set up with the same care and precautions as the international standard. Research standards are not necessarily subjected to the same extensive international collaborative assay. In some cases many become officially established as an international standard or as an international reference preparation.

International standards and reference preparations are distributed by the WHO International Laboratory for Biological Standards, National Institute for Biological Standards and Control, in London. Their distribution is not intended for routine use but for calibration of national laboratory standards or reference preparations used in BIOAs and RIAs. The materials available for BIOA purposes are: porcine corticotrophin (WHO 3rd IS), bovine growth hormone (WHO IS), ovine prolactin (WHO 2nd IS), bovine thyrotropin (WHO IS), equine serum gonadotrophin (WHO 2nd IS), human urinary menopausal gonadotrophin (2nd IRP-HMG and WHO 1st IS).[14,22] Information concerning availability and characteristics of these materials can be found in the WHO Tech. Rep. Ser., No. 413, 1969.

Some materials available through the WHO for use in RIAs have been prepared to serve as standards and reference preparations and others for use in research activities. These are: human growth hormone (WHO 66/217), human growth hormone, Raben type (Std A), human pituitary FSH (63/16 MRC Res. Std. A, and hFSH, 68/39), human pituitary LH (63/15 MRC Res. Std. A and hLH, 68/40), human pituitary FSH and LH [69/104 (derived from NPA LER 907)], human post-menopausal plasma pool (69/176), and human pituitary TSH (63/14 MRC, Std A). The characteristics of these materials, described in several publications,[23-26] can be requested from the Division of Biological Standards, National Institute for Medical Research, Mill Hill, London N.W. 7, England.

Hormone preparations of ovine, porcine, and bovine origin have been made available to research workers in the U.S. and worldwide through a program supported from 1956 till 1959 by several of the National Institutes of Health and, since 1959, by a single grant from the National Institute of Arthritis, Metabolism and Digestive Diseases, NIAMDD.[27,28] Since 1969, NIAMDD has supported a program aimed at the preparation and distribution of hormones obtained from rat pituitaries. The materials distributed through the NIAMDD programs are intended for biologic and immunological studies. These are indicated on Table 1 and can be requested from the Hormone Distribution Officer, Office of the Director, NIAMDD, Bldg. 31, Room 9A-47, NIH, Bethesda, Md. 20014.

Table 1. NIAMDD Preparations

Hormone	Ovine (o), porcine (p), bovine (b), rat (r)		Subunits
	For BIOs	For RIAs	
GH	o, b, r	o, r	
PRL	o, b, r	o, r	
FSH	o, p, r	r	
LH	o, b	o, b, r	α-LH, o, r
TSH	o	o, r	β-LH, o, r
ACTH		r[a]	β-TSH, r
Others: mouse GH (RIA), mouse PRL, Nonhuman primates FSH (RIA), rabbit PRL (RIA).			

[a]Reference preparation.

In 1963, NIAMDD initiated the activities of the National Pituitary Agency (NPA). The initial mandate of the NPA was the collection of human pituitaries for the preparation and distribution of human growth hormone for use in clinical and basic research activities. Subsequently, the scope of the Agency was expanded to provide qualified investigators with human growth hormone, human FSH, and human LH for clinical investigations as well as to provide a variety of human pituitary hormones, their subunits, and various antisera for immunological and basic research studies. These materials are indicated in Table 2, and can be requested from the National Pituitary Agency, 210 West Fayette Street, Baltimore, Md. 21201.

Table 2. NPA Materials for Use in RIAs

Hormone	Antisera	Reference preparation
hGH	Yes	
hPRL	Yes	
hFSH	Yes	Yes
hLH	Yes	Yes
hTSH	Yes	Yes
ACTH (synthetic)	Yes	
α-hTSH	Yes	
β-hTSH	Yes	
α-hFSH	Yes	
β-hFSH	Yes	
α-hLH	Yes	
β-hLH	Yes	

Ligand assays are widely used in clinical situations where accuracy and quantitation are needed. As the commercial production of assay kits and reagents has proliferated very rapidly, the need for coordination and control of quality reagent is urgent. Therefore, the manufacturers of reagents can greatly contribute to the standardization of their kits by calibrating their products in terms of internationally accepted standards or reference preparations, and by maintaining appropriate quality control procedures.

Medical science, and specially assay technology, moves very rapidly. We must expect that standards and reference preparations, and the unitage attached to them, will adapt to this rapid progress.

REFERENCES

1. E. Rosemberg, Use of standards, general considerations. *In Gonadotropins 1968,* E. Rosemberg (ed.), Geron-X, Inc., Los Altos, Calif. 1968, p. 383.

2. A. Albert, Report of the National Pituitary Agency collaborative study of the radioimmunoassay of FSH and LH: consideration of standards. *In Gonadotropins 1968,* E. Rosemberg (ed.), Geron-X, Inc., Los Altos, Calif. 1968, p. 393.

3. D.R. Baugham, Discussion. *In Gonadotropins 1968,* E. Rosemberg (ed.), Geron-X, Inc., Los Altos, Calif. 1968, p. 408.

4. A. Albert, Editorial: bioassay and radioimmunoassay of human gonadotropins. *J Clin Endocrinol Metab* **28**:1683, 1968.

5. E. Rosemberg, E.A. Solod, and A. Albert, Luteinizing hormone activity of human pituitary gonadotropin as determined by the ventral prostate weight and ovarian ascorbic acid depletion methods of assay. *J Clin Endocrinol Metab* **24**:714, 1964.

6. A. Albert, I. Derner, E. Rosemberg, and W.B. Lewis, Assay characteristics of tannate complexes of ovine gonadotropins. *Endocrinology* **76**:139, 1965.

7. E. Rosemberg, S.G. Lee, G. Bulat, G.T. Ross, and P.S. Butler, Correlation between bioassay and radioimmunoassay of FSH and LH. *In Gonadotropins,* B.B. Saxena, C.G. Beling, and H.M. Gandy (eds.), Wiley, New York, 1972, p. 616.

8. G.T. Ross, Factors governing choice of reference preparations for competitive binding assays. *In Principles of Competitive Protein-Binding Assays,* W.D. Odell and W.H. Daughaday (eds.), Lippincott, Philadelphia, 1971, p. 325.

9. W.D. Odell and G.T. Ross, Correlation of bioassay and immunoassay potencies for FSH, LH, TSH, and hCG. *In Principles of Competitive Protein-Binding Assays,* W.D. Odell and W.H. Daughaday (eds.), Lippincott, Philadelphia, 1971, p. 401.

10. Human Reproduction Unit, WHO, Assay of protein hormones related to human reproduction: problems of specificity of assay methods and reference standards. Report of a Meeting, *Acta Endocrinol (Kbh)* **71**:625, 1972.

11. G.D. Braunstein, L.E. Reichert, Jr., E.V. Van Hall, J.L. Vaitukaitis, and G.T. Ross, The effects of desialylation on the biologic and immunologic activity of human pituitary lutenizing hormone. *Biochem Biophys Res Commun* **42**:962, 1971.

12. T. Tsuruhara, M.L. Dufau, J. Hickman, and K.J. Catt, Biological properties of hCG after removal of terminal sialic acid and galactose residues. *Endocrinology* **91**:296, 1972.

13. E.V. Van Hall, J.L. Vaitukaitis, G.T. Ross, J.W. Hickman, and G. Ashwell, Immunological and biological activity of hCG following progressive desialylation. *Endocrinolgy* **88**:456, 1971.

14. WHO Tech. Rep. Ser. 384, 1968, p. 8.

15. WHO Tech. Rep. Ser. 413, 1969, p. 9.

16. R. Borth, A terminology for units of biological and immunochemical activity. *Acta Endocrinol (Kbh)* **60**:1, 1969.

17. D.R. Bangham and P.M. Cotes, Standardization and standards. *Br Med Bull* **30**:12, 1974.

18. E. Rosemberg, Immunoreactivity of standards and reference preparations used in the radioimmunoassay of follicle-stimulating and luteinizing hormones in serum. *J Clin Endocrinol Metab* **48**:163, 1979.

19. D. Rodbarb, Statistical aspects of radioimmunoassay. *In Principles of Competitive Binding Assays,* W.D. Odell and W.H. Daughaday (eds.), Lippincott, Philadelphia, 1971, p. 204.

20. D. Rodbarb, Statistical quality of control and routine data processing for radioimmunoassays and immunoradiometric assays. *Clin Chem* **20**:1255, 1974.

21. D. Rodbarb and D.M. Hutt, Statistical analyses of radioimmunoassay and immunoradiometric (labeled antibody) assays: a generalized weighted iterative least squares method for logistic curve fitting. *In Radioimmunoassay and Related Procedures in Clinical Medicine and Research.* International Atomic Energy Agency, Vol. 1, p. 165, 1974 (available from UNIPUB, P.O. Box 433, New York, N.Y. 10016).

22. P.L. Storring, H. Dixon, and D.R. Baugham, The first international standard for human urinary FSH and for human urinary LH (ICSH), for bioassay. *Acta Endocrinol (Kbh)* **83**:700, 1976.

23. D.R. Baugham and M.P. Cotes, Reference standards for radioimmunoassays. *In Radioimmunoassay Methods,* K.E. Kirkham and W.M. Hunter (eds.), Churchill Livingstone, Edinburgh, 1971, p. 345.

24. P.L. Storring, D.R. Baugham, P.M. Cotes, R.E. Gaines Das, and S.L. Jeffcoate, The international reference preparation of human pituitary luteinizing hormone, for immunoassay. *Acta Endocrinol (Kbh)* **88**:250, 1978.

25. P.M. Cotes, R.E. Gaines Das, T.B.L. Kirkwood, J.G. Bennie, and W.M. Hunter, The stability of standards for radioimmunoassay of human TSH: research standard A and the international reference preparation initially 68/38. *Acta Endocrinol (Kbh)* **88**:291, 1978.

26. R.E. Gaines Das, and P.M. Cotes, International reference preparation of human prolactin for immunoassay: definition of the international unit, report of a collaborative study and comparison of estimates of human prolactin made in various laboratories. *J Endocrinol* **80**:157, 1979.

27. L. E. Reichert, Jr. and A.E. Wilhelmi, A summary of the biological activities of the various lots of pituitary hormones prepared under the programs of the National Institute of Arthritis, Metabolism and Digestive Diseases. *Endocrinolgy* **92**:1301, 1973.

28. L.E. Reichert, Jr. and A.E. Wilhelmi, Biological activities of recent preparations of pituitary hormones produced under the programs of the National Institute of Arthritis, Metabolism and Digestive Diseases. *Endocrinology* **102**:982, 1978.

Chapter 3

Mathematics and Statistics of Ligand Assays: An Illustrated Guide

DAVID RODBARD, M.D.

INTRODUCTION

This chapter provides an introduction to the mathematical and statistical principles underlying immunoassay and ligand-assay systems in general. Much of this material is presented in the context of radioimmunoassay. However, it is equally applicable to assay systems involving non-isotopic labels for the antigen. The discussion of assay validation, dose-interpolation, and "statistics" is directly applicable to labeled antibody assays (e.g. IRMA, 2-site IRMA, ELISA, and USERIA) as well as to labeled antigen assays (RIA, EMIT).

Most of the principles presented here are much easier to present as pictures or graphs, rather than as mathematical equations. For the convenience of the reader, an outline of the major topics covered in this chapter is provided in Table I at the end of the chapter. Some readers may wish to use this outline to select special topics of interest, rather than reading the entire chapter sequentially.

Biophysical Endocrinology Section, Endocrinology and Reproduction Research Branch, National Institute of Child Health and Human Development, National Institutes of Health, Bethesda, Md. 20205

REACTION KINETICS OF IMMUNOASSAY

Figure 1a illustrates the kinetics of the reaction between an antigen (P) and a homogeneous univalent antibody (Q), which combine to form the antigen-antibody complex (PQ). The RIA reaction kinetics are as follows:

$$\mathrm{Ag} + \mathrm{Ab} \underset{k_{-1}}{\overset{k_1}{\rightleftharpoons}} \mathrm{AgAb} \qquad \text{(I)}$$

$$\text{or} \quad H + R \rightleftharpoons HR$$

$$\text{or} \quad \underset{\text{(Free)}}{P + Q} \rightleftharpoons \underset{\text{(Bound)}}{PQ}$$

The relationship between $[PQ]$ and time is obtained when there is a constant concentration of antibody present. The higher the concentration of antigen (p), the more rapid the formation of $[PQ]$. This follows directly from the *mass action law.* It is assumed that the association rate constant (k_1) and the dissociation rate constant (k_{-1}) remain constant. As the amount of P increases, the amount of $[PQ]$ formed increases. However, the total amount of $[PQ]$ cannot exceed the total concentration of antibody (q). The slope of the relationship between $[PQ]$ and time, when evaluated close to the origin, is equal to $v_0 = k_1[P]\,[Q]$. If the total concentrations of P and Q (p and q, respectively) are known, an estimate of the rate constant can be obtained by measuring the slope of the association curve at a point very close to $t = 0$. When $t = 0$, all of the

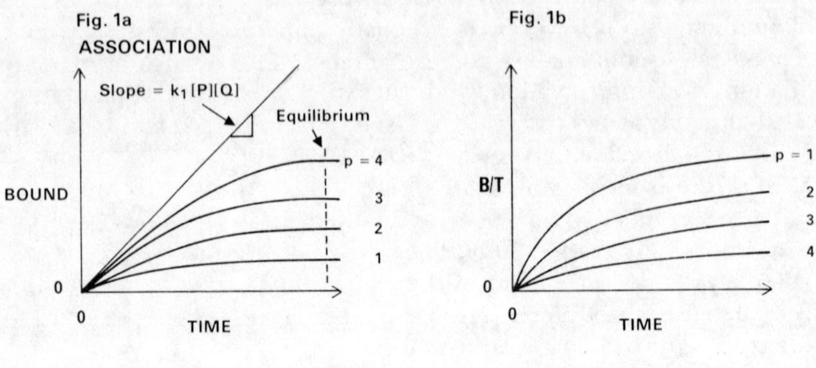

Fig. 1a. Kinetics of the reaction between an antigen (P) and a homogeneous univalent antibody (Q), which combine to form the antigen-antibody complex (PQ).

Fig. 1b. Relationship between the bound to total ratio (B/T) for the ligand and the reaction time.

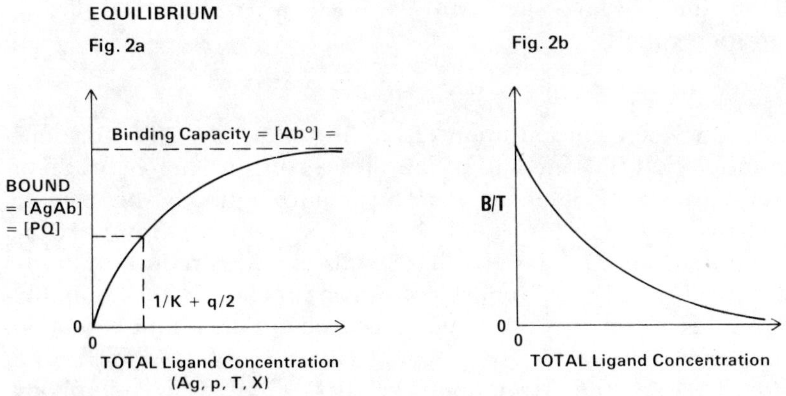

Fig. 2a. Relationship between the amount of bound antigen and total antigen at equilibrium.

Fig. 2b. Relationship between the bound to total ratio (B/T) and the total ligand concentration at equilibrium.

antigen and all of the antibody are in the free or unbound form; accordingly, the effect of the dissociation reaction may be ignored.

Figure 1b shows the relationship between the bound to total ratio (B/T) for the ligand and the reaction time. The higher the total concentrations of ligand (p), the lower the bound to total ratio. Thus although there is more [PQ] formed at any point in time (Figure 1a), the bound to free (B/F) or bound to total ratio is smaller.

Figure 2a illustrates the relationship between the amount of bound antigen and total antigen at equilibrium. Such a curve can be constructed by drawing a vertical dashed line in Figure 1a and then plotting [PQ] versus the total concentration (p), resulting in a hyperbolic relationship. This is analogous to the Michaelis-Menten hyperbola for enzyme kinetics.

Figure 2b shows the relationship between the bound to total ratio (B/T) and the total ligand concentration at equilibrium. The ordinate at each point in Figure 2a is divided by the abscissa to obtain the slope of the line emanating from the origin. As the total concentration of ligand (p) increases, the bound to total ratio decreases and ultimately approaches zero as p becomes "infinite." A similar curve would be obtained using values taken from Figure 1a or Figure 1b, at a time prior to the attainment of equilibrium. Thus the shape of the dose response curve in a radioimmunosassay is determined directly by the mass action law, irrespective of whether the assay is operating close to or far away from equilibrium.

Half of the binding sites will be filled when the total ligand concentration equals

$$1/K + q/2$$

where q is the total concentration of binding sites. Thus the hormone concentration that fills one-half of the sites is equal to the reciprocal of the affinity constant only if the concentration of antibody sites is quite small relative to the reciprocal of the affinity constant. However, the dose or concentration of antigen that results in a 50% reduction in the bound to total ratio (Fig. 2b) does not bear a simple relationship to the equilibrium constant; instead, one must solve a quadratic equation involving K, p^*, and q.

Figure 3 shows the dissociation kinetics of an antigen-antibody complex. We assume that the antigen-antibody complex is formed as in Figure 1a. Then, the system is brought to an "infinite" dilution, or the concentrations of free P and free Q are forced equal to zero and maintained at zero. Ideally, if the reaction scheme shown in Figure 1a applies, the concentration of bound ligand $[PQ]$ is a simple "negative exponential" decay curve. The equation for this is

$$[PQ] \vee [PQ]_0\, e^{-k_{-1}t}$$

$$\text{or} \quad \log_e[PQ] = \log_e[PQ]_0 - k_{-1}t$$

$$\text{or} \quad \log_{10}[PQ] = \log_{10}[PQ]_0 - \left(\frac{k_{-1}}{2.303}\right)t$$

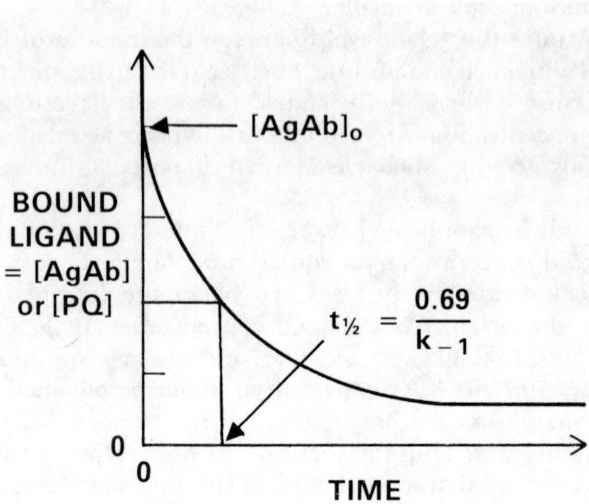

Fig. 3. Dissociation kinetics of an antigen-antibody complex.

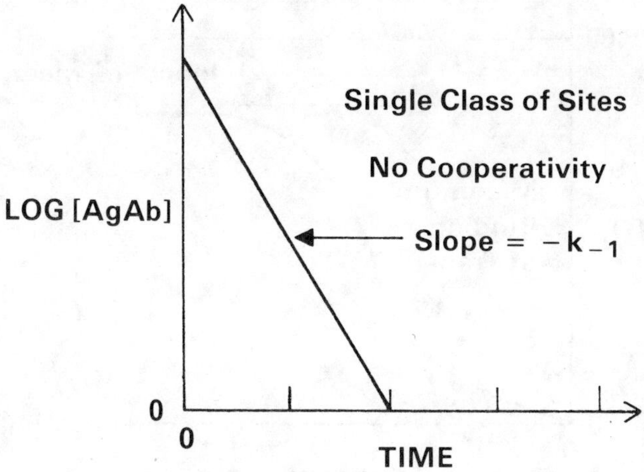

Fig. 4. The dissociation reaction, linearized by plotting the natural logarithm of the antigen-antibody complex vs. time.

The rate constant k_{-1} is the only constant that determines the shape of the curve. The half-time is given by

$$t_{1/2} = \frac{\log_e(2)}{k_{-1}} = \frac{.69}{k_{-1}}$$

Figure 4 shows the dissociation reaction, which has been linearized by plotting the natural logarithm of the antigen-antibody complex, $\log_e [PQ]$, versus time. The slope of the line is equal to k_{-1}. If the common logarithm (log to the base 10) of bound ligand is used instead, then the slope is equal to $-k_{-1}/2.303$. The factor 2.303 is the natural logarithm of 10. When dealing with a single class of antibody sites, this dissociation curve should be linear. Nonlinearity suggests (but does not establish) the presence of multiple classes of sites. Several other explanations are possible, for example, negative cooperativity, other types of interaction between sites, or failure to achieve "infinite dilution" in order to prevent the reassociation of P and Q.

Let us assume for a moment that we have a radioactively labeled antigen or "tracer" which is present in an infinitesimal concentration (Figure 5). We may then measure the bound to total ratio for this tracer, designated $(B/T)_0$ [or % $(B/T)_0$] versus antibody concentration. Since we may wish to vary the antibody concentration over several orders of magnitude, it is customary to plot the antibody concentration on a logarithmic scale. In general, a smooth symmetrical sigmoidal dose response curve will be obtained. In this case we assume that 10% of the

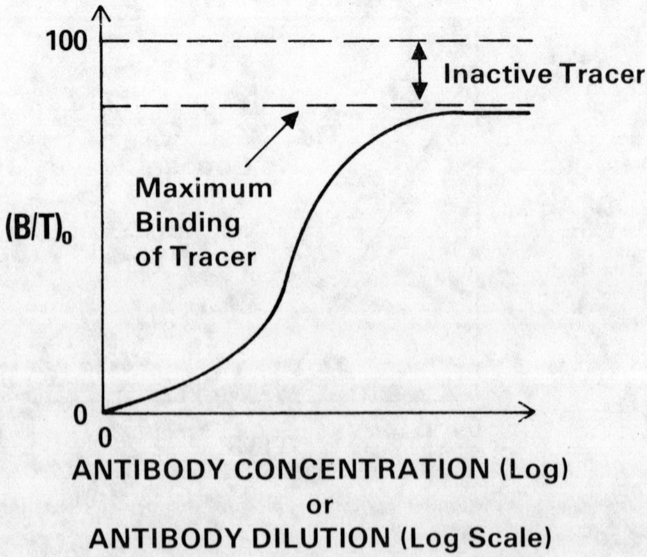

Fig. 5. The antibody dilution curve, with antibody concentration on a logarithmic scale.

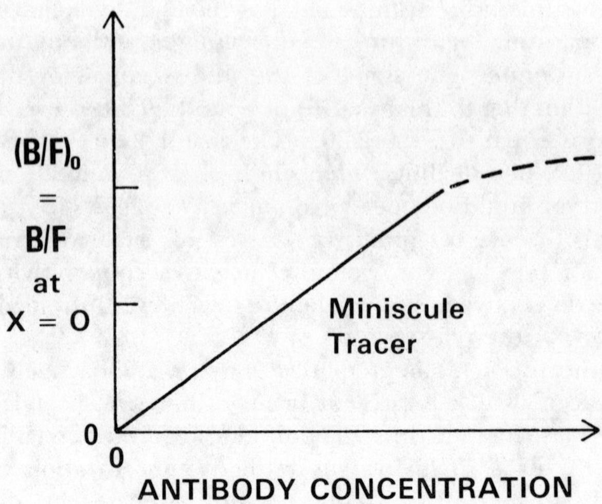

Fig. 6. The antibody dilution curve with the antibody concentration plotted on a linear scale.

tracer was damaged or immunologically inactive. Thus even with a massive excess of antibody, there is an upper limit to the fraction of tracer which can be bound. In the illustration here, it appears that only about 90% of the tracer can be bound even in the presence of an infinite antibody concentration. Systematic errors in the separation of bound and free may also produce this effect. This curve may be described by the four-parameter logistic equation (see Fig. 19, below).

Figure 6 shows the antibody dilution curve with the antibody concentration plotted on a linear scale. Again we assume that the concentration of labeled ligand is infinitesimal. Measuring the bound to free ratio, designated *B/F,* for the tracer (assuming that the user has corrected for the fact that not all of the tracer may be immunologically active, or else that the problem depicted in Figure 5 is not of great significance) results in a linear relationship between the bound to free ratio and the antibody concentration. This important result was pointed out by Berson and Yalow.[1] If not all of the tracer is immunologically active, this curve will flatten out at the right (dashed lines).

Figure 7 depicts another method frequently used for the portrayal of the relationships defined by the mass action law. *The Hill plot* is a plot of

$$\log\left(\frac{\text{Bound}}{B_{\text{max}} - \text{Bound}}\right)$$

versus the logarithm of the free ligand concentration, where B_{max} corresponds to the total binding capacity of the antibody (q in Fig. 2a). The total amount or concentration of antibody or binding protein is constant, q. If the system obeys reaction scheme I (above), a univalent homogeneous antigen reacting with a homogeneous antibody with no "cooperativity," this relationship should be linear with a slope of unity.

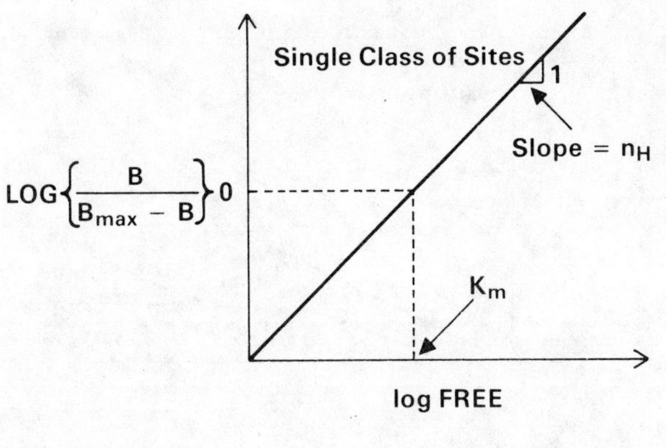

Fig. 7. The Hill plot.

Either $\log_{10}$ or $\log_e$ can be used, but the same should be used on both ordinate and abscissa. When the ordinate is zero the abscissa should be equal to $\log(K)$:

$$\text{Bound} = \frac{1}{2}B_{max} \quad \text{or} \quad \frac{B}{B_{max} - B} = 1 \quad \text{or} \log\left(\frac{B}{B_{max} - B}\right) = 0$$

The major assumptions involved in this graphical technique are (1) equilibrium, (2) perfect separation of bound and free, and (3) perfect knowledge of B_{max}. An error in the estimation of B_{max} may result in a serious distortion of the apparent Hill plot. The Hill plot, first presented by Brown and Hill in 1923, is conceptually and mathematically identical to Sip's plot later introduced into immunology following Nissonoff and Pressman's studies in the mid 1950s. Thus, the Hill coefficient and Sip's coefficient are essentially synonymous.

Figure 8 shows Hill plots in the cases of positive and negative cooperativity. In the presence of positive cooperativity, the slope of the Hill plot at its steepest point, designated $n_{H_{max}}$, will be greater than unity. Conversely, in the presence of negative cooperativity (where the binding of one molecule of ligand decreases the proclivity for binding an additional molecule of ligand), the Hill plot will have a minimum slope less than unity. In general, in the presence of either positive or negative cooperativity, there will be nonlinearity of the Hill plot in the middle region of the curves, but the curves becomes straight with a slope of unity for very high or very low free ligand concentration.

Numerous chemical and mathematical models have been developed to describe cooperativity, the phenomena occurring in the binding of oxygen to hemoglobin or in the binding of many substrates to their enzymes (Fig. 9) (3,13). The so-called "stepwise" model assumes that one

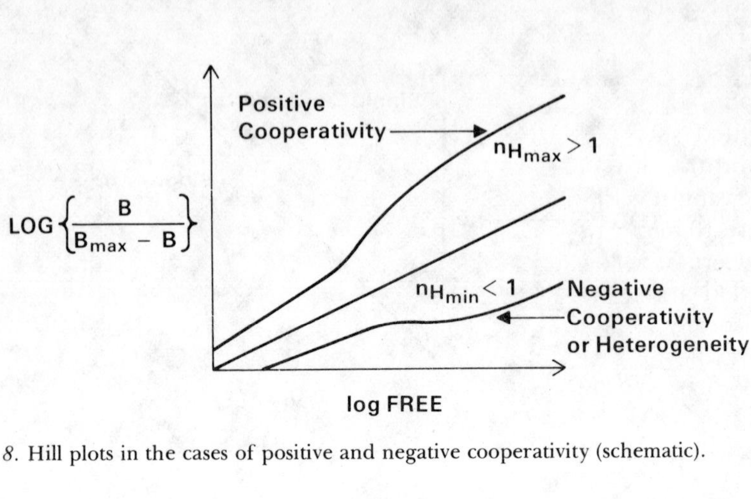

Fig. 8. Hill plots in the cases of positive and negative cooperativity (schematic).

$$P + Q \overset{K_1}{\rightleftharpoons} PQ \overset{K_2}{\rightleftharpoons} PQP \overset{K_3}{\rightleftharpoons} P_3Q \overset{K_4}{\rightleftharpoons} P_4Q \rightleftharpoons \text{etc.}$$

If $K_1 = K_2$: No cooperativity

If $K_1 < K_2$: Positive cooperativity

If $K_1 > K_2$: Negative cooperativity

Fig. 9. Cooperativity. The constants in the figure are represented by K_1–K_4 in the text.

molecule of ligand reacts with the antibody to form the complex designated *PQ* (3,13). This, in turn, may react with another molecule of ligand to form *PQP*. If the intrinsic or so-called microscopic rate constant for the binding of the first molecule of ligand (K_1) is equal to the microscopic affinity constant for the second molecule of ligand (K_2), then there is no cooperativity. If K_1 is less than K_2 there is positive cooperativity. If K_1 is greater than K_2, there is negative cooperativity. The K's in this case represent the microscopic affinity constants, and are different from the so-called stepwise affinity constants (*K*), which take geometrical (or "statistical") factors into account. These statistical factors take into account the fact that the first *P* may bind to either of two available sites, whereas the second P has only one site available. Likewise, *PQP* can dissociate in two ways, whereas *PQ* or *QP* can only dissociate in one way. Because of this, $K_1 = 2\mathrm{K}_1$, into $K_2 = \mathrm{K}_2/2$. Thus constancy of K's is not the same as constancy of *K*'s.

In our routine program for the analysis of radioimmunoassay results, the computer automatically attempts a curve-fit corresponding to Figures 10–13. The computer then decides which of these four models provides the best "fit" to the observed Scatchard plot, utilizing the weighted sum of the squares (SS) of deviations of the observtaions around the fitted curve as the criterion for determining the "best fit." Increasing the number of parameters from two (K_1, q_1) in the case of Figure 10 to five (K_1, K_2, K_3, q_2, q_2) in the case of Figure 13 should result in a decrease in the sum of the squares of deviation around the line. The question arises whether this decrease in deviations around the line is "statistically significant."

One of the most useful methods for the analysis of an antigen-antibody or protein-ligand binding system is the so-called Scatchard plot (Fig. 10). When an equilibrium between antigen and antibody is reached, there will be a linear relationship between the bound to free ratio for the

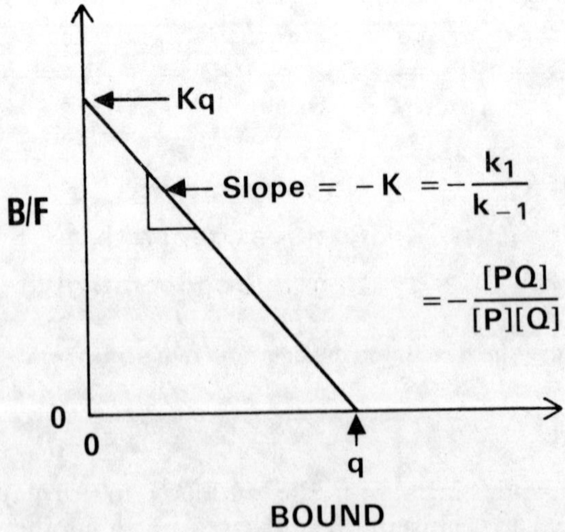

Fig. 10. Scatchard plot: equilibrium; 1 class of site; perfect separation.

ligand and the concentration of bound ligand. The slope of this line is −1 times the affinity constant (K), the intercept on the horizontal axis is the concentration of binding sites present (q), and the intercept on the vertical axis is Kq. This is the most frequently utilized method for the estimation of affinity constants. It is one of the ways to linearize the Michaelis-Menten hyperbola. Others include the Lineweaver-Burk or the "double reciprocal" plot. Although all methods proposed for the linearization of these curves introduce statistical problems, the Scatchard plot is perhaps the most generally suitable. However, the curve fitting should be performed in terms of the observed variables, e.g., B/T and T.

Figure 11 shows a Scatchard plot in the case where a small quantity of a high affinity antibody (Q_1) with equilibrium constant of association (K_1) is present. In addition, a virtually limitless or infinite amount of a second class of binding sites (or antibody), which has extremely low (or infinitesimal) affinity, is present. This occurs, for example, when a steroid such as estradiol binds with testosterone-estrogen binding globulin (TeBG) with a very high affinity (e.g., 10^9 L/mol), but a 10^3- or 10^4-fold molar excess of binding sites on albumin with an equilibrium constant four orders of magnitude lower is also present. Here the Scatchard plot (solid line) is an hyperbola, but not a rectangular hyperbola. Notice that the sum of the intercepts of the components on the vertical scale must equal the intercept of the solid line.

Figure 12 shows a Scatchard plot of a system where a single univalent homogeneous ligand is competing with two classes of binding sites (Q_1 and Q_2), present in quantities q_1 and q_2, with equilibrium constants of

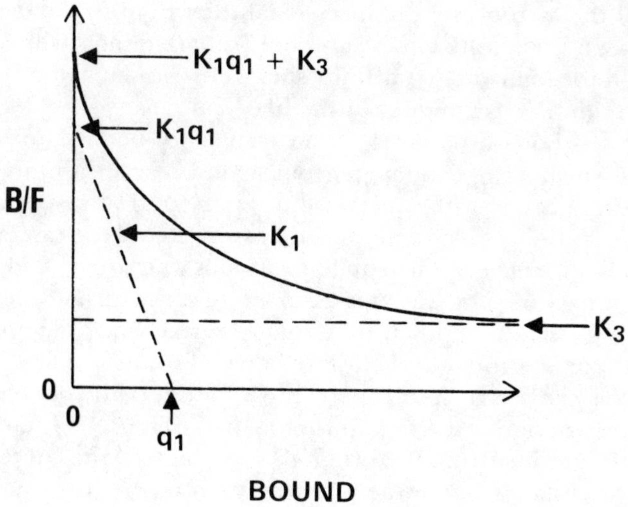

Fig. 11. Scatchard plot: 1 class saturable; 1 class unsaturable. K_3 is the B/F ratio for the horizontal asymptote.

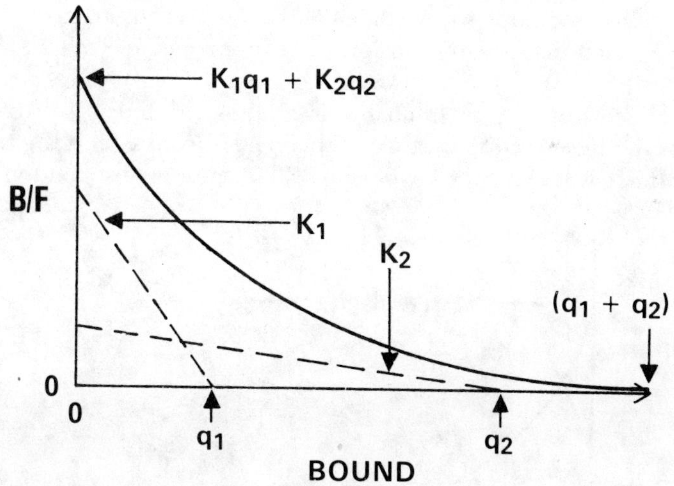

Fig. 12. Scatchard plot: 2 classes; saturable.

association K_1 and K_2, respectively. Again, the relationship is a hyperbola. The sum of the y intercepts of the dashed lines must equal the y intercept of the solid curve. Likewise, the sum of the x intercepts of the dashed lines must equal the x intercept of the solid curve. One may also draw a line emanating from the origin to any point on the solid curve. The total distance from the origin to the point on the solid curve will equal the sum of the distances from the origin to the dashed lines ($d_1 + d_2 = d$). The dashed lines show the Scatchard plots which would be obtained if the high and low affinity sites were present alone. These lines also represent the asymptotes of the hyperbola.

Figure 13 shows a nonlinear Scatchard plot obtained for a binding system in which a single homogeneous ligand reacts with three types of binding sites present with concentrations q_1, q_2, and q_3, respectively. Q_3 is effectively "infinite" relative to the other two. (Recall the case of albumin and the case of Fig. 11.) The equilibrium constants are K_1 and K_2 for the first two classes of sites, and it is assumed that the affinity for the third class of sites is infinitesimal, or virtually zero. Now the sum of the y intercepts for the three dashed lines is equal to the y intercept for the solid curve. There is no intercept on the x axis, since the intercept for the dashed line (designated K_3) is "infinite." As in Figures 11 and 12, if we draw a straight line from the origin to any point on the curve, then the sum of the distances from the origin to each of the three dashed lines should be equal to the distance from the origin to the solid curve. This relationship is useful when attempting graphical "curve peeling." However, in the case of a nonlinear Scatchard plot, graphical curve peeling is extremely hazardous! It is highly advisable to utilize computerized methods for nonlinear least squares in order to obtain an objective, quantitative description of the properties of the binding system.

Figure 14 shows a Scatchard plot that is nonlinear or "concave." Perhaps the most frequent cause of this type of concavity is the presence of multiple classes of sites, or perhaps a continuous distribution for the

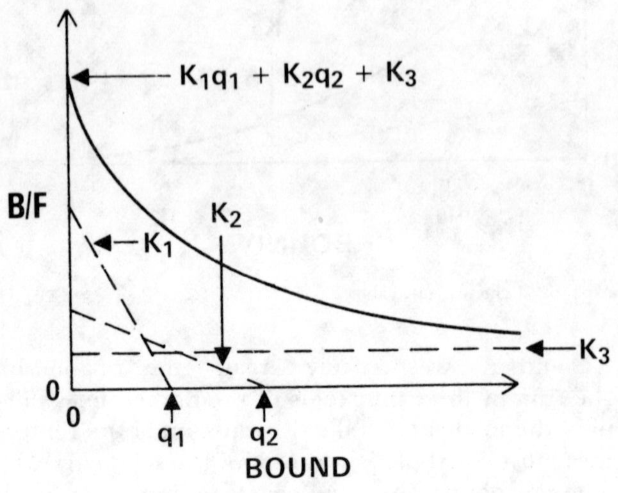

Fig. 13. Scatchard plot: 2 classes, saturable; 1 class, unsaturable.

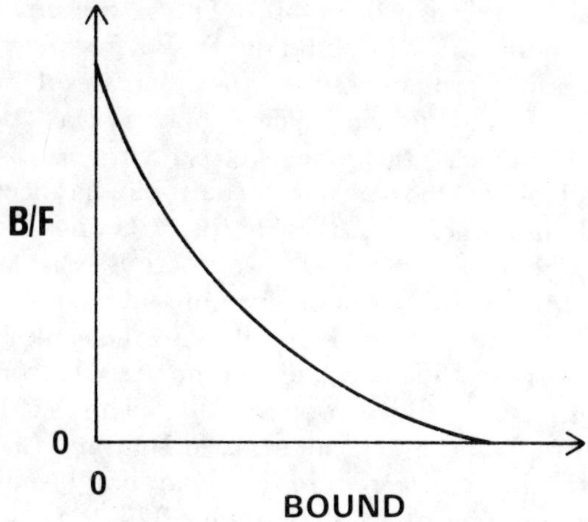

Fig. 14. Scatchard plot: nonlinear concave. Negative cooperativity, or multiple classes of sites.

equilibrium constants of the population of antibodies. Such a Scatchard plot may also be observed in the presence of negative cooperativity (see Fig. 9), and it is impossible to determine, on the basis of a Scatchard plot alone (or any equilibrium data), whether the nonlinearity is due to heterogeneity of binding sites or whether it is due to negative cooperativity. Accordingly, "kinetic studies," i.e., association and/or dissociation studies (Fig. 1 and 3) must be performed to discriminate between these two possibilities.

Figure 15 shows a Scatchard plot which is nonlinear and "convex" (or concave downward). As the amount bound increases, the bound to free

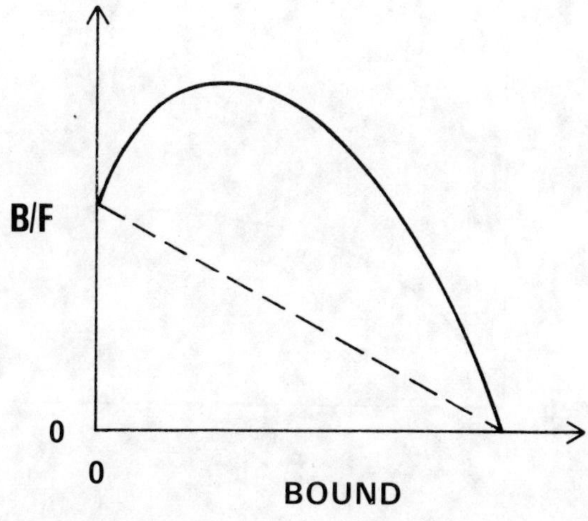

Fig. 15. Scatchard plot: nonlinear convex. Positive cooperativity — watch out for artifacts.

ratio first increases and then decresases. This is presumptive evidence for "positive cooperativity": the binding of the first few molecules of ligand to the binding protein results in an increase of propensity for other ligand molecules to do likewise. This may be due to a conformational change in the molecule, e.g., in the case of oxygen binding to hemoglobin. This type of Scatchard plot has been observed in a variety of radioimmunoassays, notably for hCG and ACTH. A small degree of "hook" has been observed in numerous other assay systems, including those for growth hormone, insulin and enkephalin. Cleavage of the divalent immunoglobulin molecule into molecules with a single binding site (Fab fragments) abolishes the hook and strongly supports the hypothesis of true positive cooperativity. (This has been demonstrated by Weintraub and by Matsukura and Imura.) However, it must be stressed that artifacts or errors in the separation of bound and free may also result in this type of a Scatchard plot. This is particularly true in the case of hormone-receptor interactions when a variable concentration of labeled ligand is used, rather than a constant concentration of labeled ligand and variable concentrations of the unlabeled ligand.

INTRODUCTION TO RIA DOSE-RESPONSE CURVES

Figure 16 shows the basis for the radioimmunoassay dose response curve. (This is the same as Fig. 2.) As the total concentration of unlabeled ligand increases, the total amount bound also increases. Here X represents the concentration of unlabeled ligand. In addition, there is

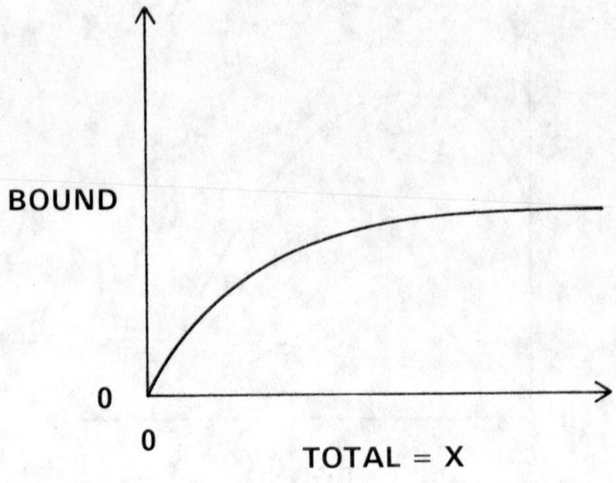

Fig. 16. The "binding isotherm."

some labeled ligand present, designated P*, in an amount which is not necessarily infinitesimal as it would be for a true tracer. The "binding isotherm" may be shown in several other coordinate systems, e.g., bound vs. log(total), bound vs. log(free), or log(bound) vs. log(free).

Figure 17 shows a plot of the bound to total (B/T) or the bound to free (B/F) ratio versus the concentration of unlabeled ligand on an arithmetic scale. Usually such a relationship appears to be "hyperbolic." Ideally, as the amount of unlabeled ligand becomes infinite, the B/T ratio should decrease asymptotically to zero. Due to methodological artifacts, or small systematic errors in the separation of bound and free, the lower asymptote is usually not zero, but rather some small nonspecific count. Baulieu and Raynaud use a related method for display of the curve: log(B/T) vs. log(total), designated a "proportion plot."

Figure 18 shows the same dose response curve as in Figure 17 with the unlabeled ligand shown on a logarithmic scale. The dose response curve, in terms of B/T (0 to 100%) versus log dose is a smooth symmetrical sigmoidal curve. In generating these curves, it is assumed that the concentration of labeled ligand, designated p^*, is inversely related to the equilibrium constant ($p^* = 4/K$). Likewise, it is assumed that the total concentration of antibody combining sites is inversely related to the equilibrium constant ($q = 3/K$). These values of p^* and q would give rise to an assay with the best possible sensitivity (smallest possible minimal detectable dose) in the very special case in which experimental errors were negligible, so that counting errors were the only sourve of variation in the response.[2] In the presence of experimental errors, optimal

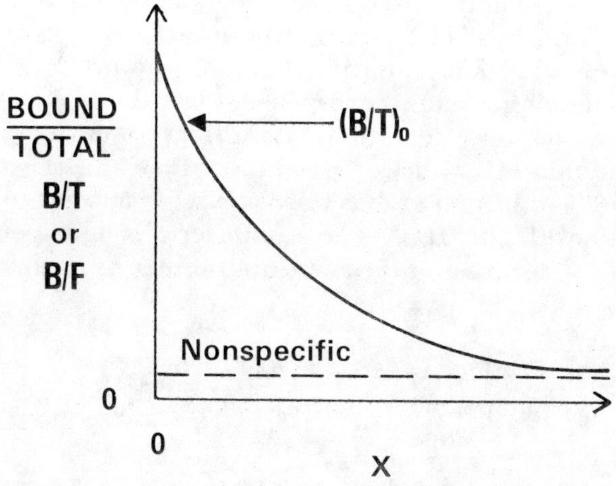

Fig. 17. Bound to total (B/T) or bound to free (B/F) ratio vs. the concentration of unlabeled ligand on an arithmetic scale.

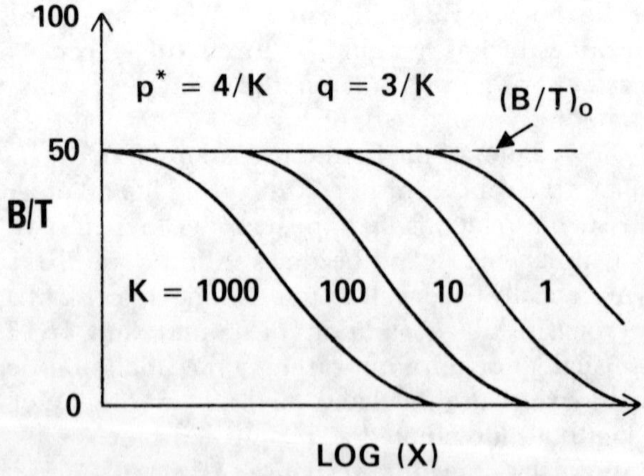

Fig. 18. Same dose response curve as in Figure 17 with the unlabeled ligand shown on a logarithmic scale.

conditions occur when there is a slightly smaller value for both p^* and q, and a $\%(B/T)_0$ which is smaller than 50%. Under these circumstances, and with the above arbitrary rules governing the amount of p^* and q present, when the concentration of unlabeled ligand is zero ($X = 0$), $\%B/T$ will equal 50%. As the equilibrium constant of association is increased, the curve "slides" to the left: A tenfold increase in the equilibrium constant results in a tenfold decrease in the concentration of unlabeled ligand, resulting in any arbitrary bound to total ratio.

Figure 19 illustrates an empirical way to describe the dose response curve in a radioimmunoassay. The equation shown is not derived directly from the first order mass action law, but is usually a good empirical approximation. This curve has four parameters: *a, b, c,* and *d.* The parameter *a* represents the response at zero dose. The parameter *d* represents the response at "infinite" dose. The parameter *c* represents the concentration of unlabeled ligand (i.e., "dose"), which results in a decrease in B/T or B/B_0 to a value which is exactly halfway between *a* and *d* (i.e., *c* is the ED_{50} or ID_{50}). The parameter *b* is an exponent which determines the steepness of the curve at its center or for that matter at any other point:

$$dy/d\,\log_e(X) = b\,(a - d)/4 \quad \text{when } X = c$$
$$dy/d\,\log_{10}(X) = b\,(a - d)(.56) \quad \text{when } X = c$$
$$\text{slope} \propto b$$

Figure 20 shows a popular method of linearizing the dose response curve shown in Figure 19. Taking the logit transformation of B/B_0 (a response variable which must of necessity range between zero and unity)

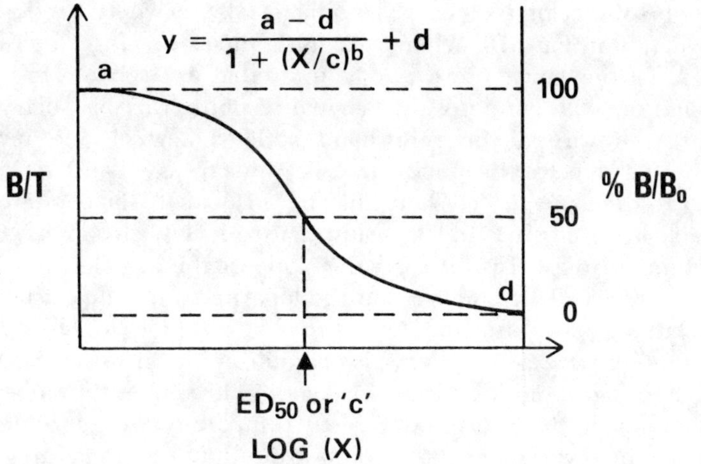

Fig. 19. Empirical way to describe the dose response curve in a radioimmunoassay.

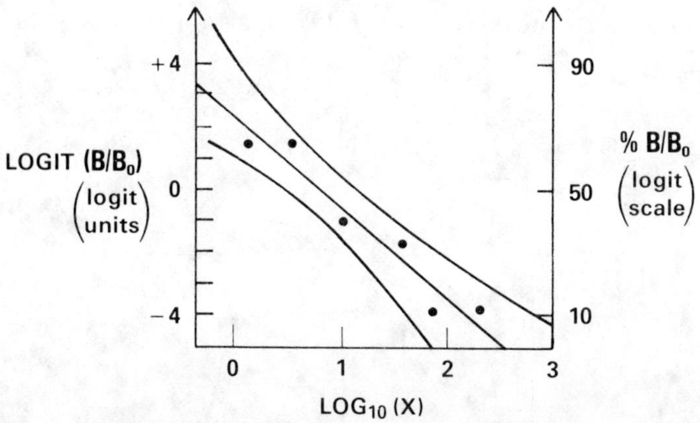

Fig. 20. Popular method of linearizing the dose response curve shown in Figure 19.

and plotting against log(dose) should result in a linear relationship. The logit transformation is defined as

$$Y' = \text{logit}(Y) = \log_e \left(\frac{Y}{1 - Y}\right) \quad \text{for } 0 < Y < 1 \text{ (decimal fraction)}$$

$$Y' = \text{logit}(Y) = \log_e \left(\frac{Y}{100 - Y}\right) \quad \text{for } 0 < Y < 100 \text{ (percentages)}$$

The slope of this logit-log curve is equal to $-1 \times b$ (where b is defined by the equation in Fig. 19). When calculating the slope of the logit-log line ($\Delta Y'/\Delta X'$), one must use the logit units that are shown here on the left-hand ordinate, and not the original response variable such as B/B_0, which is shown on the right-hand scale. Likewise, one must use logarithmic units for the abscissa (i.e., 0.1 appears as -1 and 100 appears as $+2$) to calculate $\Delta X'$. When utilizing a calculator or computer, it is advisable to utilize natural logarithms to calculate the logits and the logarithms of dose. In this case, the slope of the logit-log plot will be approximately -1. If one uses natural logarithms for the calculation of logits, but $\log_{10}$ for dose, one is likely to obtain a slope close to -2.303 in most radioimmunoassay systems. If one utilizes $\log_{10}$ instead of $\log_e$ when calculating logits and $\log_{10}$ when calculating dose, then the slope will be approximately -1. One cannot directly compare the standard deviation (or the residual variance) of the points around the line in Figures 19 and 20. In Figure 20, the deviations around the line and the corresponding residual variance or root mean square (RMS) error around the line are in logit units, whereas in Figure 19, they are in units of counts, $\%B/B_0$, etc. It would be necessary to calculate the appropriately weighted RMS error (standard error of the estimate) in the same units (B/T, or logit (B/B_0)) in order to make meaningful comparisons between the various models.

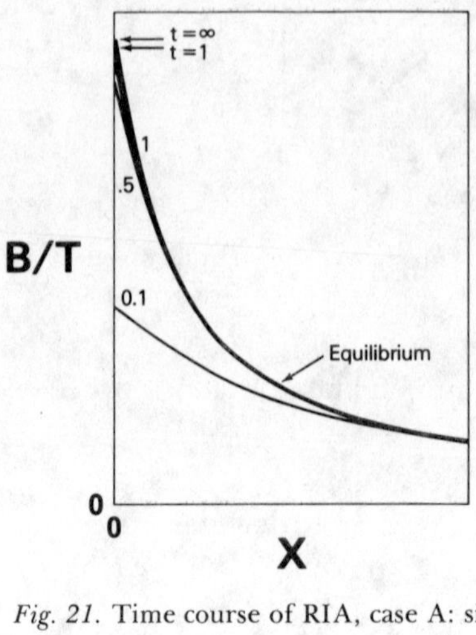

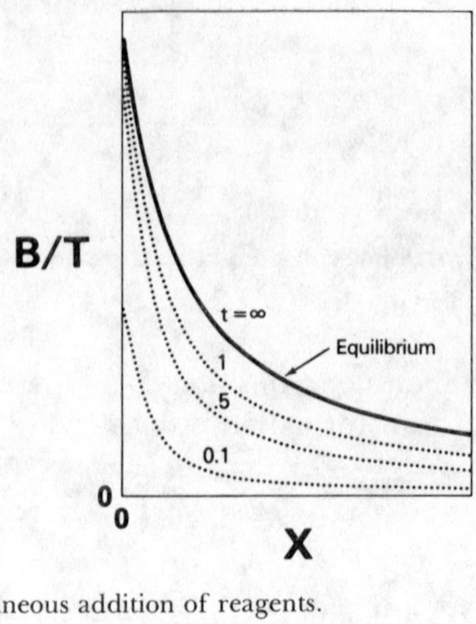

Fig. 21. Time course of RIA, case A: simultaneous addition of reagents.
Fig. 22. Time course of RIA, case B: delayed addition of labeled ligand.

OPTIMIZATION OF RIA

Figure 21–24 show the kinetics of the radioimmunosassay dose response curve under three sets of conditions: (A) Simultaneous Addition of Labeled and Unlabeled Ligand; (B) Delayed Addition of Labeled Ligand; and (C) Delayed Addition of Unlabeled Ligand.

Figure 21 shows the relationship between $\%B/T$ and dose on an arithmetic scale when the labeled or unlabeled antigen and the antibody are added simultaneously at $t = 0$. As the incubation time increases, so that equilibrium is obtained, the dose response curve "rises" and asymptotically approaches the equilibrium curve. Failure to reach equilibrium (use of a much shorter incubation time) results in a marked decrease in the $\%B/T$ observed for $X = 0$ and also in a marked decrease in the slope of the dose response curve, for any and all dose levels.

Figure 22 shows the case where unlabeled antigen, designated P, and the antibody react to (or at least nearly to) equilibrium. Then the labeled ligand, P^*, is added. This system is allowed to incubate, but the reaction is stopped prior to the attainment of equilibrium. Notice that the "clock" is started at the time that the labeled antigen is added. As in the case of Figure 21, at any given incubation time, the $\%B/T_0$ (the $\%B/T$ for $X = 0$) is considerably lower than the equilibrium value. However, in contrast to Figure 21, the slope of the dose response curve in the low dose region is

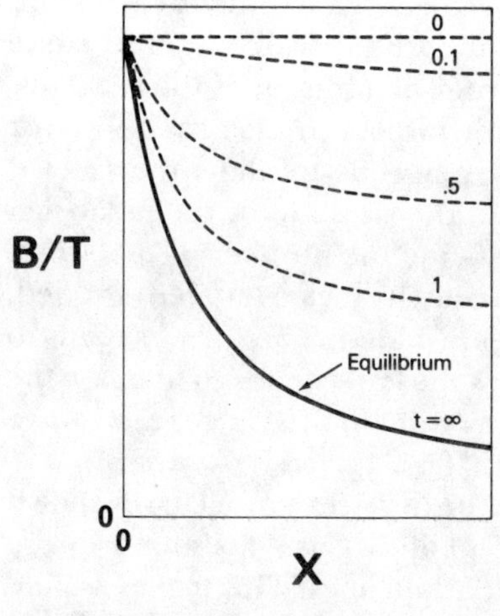

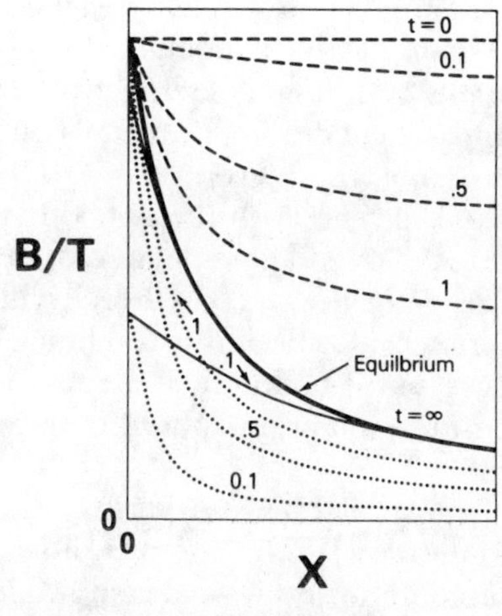

Fig. 23. Time course of RIA, case C: delayed addition of unlabeled ligand.

Fig. 24. Superimposition of the dose response curves shown in Figures 21–23.

considerably increased for any given incubation time. This is because we approach equilibrium more rapidly in the low dose region than in the high dose region. When $X = 0$, (and for low doses) the labeled antigen is simply reacting together with the antibody, exactly as for $X = 0$ in the case of Figure 21. However, for higher doses of X, in order for the labeled antigen to react with the antibody, some of the unlabeled antigen must first dissociate from the antibody. In general, for systems which have a high equilibrium constant of association, this dissociation reaction is much slower than the forward or association reaction, since $K = k_1/k_{-1}$. This increase in the slope of the dose response curve can be utilized to advantage. In many assay systems, the minimal detectable concentration may be reduced by approximately a factor of two or three, i.e., a two- or three-fold increase in "sensitivity." However, use of delayed addition of labeled ligand and nonequilibrium requires precise control of the temperature and duration of the reaction.[21]

Figure 23 shows dose response curves for a radioimmunoassay in which the labeled ligand is reacted with the antibody until equilibrium is reached (case C). Then the unlabeled hormone is added and the clock is started, so that incubation times correspond to those in Figures 21 and 22. At zero time, the percentage of labeled antigen that is bound will be the same irrespective of the dose X, which will subsequently be added to the tube. Thus at zero time we have a horizontal line. After addition of the unlabeled ligand, there will be progressive dissociation of the labeled ligand as the unlabeled hormone begins to occupy binding sites on the antibody. Thus the final equilibrium curve is approached from above and from the right. In general, this will result in a decreased slope, and a loss of sensitivity and precision in the assay.

If equilibrium is finally reached and if the antigen-antibody reactions are completely reversible, the same equilibrium dose response curve should be obtained irrespective of the order of addition of the reagents. Thus when dealing with an equilibrium radioimmunoassay (e.g., for thyroxine and steroids), it may be advantageous to allow the labeled ligand to react with the antibody prior to the addition of the unlabeled standard or unknown material, thus reducing the number of pipettings of reagents needed. Further, if a little too much labeled antigen is added, there will also be a little too much antibody added. The former tends to decrease the bound to total ratio, whereas the latter tends to increase the bound to total ratio, and these two effects will tend to cancel each other out.

Figure 24 shows a superimposition of the dose response curves shown in Figures 21–23. Case A is shown by solid lines. Case B is shown by the dotted lines, and Case C is shown by the dashed lines. This makes it quite obvious that for short times of incubation, delayed addition of labeled ligand (Case B) results in a considerable increase in the steepness of the dose response curve.

For any given combination of radioactive labeled antigen (p^*) and antibody (q) for any given equilibrium constant of association (K), there will be a uniquely defined bound to free ratio, if equilibrium is reached and perfect separation of bound and free is achieved (Fig. 25). However, any given "starting bound to free ratio" or initial $(B/F)_0$ can be achieved by an infinite number of combinations of p^* and q. For example, if we wish to start out with 50% B/T, or $B/F = 1$, then q is equal to $1/K + p/2$. Hence, one can increase the antibody concentration and make a corresponding increase in the amount of tracer, and still obtain the same B/F_0. Likewise, for 33% initial binding, the equation is

$$q = 1/(2K) + p/3$$

If we make several assumptions, viz., attainment of equilibrium, perfect separation of bound and free, homogeneity of the antibody, identity of labeled and unlabeled material, and known values for experimental and counting errors, then the combination of p^* and q that results in the optimal assay conditions (in terms of minimizing the minimal detectable dose) can be computed (Fig. 26). Then, for any lower degree of performance (in terms of minimal detectable dose or in terms of precision at any desired target dose level), there will be several combinations of values of p^* and q that will provide an assay of similar behavior. It is convenient to display these combinations on a "contour

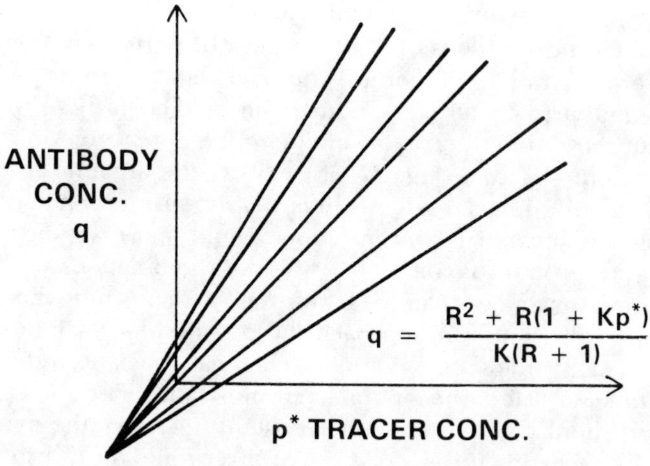

Fig. 25. Combinations of p^* and q giving the same $(B/F)_0 = R$.

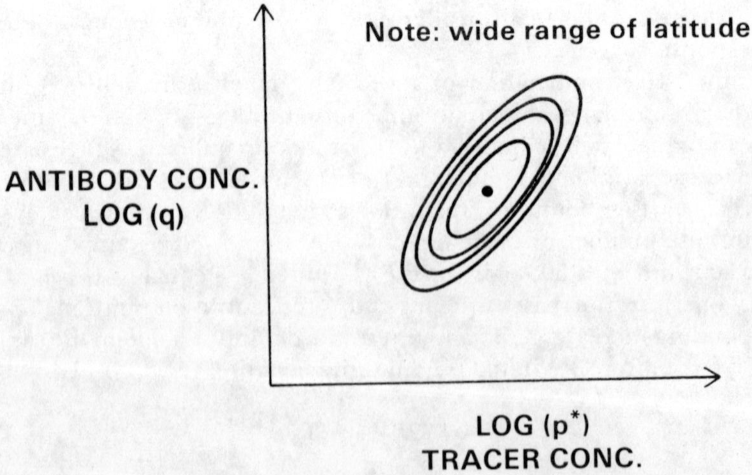

Fig. 26. Regions of p^*, q giving the same sensitivity, i.e., minimal detectable concentration.

map" in terms of $\log(p^*)$ and $\log(q)$. Increasing p^* while decreasing q results in a rapid decrease in assay performance. Likewise, decreasing p^* and increasing q also results in a rapid decline of assay performance. By comparison with Figure 25, we see that these changes would result in a marked change in the bound to free ratio, whereas when p^* and q move in the same direction, the B/F or B/T value remains essentially constant. Thus there is an optimal $(B/T)_0$. Almost any assay that gives the same B/T_0 will perform close to the "ideal" assay. An understanding of this "sensitivity surface" facilitates both experimental and theoretical approaches to optimizing a radioimmunoassay.[20]

Just as the concentrations of p^* and q must be optimized, so must the process for separation of bound and free ligand. In the charcoal methods (and virtually all other adsorption methods), there will be an optimal concentration of charcoal and an optimal reaction time for the incubation with charcoal (Fig. 27). Increasing the amount of charcoal decreases the optimal reaction time nearly proportionately, while decreasing the charcoal concentration would increase the optimal reaction time proportionately[3]. The various combinations of charcoal concentration (or amount) and reaction time are shown by the contour lines. Empirically, one can approach the optimization as follows. In a first experiment, hold the amount of charcoal constant and vary the reaction time to select the optimal reaction time. Then in a second experiment, hold the reaction time constant and vary the amount of charcoal. By repeating this process two or three times (or by using a grid of several selected values of charcoal concentration and several selected values of reaction time) one can "zero in" on the optimal concentration. It is not necessary to run an entire dose response curve for each of the combinations of charcoal and reaction time. Rather, one should examine $(B/T)_0$ and the "nonspecific" counts in the absence of antibody. Optimizing the difference in B/T for the zero dose tubes and for the tubes in the absence of antibody or in the presence of an infinite amount of ligand ($\Delta B/T$) is very nearly equivalent to optimizing the slope of the dose response curve in the low dose region. Again, there is usually a wide range of conditions providing satisfactory assays.[3]

Superimposed on the contour lines, we show one possible experimental design that might be utilized in a laboratory attempting to find the optimal combination of charcoal concentration and reaction time. Thus we might first select the charcoal concentration designated B, corresponding to the lower horizontal line. One might then try five different reaction times, designated 1 through 5 (e.g., 10, 15, 30, 45 min). We might find that we get our best result with the second choice of reaction time, namely 15 min. One might then hold the reaction time constant at 15 min and systematically vary charcoal concentration. Again we might use five values (A through E). We would be likely to find that charcoal concentrations B and C gave the best results, and that there was little difference between them, but that concentration C appeared to be slightly better than concentration B. One might then hold the charcoal concentration constant at this new level (C), and then repeat the experiment for a series of reaction times. This is shown by the black dots on the horizontal line passing through the point labeled C. Using this kind of strategy, one can usually fairly quickly optimize the concentrations of charcoal and reaction time. When selecting the combination of charcoal and reaction time, it is helpful to realize that, in general, an

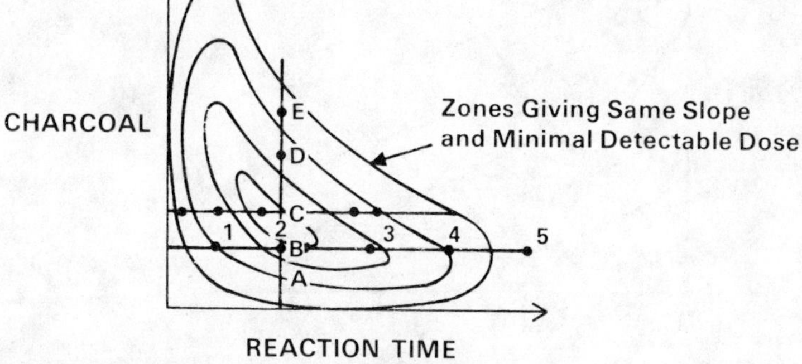

Fig. 27. Separation of bound and free; charcoal method.

increase of charcoal concentration will result in a decrease optimal reaction time, and vice versa.

A similar approach can be utilized for the optimization of any two variables in the assay. For instance, this kind of a "search" can be utilized to optimize antibody concentration and tracer concentration (cf. Fig. 26).

The "true" curve, which would be obtained with perfect separation of bound and free, is shown by the heavy solid line in Figure 28. Utilizing too little charcoal or adsorbent might result in the dose response curve shown by the dashed lines, where t represents the duration of the reaction with charcoal. A very short incubation with charcoal results in a relatively high value of the apparent $\%B/T$ for zero dose, but also in very high nonspecific counts for infinite dose. As the reaction time with charcoal increases, the apparent $(B/T)_0$ begins to decrease. This is due to the dissociation of the antigen-antibody complex during the reaction with charcoal. However, there is a gradual increase in the slope of the dose response curve as the reaction with charcoal progresses. Thus a compromise between $\%(B/T)_0$ and slope is needed. The charcoal method of separation of bound and free can result in a marked distortion of the dose response curve and a corresponding disastrous change in the nature of the Scatchard plots derived from such dose response curves.

A computerized approach to optimization of p^*, q, reaction time, and conditions for separation of bound and free is available. The computerized, "rational" approach requires reliable estimates of the rate constants and equilibrium constants. Methods for obtaining these will be discussed below.

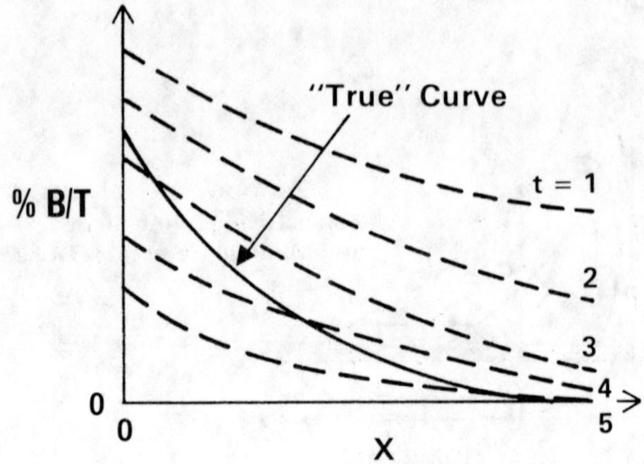

Fig. 28. Effect of too little charcoal.

ANTIBODY OR RECEPTOR HETEROGENEITY

Most of the preceding illustrations have assumed that the antiserum consists of only a single class of high affinity antibody. In practice, the antibodies are likely to be heterogeneous (e.g., within two species, Q_1 and Q_2, with differing equilibrium constants and rate constants). Likewise, the labeled and unlabeled ligand may react with different affinities. In addition, several physicochemically distinct ligands may be present, both in the tracer and in the standards or unknown materials. Accordingly, at least four simultaneous reactions between two ligands and two antibodies, each with its own equilibrium constant, must be considered (Fig. 29). Real systems may become much more complex. The mathematical theory to predict the behavior of such systems has been developed.[27] This theory is also useful for describing the reaction between T_4 and T_3 in various serum proteins and the reaction between various steroids and plasma binding proteins.

One of the most common problems involving "crossreactivity" arising in practice is in the radioimmunoassay for a hormone, designated H_1 or H^* (Fig. 30). The dose response curves are constructed not only for the unlabeled analog of H^*, but also for a variety of potentially crossreacting ligands. The usual method for characterization of these crossreacting ligands is the measurement of their relative concentration needed for 50% displacement of the radioactive label from the binding protein. This has often been called the relative binding affinity (RBA). The ratio of the ED_{50}'s for two crossreacting ligands is approximately equal to the ratio of their affinity constants. This approximation is best for low values of the B/F ratio. However, with bound to free ratios for the radioactively labeled ligand that are appreciably different from zero, a correction factor needs to be introduced utilizing the equation shown in Fig. 30.

$$P_1 + Q_1 \rightleftharpoons P_1Q_1 \qquad K_{11}$$
$$P_1 + Q_2 \rightleftharpoons P_1Q_2 \qquad K_{12}$$
$$P_2 + Q_1 \rightleftharpoons P_2Q_1 \qquad K_{21}$$
$$P_2 + Q_2 \rightleftharpoons P_2Q_2 \qquad K_{22}$$

e.g. T, DHT, E_2 for Alb, TeBG,
T_4, T_3 for Alb, TBG,
TBPA, F, Prog, 17 αOH for
Alb, CBG.

Fig. 29. Four simultaneous reactions between two ligands and two antibodies.

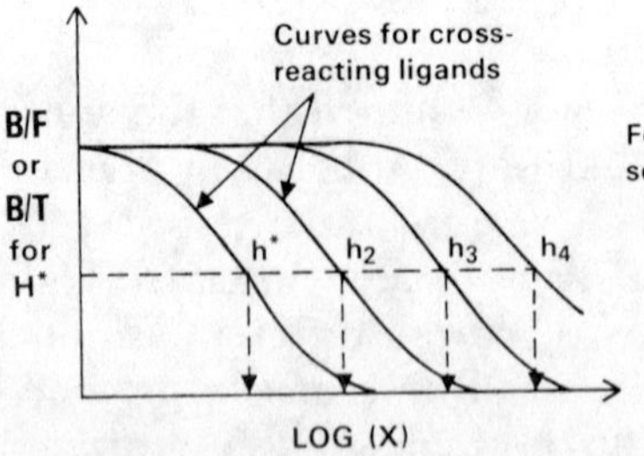

$$H^* + Q_1 \rightleftharpoons H^*Q_1$$
$$H_2 + Q_1 \rightleftharpoons H_2Q_1$$

For only one class of site, equilibrium, perfect separation:

$$\frac{h_2}{h_3} = \frac{1 + (K_2/K^*)\,R\,K_3}{1 + (K_3/K^*)\,R\,K_2}$$

$$\cong \frac{K_3}{K_2} \text{ for low } B/F \sim 0$$

where $R = B/F$ for h^*, h_2, etc.

Fig. 30. Crossreactivity.

Here K_2 and K_3 refer to the equilibrium constants of association for the unlabeled ligands. The relative binding affinity (RBA) should be measured at more than one level of B/T or B/F, and one should verify that there is no systematic relationship between the calculated ratio K_2/K_3 and the bound to free ratio for the labeled ligand (see Appendix III of ref. 8). This relationship is based on Eq. 31 of Ekins et al.[2]

LABELED ANTIBODY ASSAYS (IRMA, 2-SITE IRMA, ELISA)

An important type of radioligand assay involves antibody (rather than the antigen or hapten) labeled with a radioactive or enzymatic label i.e. the immunoradiometric assay (Fig. 31). Thus one has a reaction between the unlabeled ligand (standard or unknown) and radioactively labeled purified antibody (Q^*). After this first reaction has approached equilibrium, a solid phase immunoadsorbent (e.g., insulin bound to cellulose powder) is added. This will react with any of the remaining radioactively labeled antibody to form an insoluble precipitate (RQ^*). After the second reaction has proceeded for some time, the tubes are centrifuged and the radioactivity remaining in the supernatant is counted. The role of the immunoadsorbent R in the system is analogous to the role of the charcoal adsorbent in labeled antigen RIAs. The dose response curve that is obtained when plotting the response against the logarithm of the concentration or dose of the unlabeled ligand is sigmoidal in shape. In these assays, there is usually fairly good uniformity of variance, i.e., the error of the response variable σ_y in the vertical direction is nearly constant. These dose response curves can usually be described by a simple empirical formula of the type shown in the insert of Figure 31 (also of Figure 19).

Figure 32 shows an important variation of the immunoradiometric assay, otherwise known as the "sandwich assay" or junction test. Here the first antibody (Q_1) is solid phase. It is absorbed onto a test tube, a latex

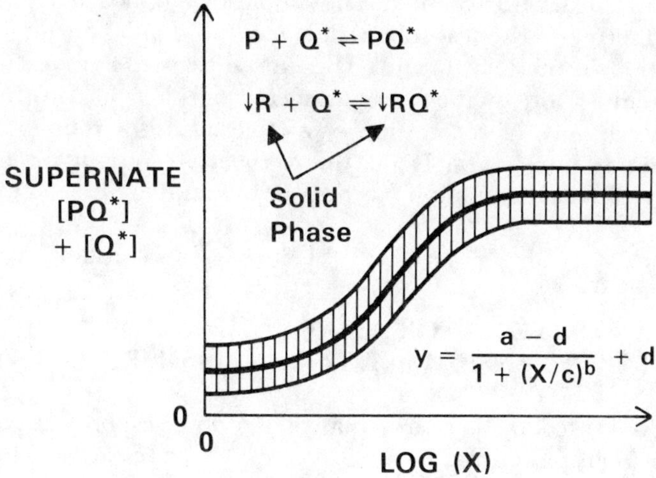

Fig. 31. Labeled antibody immunoradiometric assays (IRMA).

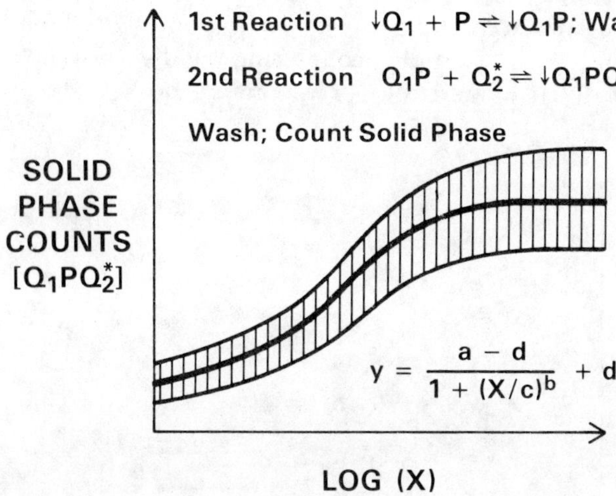

Fig. 32. "Sandwich" assay or "2-site IRMA."

bead or other support. The antigen hapten or ligand to be measured is introduced into the test tube and allowed to react toward equilibrium. The test tube is then carefully washed and a radioactively labeled antibody (Q_2*) is added. It reacts with the antigen, which is now bound to the solid phase. This results in the formation of a complex (Q_1PQ_2*). After this reaction has proceeded for a time, the tubes are again decanted, washed, and counted. The amount of radioactively labeled antigen adhering to the test tube wall is measured as a function of the concentration of the total ligand. These dose response curves may be described empirically by the four-parameter logistic equation. In these assays, the variance of the response variable increases roughly as the square of the response variable, i.e., there is nearly a constant percentage error or coefficient of variation for the counts bound to the solid phase:

$$\sigma_y \propto y, \quad \text{or } \sigma_y^2 \propto y^2, \quad \text{or } \%CV_y = \sigma_y/y = \text{constant}$$

CRITERIA FOR ASSAY VALIDATION: PRECISION, SENSITIVITY, PARALLELISM, RECOVERY

Figure 33 is a schematic representative of a dose response curve with confidence limits placed at ±1 standard errors of the response. The basis for dose interpolation is shown. For any given response level, designated by y, read over to the curve horizontally and then read down to the X axis to obtain an estimate of the potency estimate (X) for the unknown. To obtain an estimate of the lower limit (LL) for the potency estimate, read over to the curve, read up to the upper 1σ confidence limit for the curve, read over to the left until encountering the dose response curve, and then read down to find the corresponding dosage. To find the

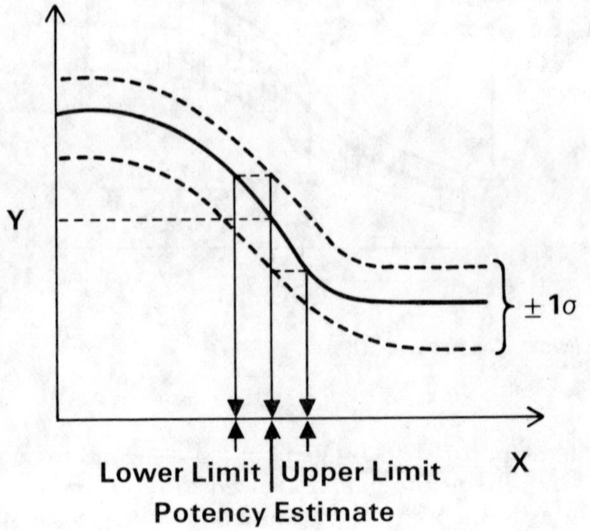

Fig. 33. Schematic representation of a dose response curve with confidence limits placed at ±1 standard errors of the response.

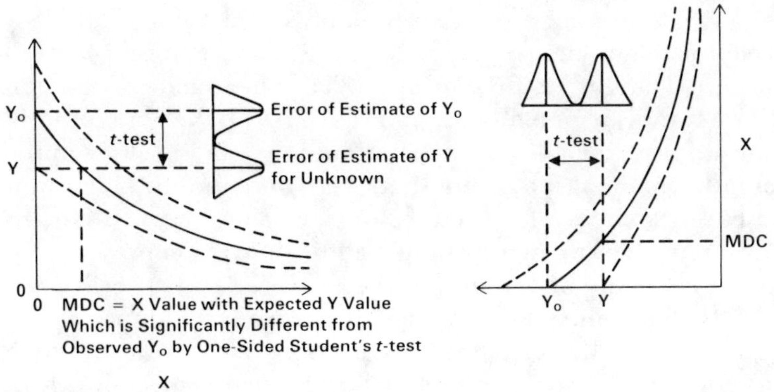

Fig. 34. Graphical representation of considerations involved in the estimation of the minimum detectable concentration. (a) Y versus X; (b) figure in panel a rotated so that the response variable is horizontal.

upper limit (UL) for the potency, read from the y value over to the curve, read down until encountering the lower confidence limit, and then read over to the right until intersecting the curve. The corresponding dose is the upper limit for the potency estimate.

For routine radioimmunoassays, it is too cumbersome to print out both the upper and lower limits for each of the hundreds of samples in an assay. Instead, it is convenient to obtain upper and lower limits by the method shown. Then an approximate coefficient of variation ($\%CV$) or "percentage error" can be calculated by utilizing the formula

$$\%CV = \frac{UL - LL}{2X} \times 100$$

where X is the potency estimate.

For this purpose it is convenient to use confidence limits calculated at ± 1 standard deviation. This estimate of precision ignores the uncertainty in the location of the dose response curve itself. Calculations that include this factor can be performed when necessary, but are much more complicated.

Figure 34 provides a graphical representation of considerations involved in the estimation of the minimal detectable concentration, one of the important measures of assay sensitivity. The calculation of the minimal detectable concentration depends on three factors. The first is the uncertainty in the estimate of the "true" response for zero dose, designated Y_0. Although the use of replicates at zero dose and/or multiple observations in the low dose region of the dose response curve allow for a fairly reliable estimate of Y_0, it is nonetheless subject to some uncertainty. The second is the uncertainty of the value of the response variable for the unknown (or for the mean of several replicates for the unknown). The third is the uncertainty in the estimate of the standard deviation for this region of the curve. The *MDD* is the dose for which the mean response for the unknown would be statistically significantly different from the mean response for zero dose (or our best estimate of Y_0 based on analysis of the entire dose response curve). Usually, for practical purposes, we may assume that the dose response curve is linear and has uniformity of variance in the small region between $X = 0$ and $X = MDD$. The minimal detectable dose depends both upon the degree of replication of the response for zero dose, and upon the degree of replication for the unknown sample being tested. Thus it is insufficient to state a minimal detectable dose for an assay. One must stipulate the number of replicates being used for the unknown (single tube, duplicates, triplicates, etc.) and the assay design utilized (number and placement of dose levels). Through the use of analysis of variance and related statistical techniques, one can improve the reliability of the calculation of the minimal detectable concentration.[10,19] Nevertheless, these values can be quite erratic between assays, because they are based on estimates of the variability in the response variable based on a small number of replicates and hence low degrees of freedom. It is desirable that the minimal detectable concentration (*MDC*) be calculated by the program utilized for routine analysis of the dose response curve. It is inadvisable to utilize a crude rule such as a response which is two standard deviations away from the response for zero dose. Such "rules of thumb" are better than no rules at all, but may be misleading, since they ignore the uncertainty in the estimate of the response for zero dose.

Figures 35 and 36 illustrate one of the requirements for testing the validity of a radioimmunoassay. As one increases the volume of serum or plasma introduced into the test tube, the calculated potency (e.g., in ng per tube) should increase in a directly linear fashion. Similarly, a "stripped" plasma containing no ligand or antigen, but to which varying amounts of standard ligand have been added, may be used. Again, one should obtain potency estimates which are directly proportional to the amounts added.

In most RIAs, the standard error of the potency estimate increases roughly in proportion to the magnitude of the potency estimate. Thus severe "nonuniformity of variance" is present. This problem is usually so severe that use of an unweighted least squares linear regression between potency and the amount of serum (or plasma, or ligand) added (Figure 35) may yield seriously biased results, with an intercept that is spuriously "significantly different from zero." Many of these problems are rectified in Figure 36, where the recovery experiment is portrayed using a log scale for both axes. This is useful, since it is usually desired to show that

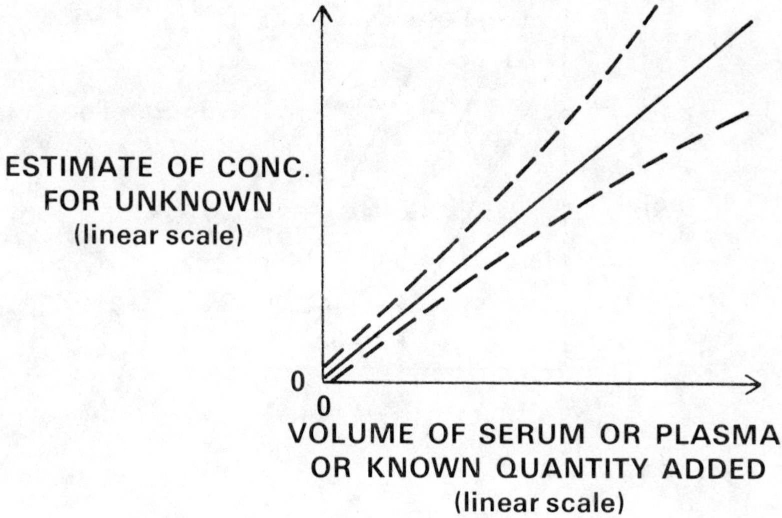

Fig. 35. Testing of "recovery", using linear scales.

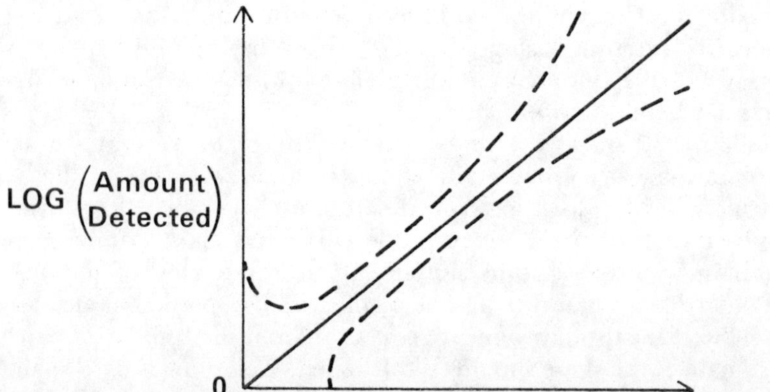

Fig. 36. Testing of "recovery", using logarithmic scales for both axes.

the assay is providing satisfactory "recoveries" over at least two orders of magnitude. Use of the logarithm of potency also results in approximate "uniformity of variance," with the scatter of the points around the line nearly constant over quite a wide range. This breaks down as the dose levels approach zero, in which case reverting back to the use of the linear coordinate system (Figure 35) is helpful. Thus a least squares linear

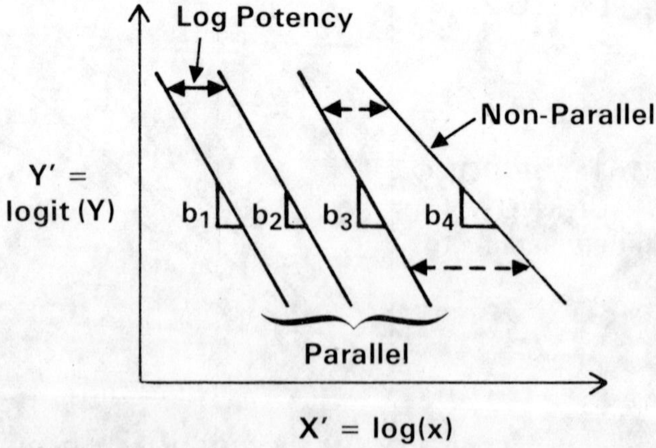

Fig. 37. Parallel line analysis.

regression should be calculated between the logarithm of the estimated concentration of the ligand and the logarithm of the volume of serum (or plasma, or the quantity of known ligand added to the reaction mixtures). This line should have a slope of unity. Any departure from linearity or from a slope of unity would be indicative of an "invalid assay," corresponding to nonparallelism of the dose response curves for standard and unknown.

Figure 37 shows the dose response curves for several standards or unknowns, each with its own slope (b_1, b_2, b_3, b_4). One of the primary virtues of the logit-log coordinate system is that it provides for linearization of the dose response curves for most (although not all) radioimmunoassays, thus simplifying the evaluation of parallelism of standard and unknown. The slope of each line should be calculated by a weighted least squares linear regression, and the standard error of the estimate of the slope should be calculated. Weighting is used so that very precise points (usually in the center of the curve) are given a lot of weight, while very imprecise (or "fuzzy") points (usually at the ends of the curve) are given relatively little weight. Each point should be given weight in proportion to the "information" that it contains. This permits the use of the Student's t test for parallelism of standard and unknown. This analysis can be applied whenever the unknown samples have been analyzed at two or more dose levels. If one assumes that the scatter around the curve for the unknown is the same as that for the standard, then tests of parallelism are possible even when there are only two points on a dose response curve for the unknown.[7] "Parallelism" may be tested when utilizing other types of analysis of dose response curves, but this becomes less efficient. However, a graph and regression analysis of the form shown in Figure 36 may be used to test parallelism of standard and unknown, even in the case where the dose response curve is nonlinear. Use of the analysis given in Figure 36 is readily adaptable to small desk-top calculators, and involves nothing more than linear regression analysis, irrespective of the complexity of the dose response curve.

CONFIDENCE LIMITS FOR IMMUNOASSAY DOSE RESPONSE CURVES

Figures 38–43 show the dose response curve for RIAs in a variety of coordinate systems. It is important to consider not only the shape of the dose response curve, but also the shape of the 95% confidence region around the dose response curve. One should note that curves such as these may be obtained empirically, in practice, by running 10 replicates at each of 10 dose levels. Next plot the dose response curves in each of the coordinate systems, showing each observation, and the range. Then construct the approximate 95% confidence limits for the response, by calculating the mean, $\pm 2\sigma$ limits, and "smoothing" the size of the confidence limits, to reduce the effect of random sampling error in the sample standard deviations (which are quite unstable, due to the low number of degrees of freedom).

Figure 38 shows a graph of bound over total versus dose of unlabeled ligand on an arithmetic scale. Similar curves are obtained whether one uses *B/T*, *B/F*, or counts bound. A similar (though inverted) hyperbola is obtained if one measures free/total, free/bound, or free counts. This curve is a hyperbola and is severely nonlinear. There is a moderate

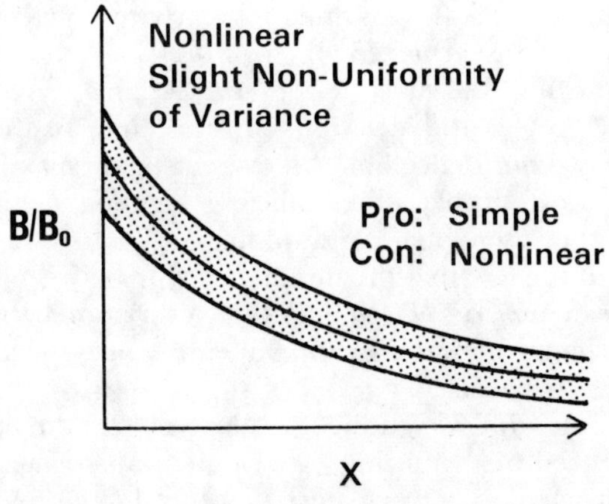

Fig. 38. Graph of bound over total versus dose of unlabeled ligand on an arithmetic scale.

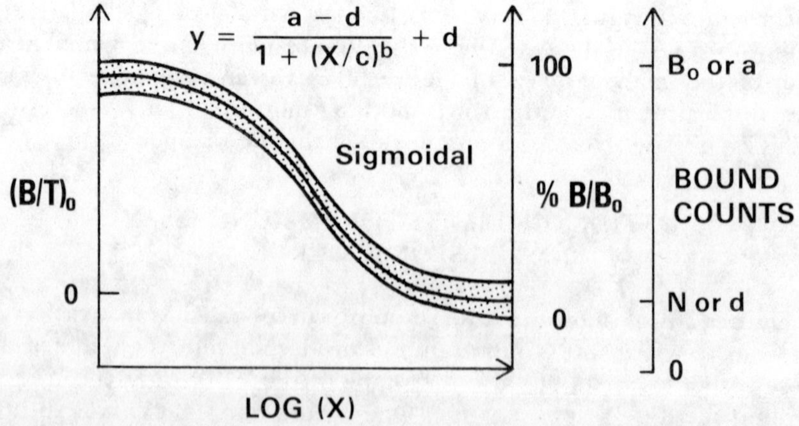

Fig. 39. Typical dose response curve in terms of bound over total (B/T) vs. logarithm of dose.

degree of nonuniformity of variance, illustrated by the tapering of the confidence limits in the vertical direction. Notice that larger counts usually have a larger standard deviation whether one is using bound counts or free counts.

Figure 39 shows a typical dose response curve in terms of bound over total (B/T) versus logarithm of dose. This results in a sigmoidal dose response curve, which is usually symmetrical. Similar curves are obtained using $\%B/T$, normalized B/T, or $\%B/B_0$, bound counts, or B/F. A similar curve, although rising, is obtained when utilizing free over total (F/T), free over bound (F/B), or free counts.

Figure 40 is an important representation of the dose response curve with the logit(B/B_0) on the vertical scale and logarithm of unlabeled ligand on the horizontal scale, resulting in nearly complete linearization of the function. This is achieved by "compressing" the curve in the middle and "stretching" the curve at its extremes. This also has the effect of squeezing the 95% confidence limits in the center of the curve and stretching the 95% confidence limits at the extremes, making weighted regression analysis desirable when utilizing logit-log methods. When fitting a curve by "eye" on logit-log graph paper, the investigator readily takes into account the fact that the minor variation between 90 and 95% is much more severe *in terms of logit units* than a variation between 50 and 55%. Indeed, a change between 95 and 96% influences the logit about as much as a change between 50 and 60%!

Accordingly, rules for weighting the analysis should be built into curve-fitting procedures utilizing the logit transformation, unless attention is restricted to a very narrow central region of the dose response curve, where there is uniformity of variance.

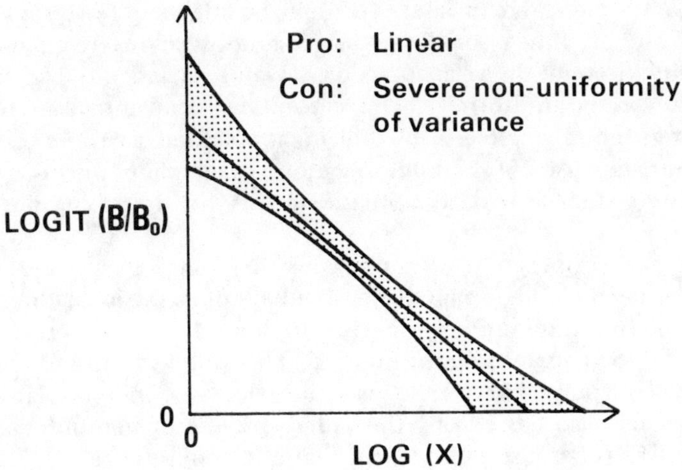

Fig. 40. Representation of the dose response curve with the logit (B/B_0) on the vertical scale and logarithm of unlabeled ligand on the horizontal scale.

Figure 41 shows a popular attempt to linearize the hyperbola shown in Figure 38. Plotting the reciprocal of B/T, the reciprocal of B/B_0, or the reciprocal of bound counts against arithmetic dose results in nearly perfect linearization of the dose response curve, under certain limiting assumptions. This will work well if one is dealing with "saturation conditions," so that essentially all binding sites are filled. This is the case for a simple displacement or isotope dilution assay. Two problems arise, however. First, these curves are usually linear only over a very limited

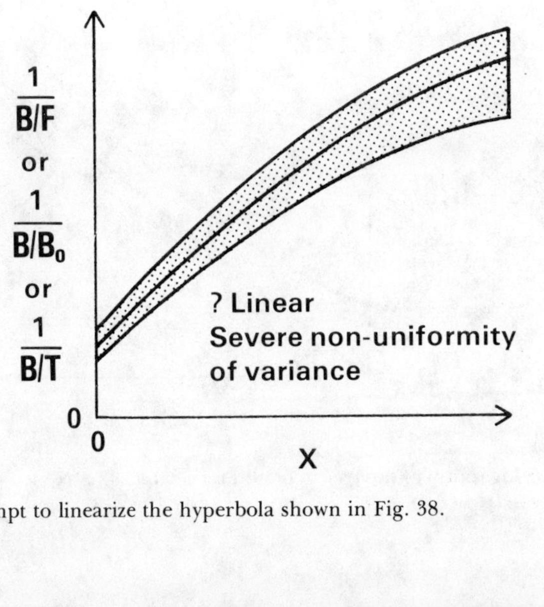

Fig. 41. Attempt to linearize the hyperbola shown in Fig. 38.

region (a 10-fold range or less). This may be adequate for assays which require use of only a small range of concentrations (e.g., digoxin, thyroxine). Second, the reciprocals of B/T and related variables usually involve severe nonuniformity of variance. One can compensate for this by adept graphical analysis or by utilizing a weighted least squares linear regression. The use of (weighted) polynomials or spline functions in this coordinate system should be quite satisfactory for describing the curve empirically.

Ekins has proposed a variation on the logit-log method which avoids the need for logit paper (Fig. 42). One plots the logarithm of the free to bound ratio minus the free to bound ratio for zero dose, $\log[F/B - (F/B)_0]$ against logarithm of X. This will result in linearization of the dose response curve exactly as in the logit-log method. However, this approach also has exactly the same problem of nonuniformity of variance. Ekins has also pointed out that one could utilize

$$\operatorname{logit}\left(\frac{B/F}{(B/F)_0}\right)$$

rather than

$$\operatorname{logit}\left(\frac{B/T}{(B/T)_0}\right) = \operatorname{logit}(B/B_0)$$

This results in a shift in the dose response curve, but since this shift is the same for both standards and unknowns, one still has a valid method for representing the dose response curve.

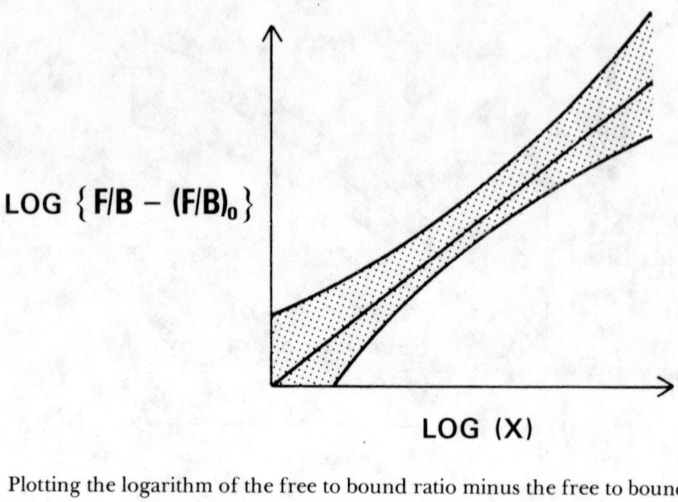

Fig. 42. Plotting the logarithm of the free to bound ratio minus the free to bound ratio for zero dose against the logarithm of X.

Several authors have pointed out that there is an approximately linear relationship between the logarithm of (B/T) or the logarithm of bound counts and the logarithm of total ligand present (labeled plus unlabeled antigen) (Fig. 43). This relationship is derived from the first-order mass action law, and becomes asymtotically correct as the saturation of all binding sites is approached. Indeed, this method may be regarded as a log-log representation of the relationship shown in Figures 38 or 41. Gilman noticed that this relationship follows from the results given by Berson and Yalow.[1] (In contrast to almost all other methods involving the logarithm of dose on the arithmetic scale, this approach uses the logarithm of the *total* concentration of labeled and unlabeled ligand rather than logarithm of the concentration of unlabeled material.) This provides fairly good linearization of the dose response curve. Also, the $\log(B/T)$ or the log(bound counts) shows fairly good uniformity of variance. However, as the counts become small, the uniformity of variance may no longer apply.

The major difficulty of this method is that it requires a reasonably reliable estimate of the mass of radioactively labeled ligand that is present. This information is often available for ^{3}H-labeled steroids, drugs, prostaglandins, etc., for which the specific activity is accurately known. This requirement does not appear in any of the "empirical" methods shown in Figures 38–42, although this requirement is shared

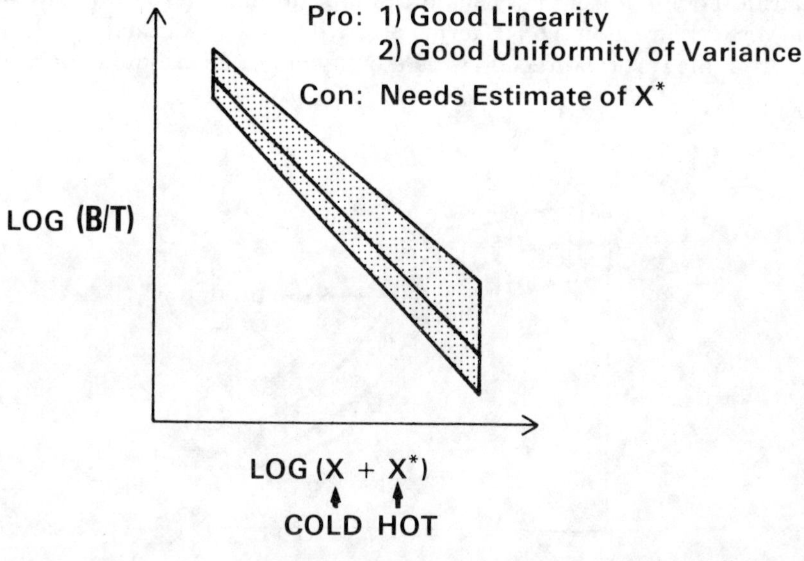

Fig. 43. Showing the approximately linear relationship between the logarithm (B/T) or the logarithm of bound counts and the logarithm of total ligand present (labeled plus unlabeled antigen).

by methods based on the mass action law. Another implicit assumption of this method is that the affinity of the antibody for the labeled material is (about) the same as the affinity of the antibody for the unlabeled material. This method may be summed up as "pretty good, when it works." Alternatively, the parameter X^* may be regarded as an empirically derived or fitted parameter, in order to give the best linearization of the dose response curve. This method is likely to break down when dealing with assays that are operating under conditions where only a small fraction of the binding sites of the antibody (or other binding protein) are occupied.

We shall confine our attention primarily to the use of the sigmoidal relationship between B/T (and related methods) versus log(dose), and the related logit-log method. We now consider the size and shape of the confidence limits for X and Y. When reporting radioimmunoassay results, it is necessary to provide an estimate of the precision or confidence limits for the results. However, there is considerable confusion in the literature regarding the methods for doing this. Many authors have confused considerations of the error in the response variable (Y) and errors in the potency estimate, X, or its logarithm log(X). Thus we must distinguish the errors or uncertainties in the vertical direction from those in the horizontal direction. Figures 44, 46, and 48 show the errors in the response in the vertical (Y) direction. Figures 45, 47, and 49 show the errors in the horizontal (X) direction. From a statistical point of view, it is usually desirable to characterize the errors in the vertical direction, i.e., in terms of the dependent variable. First, the errors in the vertical direction should, in theory, be distributed normally.

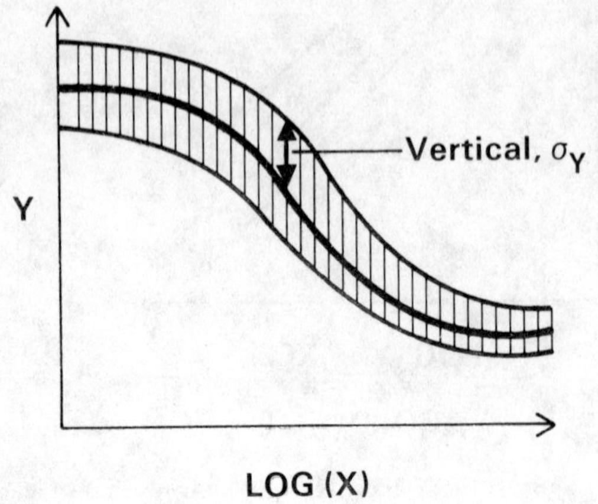

Fig. 44. Confidence limits for X and Y: error in Y, given X or log(X).

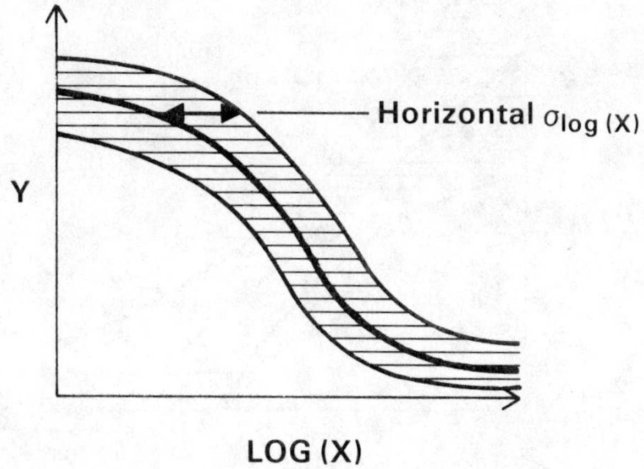

Fig. 45. Confidence limits for *X* and *Y*: error in log(*X*), given *Y*.

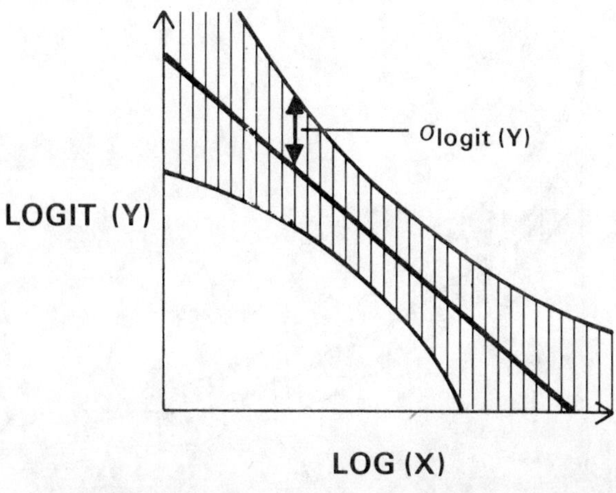

Fig. 46. Confidence limits for *X* and *Y*: error in logit(*Y*), given *X* or log(*X*).

This has been verified in practice. Second, least squares regression analysis (whether linear or nonlinear, weighted or nonweighted) seeks to minimize the deviations of the points around the fitted curve in the vertical direction. Accordingly, it is the error in the response variable that is of primary concern in statistical curve-fitting procedures.

In contrast, when reporting results, we are usually interested in the error in the potency estimate, i.e., in the value of *X*, given *Y*. In general, these errors are not subject to a Gaussian distribution. Furthermore,

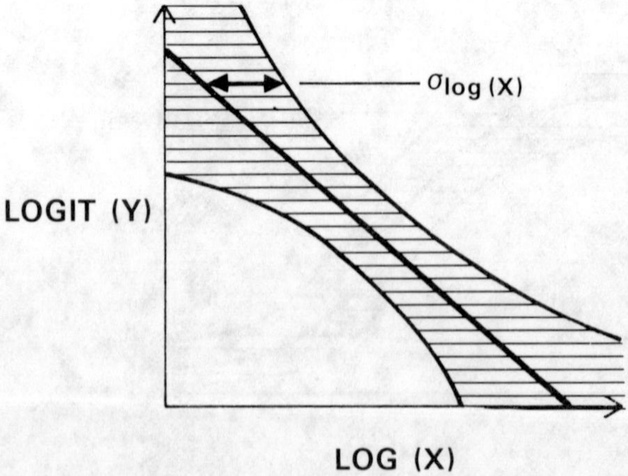

Fig. 47. Confidence limits for *X* and *Y*: error in log(*X*), given *Y* or logit(*Y*).

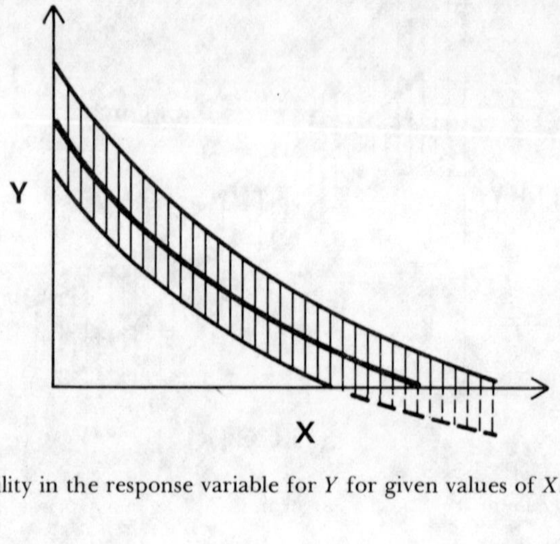

Fig. 48. Variability in the response variable for *Y* for given values of *X*.

these errors are usually unequal as one moves up and down the dose response curve. In Figures 44–49 we show the same dose response curve (and its 95% confidence limits) in three coordinate systems. Although the logit transformation (Figure 46) augments the error in the vertical direction at the extreme ends of the dose response curve, the errors in terms of log(*X*) should be exactly the same in Figure 47 as in Figure 45. We may regard Figures 46 and 47 as equivalent to Figures 44 and 45, except for the nonlinear distortion of the vertical axis. This, however, does not effect the values of *X* corresponding to any given value of *Y*.

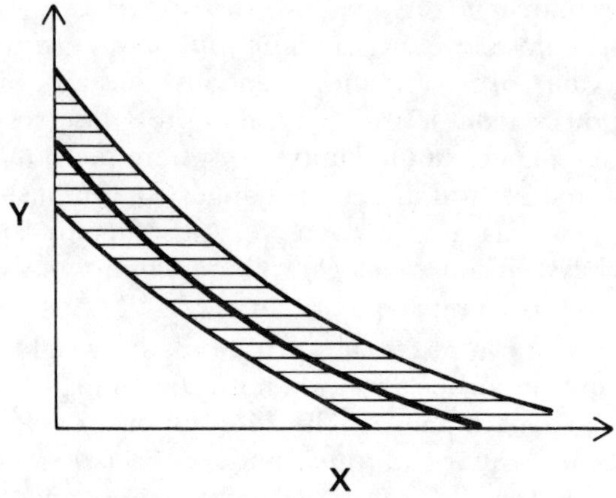

Fig. 49. Variability in (arithmetic) X for any given value of Y.

Figure 48 shows the variability in the response variable (Y) for given values of X. Figure 49 gives an impression of the magnitude of the errors in (arithmetic) X for any given value of Y. This is quite a different picture than Figures 45 or 47, since we are now on a linear, rather than a logarithmic scale. Here, as the X value increases, the size of its error also increases. Usually, we are interested in the percentage error in X. As an approximation, the percentage (or relative) error in the estimate of dose corresponds to the length of the horizontal lines in Figures 45 or 47, which utilize a logarithmic scale for dose.

If the equation for the dose response curve is known, (in particular, if its slope is known), then estimates of the error in Y may be converted to estimates of the error in X. Conversely, estimates of the error in X may be converted to estimates of the error in Y. If the dose response curve is regarded as linear in any local region, and if it is assumed that the magnitude of the error remains essentially constant in this local region, then the error in X is equal to the error in Y divided by the slope:

$$\sigma_X = \frac{\sigma_Y}{\text{slope}} = \frac{\sigma_Y}{\Delta Y / \Delta X}$$

The index of precision (λ) is usually defined as the standard error of the response variable divided by the slope. Usually this refers to the slope of the response versus $\log_{10}$ of dose. As a rough approximation, when λ is small, the percentage error in the potency estimate is approximately equal to $\lambda \times 2.303$. Thus a lambda of 0.01 would correspond to a fractional error of 0.023, or approximately a 2.3% error in the value for X, given a single observation of Y. This approximation breaks down as λ

becomes larger than 0.05. In general, the apparent λ value changes depending on the dose level in a radioimmunoassay. In the context of Figure 44, the value of σ_Y remains essentially constant, but the slopes change continuously from left to right along the dose response curve. Alternatively, one may examine Figure 46, where the slope is constant, but the error in the vertical direction changes continuously. Use of the lambda coefficient has not proven very useful for characterizing radioimmunoassays, since lambda (λ) changes continuously, depending on the position on the dose-response curve.

Figure 50 shows an approximate profile of the weights assigned to points on the dose response curve, when utilizing a logit-log regression. The weights given to each point on the dose response curve are inversely proportional to the square of the standard deviation of logit of Y (vertical lines in Figure 46). Very high weights are assigned to the center of the curve (B/B_0 between 30–60%). As one approaches B/B_0 = 0% or B/B_0 = 100%, the weights fall off precipitously. However, the weights do not go to zero. Even observations which, by accident or due to the random sampling error have an apparent response variable less than zero percent or greater than 100% B/B_0, are still counted and given a weight, by the use of "working logits" defined according to Finney.[7,8]

Figure 51 shows the approximate percentage error, relative error or percent coefficient of variation (%CV) versus position on the dose response curve in terms of the response variable on the horizontal scale. This graph allows one to make statements of the following type: "a point falling with B/B_0 equal 50% should have an expected error in the

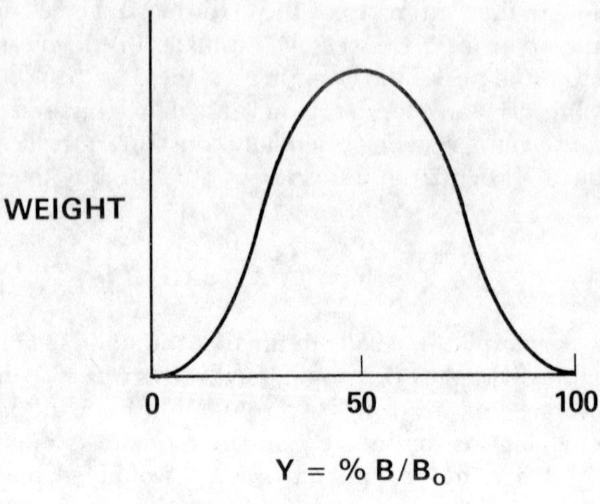

Fig. 50. Weighting profile.: Weights versus $\%B/B_0$.

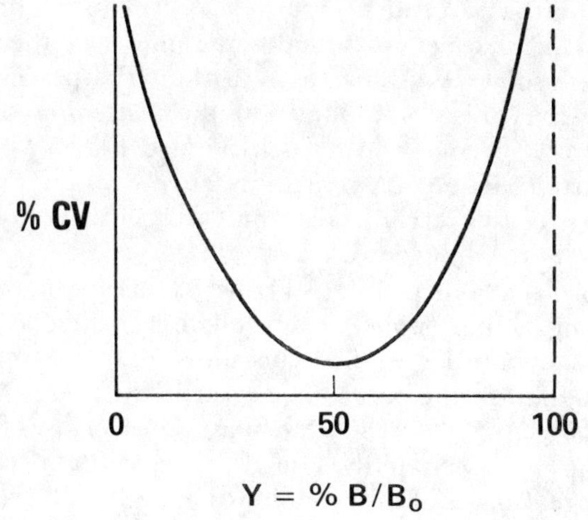

Fig. 51. Error profile: $\%CV_x$ versus $\%B/B_0$.

potency estimate of ± say 5%". This is a smooth curve and as B/B_0 approaches zero or 100%, the percentage error in the estimate of the potency for the unknown becomes astronomically large. However, in the central region between approximately 30 and 70%, the percentage error for the unknown remains approximately constant. The profile shown in Figure 51 is quite similar to that shown in Figure 50, rotated 180 degrees. The profile in Figure 51 may be derived by considering either Figure 45 or 47 and recalling that the percentage error in the answer is approximately proportional to the error in the logarithm of the potency.

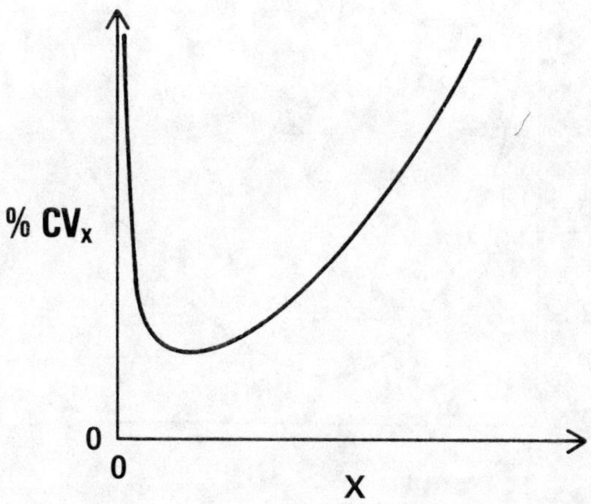

Fig. 52. Percentage error($\%CV_X$) versus the dose, X, with dose shown on a linear scale.

Figure 52 shows the percentage error ($\%CV_X$) versus the dose, X, with dose shown on a linear scale. For a moderate range of X, the percentage error remains constant. As X increases further, the percentage error increases somewhat; this corresponds to the flattening of the dose response curve as X becomes large, as in Figure 49. As X approaches zero, the standard deviation of X remains relatively constant (see Fig. 55, below), but the relative error starts increasing drastically since the denominator is approaching zero.

Figure 53 shows the same profile as Figure 52, except that now dose is displayed on a logarithmic scale. This results in a parabolic-like profile not unlike that shown in Figure 51. This shows that for approximately one order of magnitude, the percentage error in the potency estimate is essentially constant. As the dose level increases or decreases further, the percentage error increases rapidly. Use of the logarithmic scale appears to be of advantage. Curves of the type shown in Figure 53 will vary from assay to assay, depending upon the slope and position of the dose response curve.

From a statistical point of view, the simplest and easiest way to characterize the errors in the RIA dose response variable is to consider the relationship between the variance of the response variable, σ_Y^2 and the response variable itself (Y = bound counts, free counts, B/T, B/F, etc.) (Fig. 54). I prefer use of B/T, B/B_0, or of raw counts. This usually results in a relationship such as the one shown here. As the Y value increases, the variance increases. This relationship may be approximated by a linear function. For special cases such as two-site IRMA (sandwich assays) and certain types of bioassays, the variance of the response increases roughly in proportion to the square of the response. Finney

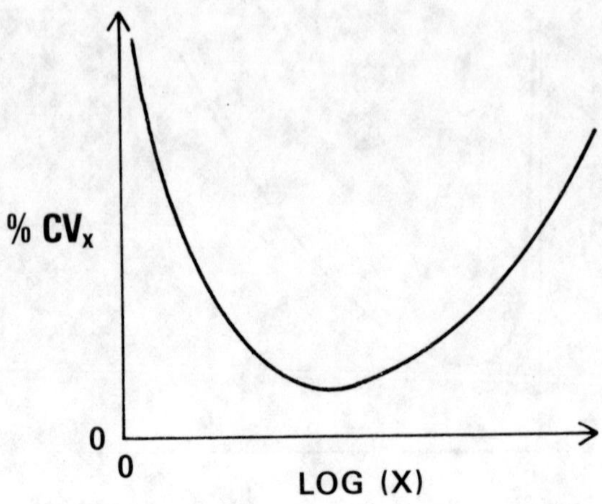

Fig. 53. The same profile as in Fig. 52, with the dose displayed on a logarithmic scale.

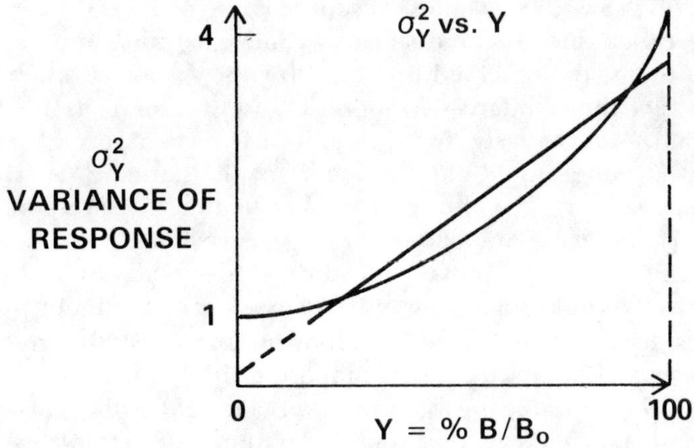

Fig. 54. (Error in Y) vs. Y. Either σ_Y or σ_Y^2 may be used on the vertical axis.

has stressed the desirability of performing this analysis in terms of raw counts rather than a derived variable such as B/T or B/B_0 (personal communication). Many users would find these graphs easier to interpret when the standard deviation of the response variable, σ_Y, is plotted versus the response variable (not shown).

Figure 55 shows the relationship between the standard deviation of the potency estimate for an unknown, σ_X, and the potency estimate, X. σ_X is essentially constant for small values of X, and thereafter increases roughly in proportion to X. This latter portion corresponds to the region of Figure 53 where the percentage error (CV_X) remains constant.

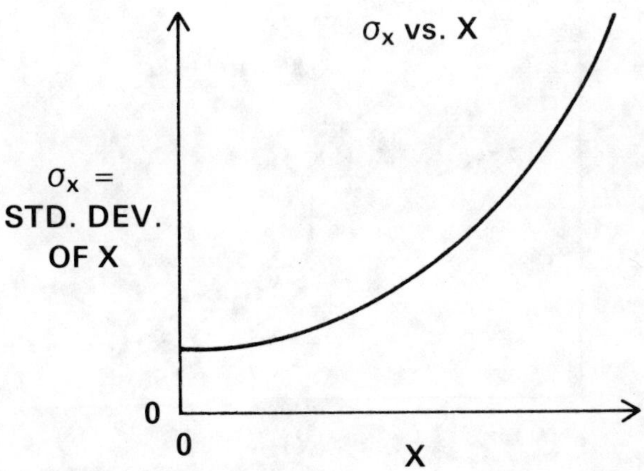

Fig. 55. (Error in X) vs. X.

Figure 56 shows a typical dose response curve of Y versus log(X). For any given dose value, we can calculate the mean (Y) and sample standard deviation (s_Y) of the observed replicates for the response variable. One can then plot the standard deviation of Y (s_Y) versus Y, resulting in a scattergram. Alternatively and preferably from a rigorous statistical point of view, one should plot the square of the standard deviation (s_Y^2, the sample variance) for the response versus the mean response level (Figures 7). Linear, parabolic or log-log regressions may be used to describe this relationship (or, one can draw a smooth curve "by eye"). Unfortunately, the results from any one assay may be uninterpretable.

The results for standards and unknowns from several assays of the same type may be pooled by superimposing the graphs for each assay (e.g., Fig. 57), resulting in a scattergram (Fig. 58) with many points. These points may appear to be totally random. However, we can make sense out of this "snowstorm," by dividing the curve into between 5 and 10 equal regions or "bins." The median variance in each local region of the curve is then plotted, and the relationship shown by the crosses (local medians) may be examined. Usually this relationship will be very clear-cut: it may be a straight-line, parabolic, or power-function relationship. This may then be described mathematically by one of the models given by the formulas below:

$$\sigma_Y^2 = a_0 + a_1 Y \quad \text{(linear)}$$

$$\text{or} \quad \sigma_Y^2 = a_0 + a_1 Y + a_2 Y^2 \quad \text{(quadratic)}$$

$$\text{or} \quad \sigma_Y^2 = a_0 Y^J \quad \text{(power function)}$$

$$\text{or} \quad \log(\sigma_Y^2) = \log(a_0) + J \log(Y)$$

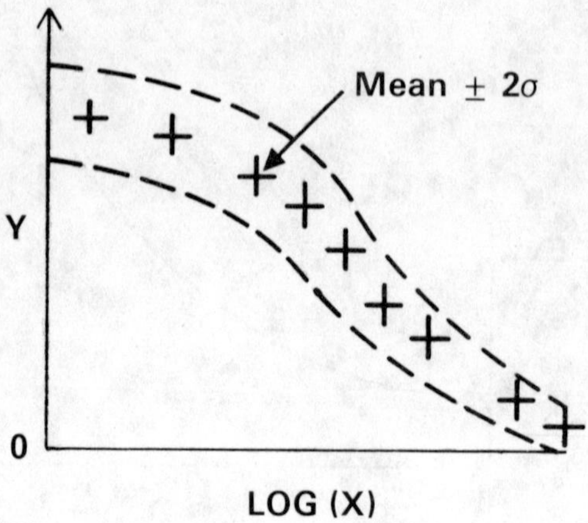

Fig. 56. Typical dose response curve of Y vs. log(X).

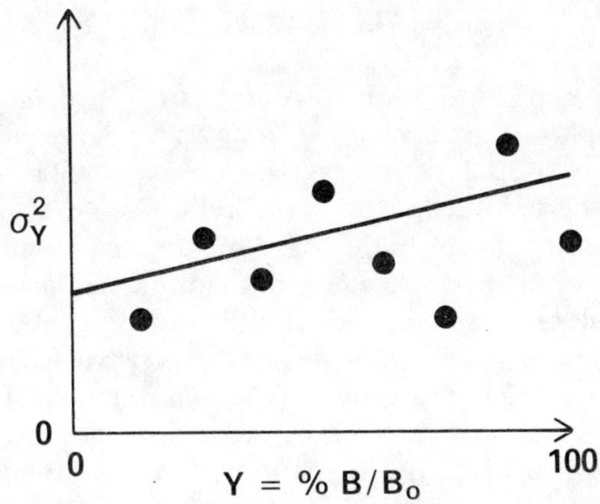

Fig. 57. Variance of Y (σ_Y^2) versus: one assay.

The values of a_0, a_1, a_2, and/or J are found by the least squares or maximum likelihood methods. Use of the medians in each region rather than the means takes the asymmetry of the chi-square distribution into account and also compensates for possible outliers. The relationship shown in Figure 58 should be examined for both the standards and the unknowns. This should provide evidence that the unknowns are behaving in a manner similar to the standards, not only with respect to parallelism of the standard curve, but also with respect to the magnitude of the errors in the response variable. Plots of σ_Y^2 or σ_Y versus Y (such as that shown in Figure 57) are provided for both the standards and for the unknowns in our current version of the logit-log method for the analysis of radioimmunoassay results.[7,9]

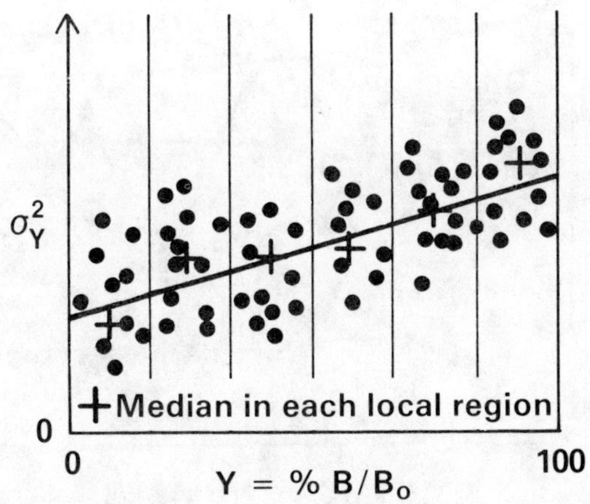

Fig. 58. Variance of Y versus Y: pooled results.

QUALITY CONTROL

Another crucial aspect of RIA statistics is *quality control.* An indispensable part of quality control analysis is a large plasma pool or a large bulk of material that is as similar as possible to the typical unknowns to be analyzed. This large pool should be aliquoted and frozen in a manner similar to that used for the unknowns. The material should be analyzed in duplicate or triplicate in each assay. A graph showing the values obtained for each individual test tube, and the mean of the replicates for each assay should be constructed (Figure 59) in order to obtain a visual impression of the magnitude of the within-assay variability (the vertical distance between the dots for each assay) and the between-assay variability (the magnitude of the changes between the means for consecutive assays). The cumulative average (the grand mean of all the values obtained to date) for a given sample and control limits at $\pm 2\sigma$ or $\pm 3\sigma$ may also be indicated. The σ used here is the standard error of the assay means. There is more than one way to construct the control limits. This is a somewhat arbitrary decision, which must be settled individually in each laboratory. The within- and between-assay variability should also be calculated using an analysis of variance (ANOVA) with a "components of variance" breakdown to separate the contributions of within and between-assay variability.[15-17] Likewise, one should use an analysis of variance to estimate the "between laboratories" component of variance in regional and international studies of assay reliability.[16]

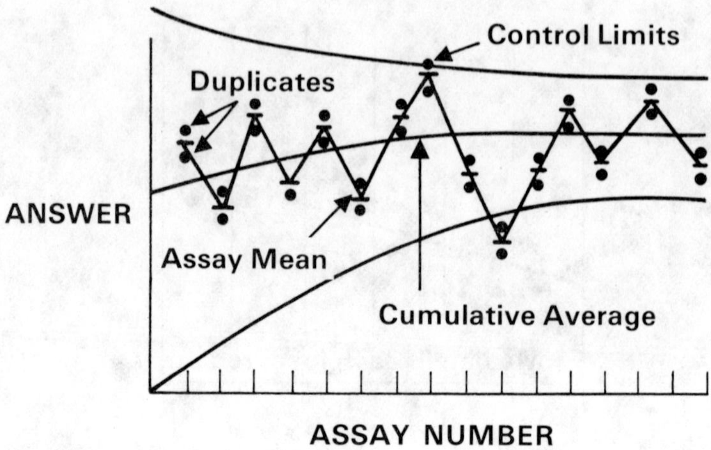

Fig. 59. Quality control charts.

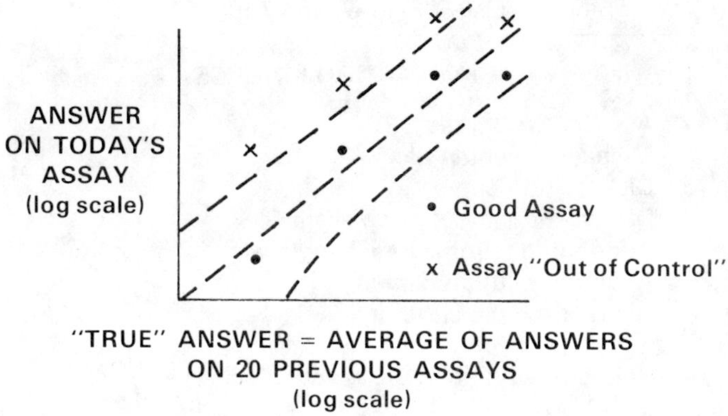

Fig. 60. Quick check for bias in current assay.

The analysis shown in Figure 59 should be repeated for at least three of four "dose levels." This makes it possible to perform the type of analysis shown in Figure 60. After each assay is completed, the local mean for the replicates for each of the quality control (*QC*) specimens may be calculated and plotted on the vertical scale versus the mean of the values for the same samples on the 10 or 20 previous assays (or the true value, if it is known) on the horizontal scale. A regression line may then be constructed relating the current values to the "true" or "best estimate" values. Ideally, this should be a straight line with a slope of unity (on log-log coordinate paper). With four or more points, a test for linearity may be performed. With three or more points, the slope may be tested to see if it is with unity (slope = 1.000). Control limits may then be constructed to indicate when an assay is "out of control." If the curve has a slope of unity, but is shifted moderately upward from the line of identity, the use of a "correction factor" may be considered to convert the values from the current assay into values more consistent with the results from previous assays. Obviously, the use of any such correction factor entails great risk! The use of such factors will very effectively reduce and obscure the magnitude of between-assay variability, but this does not alter the fact that the values are changing dramatically. The use of such correction factors seems justifiable only in cases in which *ten* or more quality control samples have been analyzed within each assay. In effect, then, the battery of quality control samples can serve as a "secondary standard" in the event that there appears to be something the matter with the primary standards. In this case, the quality control samples are, in effect, being used as the basis for constructing the dose response curve.

Table I. List of Figures and Topics Presented

	RIA REACTION KINETICS
Fig. 1	Association curves
Fig. 2	Michaelis-Menten plot
Fig. 3	Dissociation curve
Fig. 4	Dissociation curve (log scale)
Fig. 5	Antibody dilution curve (log scale)
Fig. 6	Antibody dilution curve
Fig. 7	Hill plot: single class of sites
Fig. 8	Hill plot: cooperativity
Fig. 9	Cooperativity: stepwise reaction scheme
	SCATCHARD PLOT
Fig. 10	2 parameter model: single class of sites
Fig. 11	3 parameter model
Fig. 12	4 parameter model: two independent classes of sites
Fig. 13	5 parameter model
Fig. 14	negative cooperativity
Fig. 15	Positive cooperativity
	DOSE RESPONSE CURVES
Fig. 16	Michaelis-Menton hyperbola: bound vs. total
Fig. 17	B/T or B/F vs. X
Fig. 18	B/T vs. log(X) : effect of K
Fig. 19	B/T vs. log(X)
Fig. 20	Logit(B/B_0) vs. log(X)
	KINETICS OF DOSE RESPONSE CURVES
Fig. 21	Case A: All reagents added simultaneously
Fig. 22	Case B: Delayed addition of labeled antigen
Fig. 23	Case C: Delayed addition of unlabeled antigen
Fig. 24	Superimposition of Cases A, B, and C
	OPTIMIZATION OF RIA CONDITIONS
Fig. 25	Combinations of p*, q giving same starting $(B/T)_0$
Fig. 26	Combinations of p*, q giving same mineral detectable dose
Fig. 27	Combinations of charcoal and reaction time giving same slope and sensitivity
Fig. 28	Effects of "too little" charcoal on the dose response curve
	CROSSREACTIVITY
Fig. 29	Reaction scheme
Fig. 30	Dose response curves

Table I (continued)

	IMMUNORADIOMETRIC ASSAYS (Labeled Antibody Assays)
Fig. 31	Use of immunoadsorbent
Fig. 32	"Sandwich Assay", Two-site IRMA, RAST, or ELISA
	STATISTICAL VALIDATION
Fig. 33	Precision
Fig. 34	Sensitivity: minimal detectable concentration
Fig. 35	Recovery experiment
Fig. 36	Recovery experiment (log scales)
Fig. 37	Parallelism of standard and unknown
	DOSE RESPONSE CURVES WITH THEIR 95% CONFIDENCE LIMITS
Fig. 38	B/T vs. X
Fig. 39	B/T vs. log(X)
Fig. 40	Logit(B/B_0) vs. log(X)
Fig. 41	1/B/T) vs. X
Fig. 42	Log($F/B - (F/B)_0$) vs. log(X)
Fig. 43	Log(B/T) vs. log(total ligand)
	CONFIDENCE LIMITS FOR X AND Y
Fig. 44	Error in Y given log(X)
Fig. 45	Error in log(X) given Y
Fig. 46	Error in logit(Y) given log(X)
Fig. 47	Error in log(X) given logit(Y)
Fig. 48	Error in Y given X
Fig. 49	Error in X given Y
	DEPENDENCY OF CONFIDENCE LIMITS FOR X AND Y UPON POSITION ON THE DOSE RESPONSE CURVE
Fig. 50	Weight vs. $\%B/B_0$
Fig. 51	%CV vs. $\%B/B_0$
Fig. 52	$\%CV_x$ vs. X
Fig. 53	$\%CV_x$ vs. log(X)
Fig. 54	Variance of Y vs. response level $\%B/B_0$
Fig. 55	Standard deviation of X vs. X
	HOW TO ESTIMATE THE TAPER OF THE CONFIDENCE LIMITS FOR THE DOSE RESPONSE CURVE
Fig. 56	Plot the mean of Y + 2 standard deviations vs. log(X)
Fig. 57	Plot the standard deviation or variance of Y vs. mean Y for one assay
Fig. 58	Pool results over assays, and pool for standards and unknown

Table I (continued)

QUALITY CONTROL CHARTS	
Fig. 59	Quality control chart for one quality control sample
Fig. 60	Combination of results from several quality control samples, to test for assay bias.

GLOSSARY

B/T	$(B-N)/(T-N)$
B/B_0	$(B-N)/(B_0-N) = (B/T)/(B/T)_0$
$(B/T)_0$	$(B_0-N)/(T-N)$
B/F, R, R_{bf}	bound over free ratio
F/T	free over bound ratio
logit(Y)	$\log_e\left(\frac{Y}{1-Y}\right) = 2.303 \times \log_{10}\left(\frac{Y}{1-Y}\right)$ for $0 < Y < 1$
s	sample standard deviation
σ	true standard deviation
s^2	sample variance for finite "sample" of data
σ^2	true variance
s_a	standard error of the parameter a
t	Student's t
p, [Ag], [H]	total hormone concentration (M/L)
q, [Ab^0]	total antibody concentration (M/L)
[P], [Ag]	free antigen
[P^*], [Ag^*]	free labeled antigen
[Q], [Ab]	free antibody
[PQ], [AgAb]	antigen-antibody complex
K	equilibrium constant of association (L/M), affinity constant
k_1	association rate constant (L/M/s)
k_{-1}	dissociation rate constant ($_{-1}$)
CV	coefficient of variation = standard deviation divided by mean
%CV	percent coefficient of variation = 100 × CV
n_H	Hill coefficient
b	slope
$s_0{}^2$	residual variance
QC	Quality Control
ANOVA	Analysis of variance

$\%B/T$	$100\ B/T$
$\%B/B_0$	$100\ B/B_0$
$\%(B/T)_0$	$100\ (B/T)_0$

ACKNOWLEDGMENT

Earlier editions of this material have been presented at the Radioimmunoassay Training Course of The Endocrine Society, Bethesda, Md. (1977, 1978) at the National Meeting of the Clinical Radioassay Society, Washington, D.C. (1979) and appears in syllabus material of these societies. A translation of an earlier version into Italian has been published in F. Fraioli and A. Isidori (eds.), Sistemi a Radioligandi in Endocrinologia, Societa Editrice Universo, Roma, 1977, pp. 2–75.

REFERENCES

Classical Papers

1. S.A. Berson and R.S. Yalow, Quantitative aspects of the reaction between insulin and insulin-binding antibody. *J Clin Invest* **38**:1996, 1959.

2. R.P. Ekins, G.B. Newman, and J.L.H. O'Riordan, Theoretical aspects of "saturation" and radioimmunoassay. *In Radioisotopes in Medicine: In Vitro Studies,* R.L. Hayes, R.A. Goswitz, and B.E.P. Murphy, (eds.), U.S. Atomic Energy Comm., Oak Ridge, Tenn., 1968, pp. 59–100.

General Introductory

3. D. Rodbard and R.C. Rodgers, The kinetics of radioligand assays. *In Hormones in Human Blood: Detection and Assay,* H.N. Antoniades (ed.), Harvard University Press, Cambridge, MA, 1976, pp. 92–114.

4. D. Rodbard, Statistical quality control and routine data processing for radioimmunoassays (RIA) and immunoradiometric assays (IRMA). *Clin Chem* **20**:1255–1270, 1974.

5. D. Rodbard and G.R. Frazier, Statistical analysis of radioligand assay data, *Methods Enzymol* **37**:3–22, 1975.

6. D. Rodbard, Dose interpolation for radioimmunoassays: an overview. *In Clinical Immunochemistry, Chemical and Cellular Bases and Applications in Disease, Current Topics and Clinical Chemistry,* Vol. 3, S. Natelson, A.J. Pesce, and A.A. Dietz (eds.), American Association for Clinical Chemistry, Washington, DC 1978, pp. 477–494.

Logit-Log Program

7. V.B. Faden and D. Rodbard, Radioimmunoassay Data Processing, Listings and Documentation, 3rd edn., Vols. 1 and 2, and Programs (PB 246 222-4). National Technical Information Service, Springfield, VA, 1975 (Computer Programs and Documentation). (1980 Edition available directly from author).

8. D. Rodbard and J.E. Lewald, Computer analysis of radio-ligand and radioimmunoassay data. *Acta Endocrinol* **64**(Suppl. 147):79–103, 1970.

Four Parameter Logistic

9. D. Rodbard and D.M. Hutt, Statistical analysis of radioimmunoassays and immunoradiometric (labeled antibody) assays: a generalized, weighted, iterative, least-squares method for logistic curve fitting. *In Radioimmunoassay and Related Procedures in Medicine,* Vol. 1, International Atomic Energy Agency, Vienna, 1975 (Unipub, NY).

10. D. Rodbard, P.J. Munson, and A. De Lean, Improved curve-fitting, parallelism testing, characterization of sensitivity and specificity, validation, and optimization for radioligand assays. *In Radioimmunoassay and Related Procedures in Medicine,* Vol. 1, International Atomic Energy Agency, Vienna, 1978, pp. 469–504 (see also, discussion, pp. 505–509).

11. A. De Lean, P.J. Munson, and D. Rodbard, Simultaneous analysis of families of sigmoidal curves: application to bioassay, radio-ligand assay and physiological dose response curves. *Am J Physiol Endocrinology, Metabolism and Gastrointestinal Physiology,* 1978.

Mass-Action Law

12. D. Rodbard, Mathematics of hormone-receptor interaction, I. Basic principles. *In Receptors for Reproductive Hormones,* B.W. O'Malley and A.R. Means (eds.), Plenum, New York, 1973, pp. 289–326 (*Adv Exp Med Biol* **36**).

13. D. Rodbard and R.E. Bertino, Theory of radioimmunoassays and hormone-receptor interactions: II. Simulation of antibody divalency, cooperativity and allosteric effects. *In Receptors for Reproductive Hormones,* B.W. O'Malley and A.R. Means (eds.), Plenum, New York, 1973, pp. 327-341 (*Adv Exp Med Biol* **36**).

14. D. Rodbard and R.L. Tacey, Radioimmunoassay dose interpolation based on the first order mass action law with antibody heterogeneity: exact correction for variable mass of labeled ligand. *Anal Biochem* **90**:13–21, 1978.

Quality Control

15. B.F. McDonagh, P.J. Munson, and D. Rodbard, A computerized approach to statistical quality control for radioimmunoassay in the clinical chemistry laboratory. *Computer Programs Biomed* **7**:179–190, 1977.

16. P.J. Munson and D. Rodbard, An elementary components of variance analysis for multi-center quality control. *In Symposium on Radioimmunoassay and Related Procedures in Medicine 1977,* Vol. 2, International Atomic Energy Agency, Vienna, 1978, pp. 105–125.

17. D. Rodbard, Quality control for RIA: recommendations for a minimum program. *In Symposium on Radioimmunoassay and Related Procedures in Medicine 1977,* Vol. 2, International Atomic Energy Agency, Vienna, 1978, pp. 21–38. See also: Roundtable discussion on external quality control, pp. 159–167.

Weighting

18. D. Rodbard, R.H. Lenox, H.L. Wray, and D. Ramseth, Statistical characterization of the random errors in the radioimmunoassay dose response variable. *Clin Chem* **22**:350–358, 1976.

Optimization and Sensitivity

19. D. Rodbard, Statistical estimation of the minimal detectable concentration ("sensitivity") for radioligand assays. *Anal Biochem* **90**:1–12, 1978.

20. M. Yanagishita and D. Rodbard, Computer optimization of radioimmunoassays for hCG and estradiol: An experimental evaluation. *Anal Biochem* **88**:1–19, 1978.

21. D. Rodbard, H.J. Ruder, J. Vaitukaitis, and H.S. Jacobs, Mathematical analysis of kinetics of radioligand assays: Improved sensitivity obtained by delayed addition of labeled ligand. *J Clin Endocrol* **33**:343–355, 1971.

Adaptation to Small Computers

22. H.E. Grotjan and E. Steinberger, Radioimmunoassay and Bioassay data processing using a logistic curve fitting routine adapted to a desk top computer. *Computers Biol Med* **7**:159–163, 1977.

23. S. Cernosek and R.M. Gutierez-Cernosek, Use of a programmable desk-top calculator for the statistical quality control of radioimmunoassays. *Clin Chem* **24**:1121–1125.

24. S.E. Davis, M.L. Jaffe, P.J. Munson, and D. Rodbard, Radioimmunoassay Data Processing with a Small Programmable Calculator, *J Immunoassay* **1**(1), 15–25, 1980.

Elisa, IRMA, and EMIT

25. D. Rodbard and S.W. McLean, Automated computer analysis for enzyme multiplied immunological techniques, *Clin Chem* **23**:112–115, 1977.

26. D. Rodbard and Y. Feldman, Kinetics of two-site immunoradiometric assays: I. Mathematical models for simulation, optimization, and curve-fitting, immunochemistry **15**:71–76, 1978 (See also, pp. 77–82).

27. H. Feldman, D. Rodbard, and D. Levine, Mathematical Theory of Crossreactive Radioimmunoassay and Ligand Binding Systems of Equilibrium. *Anal. Biochem.* **45**:530–556, 1972.

APPENDIX: AVAILABILITY OF COMPUTER PROGRAMS

I. Routine Programs

All programs are available directly from the author, on request.

1. The logit-log RIA program "RIAPROG," its documentation and operating instructions, a guide to the interpretation of results, and sample input-sample output. FORTRAN IV, IBM-370.
2. The four-parameter logistic RIA program "SIGMOID". Also FORTRAN IV, IBM-370.
3. "NIHRIA": Four parameter logistic model for RIA, IRMA, EMIT, ELISA, bioassays, and radioreceptor assays. This program provides RIA dose interpolation, with testing of parallelism of standard and unknown. Similar to program "SIGMOID" for the IBM 370, but is in BASIC for the DEC-10.
4. Quality Control Programs. One for routine, "Internal" QC, and a second program for between-laboratory, collaborative QC. PL/I for IBM 370. Also available for TI/59.
5. "TI-59 program package": Logit-log, four parameter logistic and quality control programs for the TI-59 calculator and PC-100 printer.

II. Research Programs

In addition to the above "routine" programs, we have several new programs available on special request.

1. "ALLFIT": Four parameter logistic fitting, with constraints, and more sophisticated testing of parallelism. BASIC for DEC-10.
2. "SCATFIT": This program fits parameters of a nonlinear Scatchard plot, for one, two, or three classes of independent variable, and allows for weighting. Useful for RIA dose interpolation based on the mass action law, when used in conjunction with "POTENT," described below. FORTRAN IV-G, for IBM 370.
3. LIGAND: A program to calculate parameters in the "n ligand–m binding site" case, i.e., multiple ligands interacting simultaneously with multiple independent classes of sites and nonspecific binding. BASIC for DEC-10.
4. SCAT1.FIT: Calculates parameters for Scatchard plot for 1 ligand and any number of sites and nonspecific binding. Also provides curve fitting for "discrete affinity distribution" and for the stepwise Adair Model. BASIC, for DEC-10.
5. "POTENT": Dose interpolation for RIAs using mass action law (to be used in conjunction with SCATFIT, LIGAND, or SCAT1.FIT, above. BASIC DEC-10.

6. "RIAOPT": Program for optimization of conditions for an equilibrium RIA, given the affinity constant. "RRVJOP": Program for optimization when using delayed addition of labeled ligand. BASIC, DEC-10.

7. "KINFIT": Program to fit k_{on}, k_{off}, K, and binding capacity for association curves. Extended BASIC for DEC-10.

8. "QKDFIT": Describes Scatchard plot in the case of a single class of sites obeying De Meyts' model for cooperativity, with K_d a linear function of occupancy. BASIC, DEC-10.

9. "EXPFIT": This program fits sums of negative exponential decay curves, using up to three "compartments" (six parameters), and picks the "best" model. Useful for dissociation curves, metabolic clearance rates, radiation inactivation, etc. FORTRAN IV-G, for IBM 370.

10. "BIOPROG": Program for classical (Finney-style) parallel line bioassay analysis, for linear-log dose response curves. FORTRAN, IBM 370.

Chapter 4

Coupling of Enzymes to Proteins and Haptens

BAUKE K. VAN WEEMEN, EBO S. BOS, TOM C. J. GRIBNAU, and ANTON H.W.M. SCHUURS

INTRODUCTION

Proteins have been coupled to themselves (either intra- or intermolecularly), and to a wide variety of substances, such as other soluble proteins, small organic molecules, and solid carriers. There have been many reasons for these procedures, such as functional studies, structure elucidation, stabilization, ease of (re)utilization, and labeling for easy identification, localization, or quantitation.

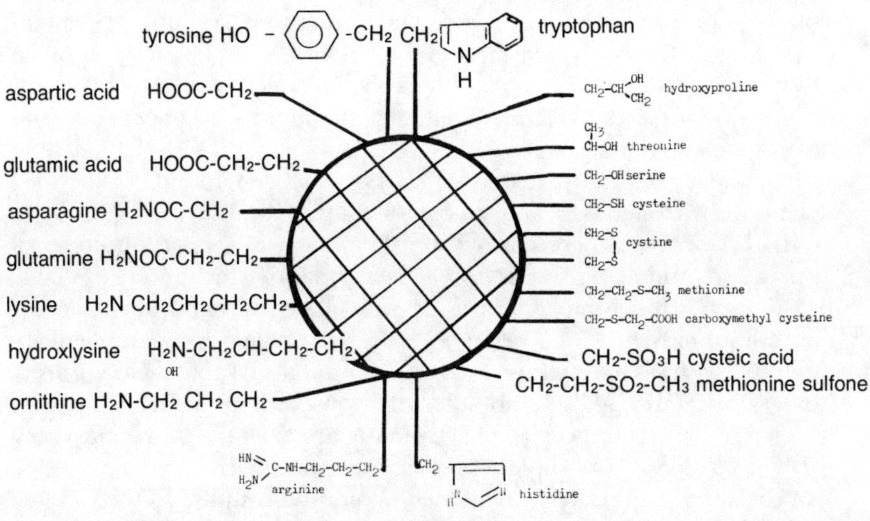

Fig. 1. Potentially reactive amino acid side chains in proteins.

Organon Scientific Development Group, Oss, The Netherlands

Fortunately, proteins are usually equipped with many groups that allow coupling. The suitable amino acid side chains are shown in Figure 1; besides, glycoproteins offer possibilities for coupling via their sugar moieties. The number of coupling reagents described in the literature is a good reflection of the wide variety of purposes and substances for coupling. In principle, most methods developed for one purpose and/or protein are equally well applicable to other problems. The scope of this chapter will be restricted to one relatively small area: coupling of enzymes to antigens, antibodies, and haptens for use in immunoassays.

BEFORE COUPLING

Before coupling, we should consider to what extent we want and are able to influence the properties of the conjugate. The ideal conjugate is stable and results in an assay that is sensitive, specific, precise, and easy to perform. Of course, the assay characteristics mentioned are determined to an important extent as well by the choice of the assay system: homogeneous or heterogeneous, competitive or of the sandwich type, and photometric or fluorometric in its endpoint determination. However, since the properties of the conjugate often directly influence which options are available, their importance for the eventual assay can hardly be overestimated.

The choice of an enzyme is the first point of consideration. Ideally, the enzyme should be (1) detectable in minute amounts; (2) detectable by simple photometric and/or fluorometric methods; (3) not present in physiological fluids; (4) not inhibited or activated by factors present in physiological fluids; (5) stable; (6) easily linkable to other molecules, without loss of activity; and (7) equally suitable to homogeneous and heterogeneous immunoassay.

This ideal enzyme, if it exists, has not yet been found. Lysozyme,[1] malate dehydrogenase,[2] and glucose-6-phosphate dehydrogenase[3] can be used for homogeneous assays, but fail in sensitivity for a number of applications and may present problems with sample interference (which, by the way, is much more serious in homogeneous than in heterogeneous immunoassays). The other enzymes that have been applied are limited to use in heterogeneous immunoassays. Of this group, horseradish peroxidase[4] and alkaline phosphatase[5] have been most widely used; they are well suited for many applications. In recent years, β-D-galactosidase[6] has rapidly been gaining popularity.

What antigen, antibody, or hapten should be coupled to the enzyme obviously depends primarily on which substance has to be assayed. Nevertheless, some options are open. If one wants to assay an antigen, either antigen or antibody can be labeled. The latter possibility (sandwich or immunometric assay) has a number of advantages as far as sensitivity, specificity, and safety (in case of assay of infectious agents) are concerned. Moreover, labeling of antibodies is a much more general procedure, presenting less problems than antigen labeling. It may be advantageous to label Fab or $F(ab')_2$ fragments rather than whole antibodies; this can increase sensitivity[7] and will avoid rheumatoid factor interference.

Antigens to be coupled should be of adequate purity. It has been advocated that antibodies or antibody fragments should be purified by affinity chromatography to avoid nonspecific reactions[8]; many authors, however, appear satisfied when using the immunoglobulin fraction. If a hapten is to be assayed, a hapten derivative containing a carboxyl group will usually be coupled to the enzyme; this usually works well, although it may be necessary to take special care in selecting the derivative.[9]

Ideally, both substances should retain their full *activity* in the conjugate. This aspect of conjugate characteristics, however, has only sparingly been investigated. In some studies, it was shown that K_M and V_{max} of β-galactosidase,[10] malate dehydrogenase,[2] and acetylcholine esterase[11] did not change very much upon coupling to other substances. Nevertheless, it is obvious that some steric hindrance will occur, which may lead to reduced activity. Whether this will still allow for the desired sensitivity of the eventual assay remains to be determined empirically. No data are available on the degree of remaining immunochemical activity.

Although a wide variety of conjugates of different composition and purity have been prepared and used, it is still fairly difficult to give definite rules about the desired properties of conjugates in these respects. It will be clear that a conjugate preparation should ideally contain neither free enzyme nor immunoreactant that is not bound to active enzyme. The latter condition is of special importance, since the presence of nonlabeled immunoreactant reduces the sensitivity. Ideal size and enzyme/immunoreactant ratio of the conjugate are much more open to dispute; contradicting data have been published.[12,13] An empirical approach still seems the best strategy, until more clear-cut data are available. In conclusion, before actual coupling experiments are started, the requirements for the desired conjugate should be defined.

COUPLING AGENTS AND PROCEDURES

Agents and methods can be subdivided into several classes, such as (1) homobifunctional vs. heterobifunctional reagents, (2) one-step vs. two-step methods, and (3) cleavable vs. noncleavable conjugates. Sometimes these classes are interrelated, e.g., a heterobifunctional reagent is used in a two-step procedure only. Therefore, a logical classification of agents is difficult to make. Instead, we shall present a personal selection of agents and methods that we consider worthwhile; these will include the most widely used ones. We shall refrain from dealing with specific reaction conditions; details can be found in the original publications, or in the useful review articles that have appeared in recent years.[12,14,15,26]

Protein-Protein Coupling

Structures of the various reagents are given in Figures 2 and 3.

GLUTARALDEHYDE

Glutaraldehyde (I) is used to crosslink protein amino groups, with initial Schiff-base formation, followed by rearrangements that make the link extremely stable toward changes in pH and/or temperature. Data about the possible nature of these rearrangements and the final link have been published recently.[27] The procedure usually leads to ill-defined high-molecular-weight preparations, especially if enzyme and immunoreactant are simultaneously mixed with the reagent (one-step procedure). Nevertheless, we have obtained quite useful conjugates using glutaraldehyde, particularly using the two-step procedure.

SODIUM PERIODATE

Sodium periodate[16] is used for coupling glycoproteins (e.g., horseradish peroxidase and immunoglobulins) to protein amino groups, by oxidizing the sugar residues in a first reaction step and coupling these to the other protein in a second step.[16] Usually, heterogeneous conjugates of high molecular weight arise; it has been reported that these are more suitable for enzyme immunoassay than smaller glutaraldehyde conjugates.[13] As with glutaraldehyde, we have prepared satisfactory conjugates. However, we have indications that they are less stable than conjugates prepared with glutaraldehyde.

O-PHENYLENE DIMALEIMIDE (OPDM) (XIII)

OPDM is advocated for coupling protein SH groups.[7] It has primarily been used for conjugating β-D-galactosidase, which contains free sulphydryl groups, to Fab fragments of antibody molecules; non-SH containing proteins can be used after prior mercaptosuccinylation.[18] Our personal experience is that the method is difficult to control, probably due to hydrolysis of the remaining maleimide group after the first reaction step.[28]

Other Reagents

As neither of the three reagents mentioned above yields well-defined products in an easily controlled way, it appears worthwhile to look at other reagents. Most homobifunctional reagents (Figure 2) show little promise, with the possible exception of halodiazines (VIII), halotriazines

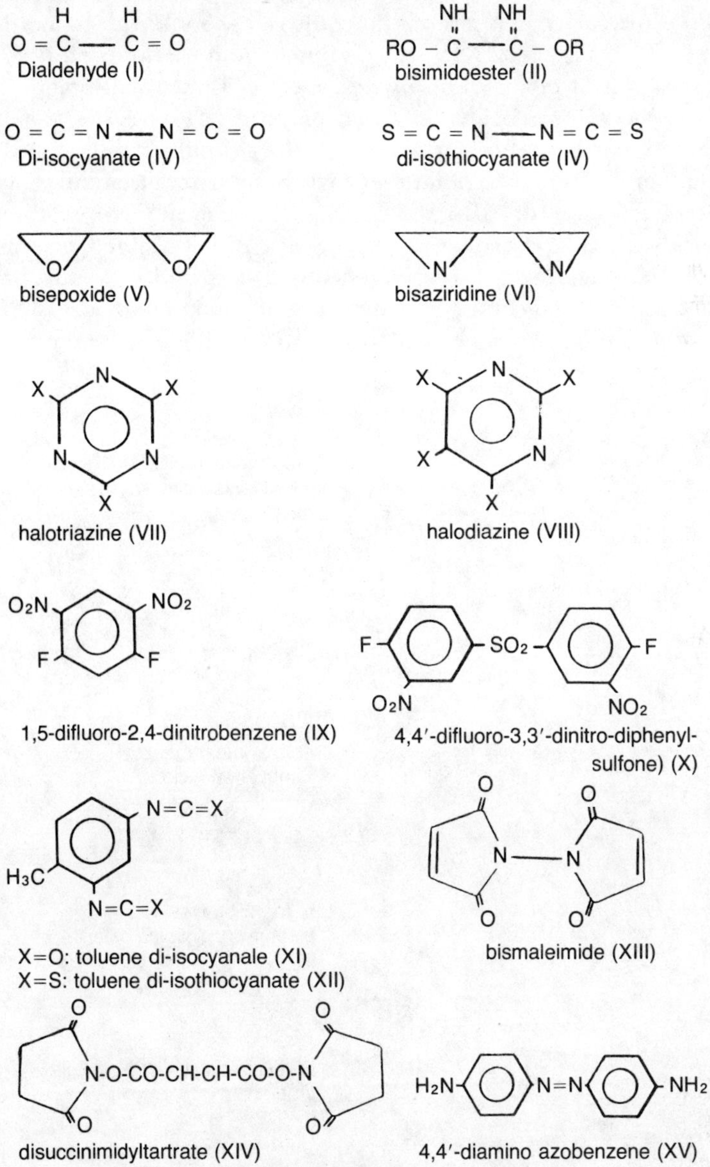

Fig. 2. Some homobifunctional protein-coupling reagents.

(VII) and toluenediisothiocyanate (XII).[20] With these reagents, the reactivity of the second group is clearly reduced as soon as the first group has reacted; this requires different reaction conditions and allows for a more easily controlled conjugation procedure. Early experiments with these reagents in the 1960s were not particularly successful, but further investigation may be fruitful. Cleavable homobifunctional reagents allow easier analysis of the conjugates. Some substances have been described (Figure 2: XIV, XV),[21] but these have not been used for the preparation of enzyme conjugates. Heterobifunctional reagents, of which a variety have been described (Figure 3), have the potential advantage of easier and better control of the coupling reaction and the resulting conjugates. Maleimidobenzoyl N-hydroxysuccinimide ester (XVI) has been used for β-D-galactosidase conjugation.[22] N-succinimidyl 3- (2-pyridyldithio) propionate (XX), or SPDP, has yielded promising data.[23] Both reagents have given encouraging results in our hands recently. Well-defined conjugates could be obtained in high yields. SPDP has the additional advantage that the reaction can easily be monitored spectrophotometrically.

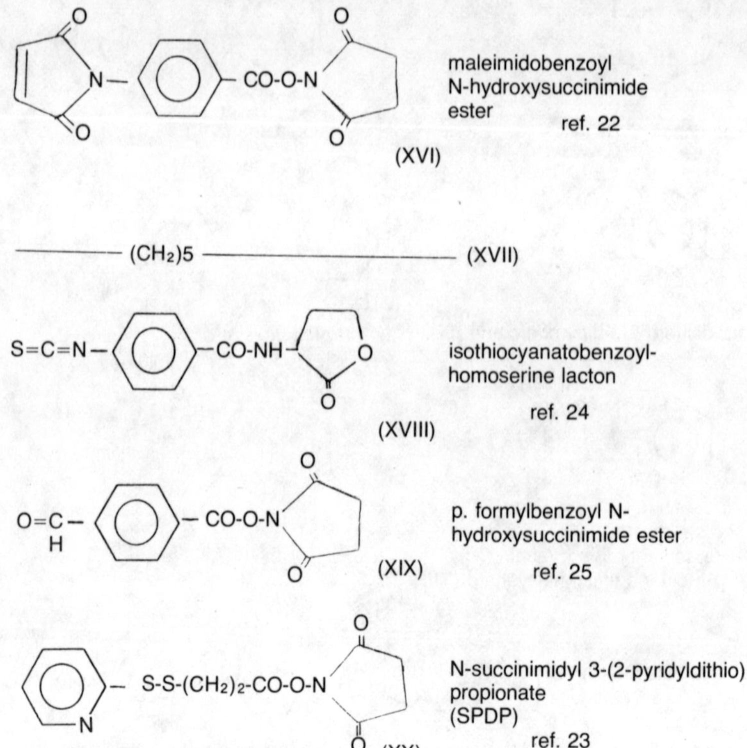

Fig. 3. Some heterobifunctional protein-coupling reagents.

Hapten-Protein Coupling

Preparation of hapten-enzyme conjugates is relatively easy, since haptens are well-defined organic molecules, usually with one functional group. Mixed anhydride or carbodiimide methods are mostly used for coupling hapten carboxyl groups to enzyme amino groups; the methods are outlined in Figure 4. Incorporation of haptens can be controlled to a certain degree by selection of the hapten/enzyme ratio during the reaction.

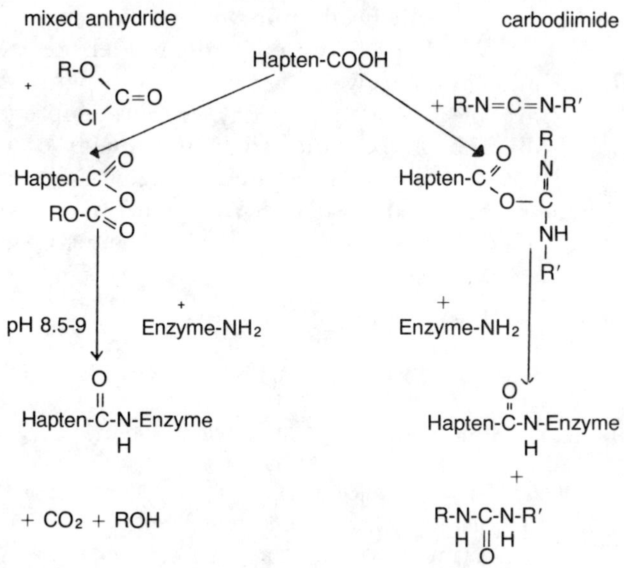

Fig. 4. Hapten-enzyme coupling.

CONJUGATE PURIFICATION AND CHARACTERIZATION

Purification of the conjugate after the coupling procedure is often required. Removal of nonconjugated enzyme and immunoreactant is important. Selection of a certain population of conjugate may be advantageous. The usual physicochemical methods (gel filtration, ion exchange chromatography, etc.) have often been applied. Affinity chromatography, either during or after the coupling procedure, appears the ideal solution in the end, provided elution conditions can be found that damage neither the enzyme activity nor the immune activity of the conjugate. Characterization of the conjugates with respect to composition, molecular weight, activity of the component parts, etc., is important for standardization. The eventual criterion, however, is the performance of the conjugate in the assay system it was designed for. WHO/IUIS is at present attempting to establish reference preparations for enzyme conjugates, very similar to the existing ones for immunofluorescence.

CONCLUSIONS

A wide variety of methods for production of enzyme conjugates are known. For enzyme-hapten conjugates, the available methods give satisfactory results and hardly need improvement. For enzyme-protein conjugates, the most widely used reagents (glutaraldehyde, periodate) give ill-defined conjugates, mostly of high molecular weights. Although such conjugates are of use in many assay systems, improvement is advisable, and will probably be reflected in the quality of the assay systems in which the conjugates are used. Reagents that may give superior conjugates are already available. We predict that in the future glutaraldehyde and periodate will be replaced by better reagents and methods.

REFERENCES

1. K.E. Rubenstein, R.S. Schneider, and E.F. Ullman, *Biochem Biophys Res Comm* **47**:846, 1972.
2. G.L. Rowley, K.E. Rubenstein, J. Huisjen, and E.F. Ullman, *J Biol Chem* **250**:3759, 1975.
3. J.J. Chang, C.P. Crowl, and R.S. Schneider, *Clin Chem* **21**:967, 1975.
4. B.K. van Weemen and A.H.W.M. Schuurs, *FEBS Lett* **15**:232, 1971.
5. E. Engvall and P. Perlmann, *Immunochemistry* **8**:871, 1971.
6. R.C. Lauer and B.F. Erlanger, *Immunochemistry* **11**:533, 1974.
7. K. Kato, H. Fukui, Y. Hamaguchi, and E. Ishikawa, *J Immunol* **116**:1554, 1975.
8. E. Engvall and I. Ljungström, *Acta Pathol Microbiol Scand (c)* **83**:231, 1975.
9. B.K. van Weemen, A.M.G. Bosch, E.C. Dawson, H. van Hell, and A.H.W.M. Schuurs, *Scand J Immunol* **8**(Suppl. 7):73, 1978.
10. F. Comoglio and S. Celada, *J Immunol Methods* **10**:161, 1976.
11. M. van der Waart and A.H.W.M. Schuurs, unpublished observations, 1976.
12. S. Avrameas, T. Ternynck, and J.L. Guesdon, *Scand J Immunol* **8**(Suppl. 7):7, 1978.
13. D.M. Boorsma and J.G. Streefkerk, *J Immunol Methods,* **245**, 1979.
14. J.H. Kennedy, L.J. Kricka, and P. Wilding, *Clin Chim Acta* **70**:1, 1976.
15. A.H.W.M. Schuurs and B.K. van Weemen, *Clin Chim Acta* **81**:1, 1977.
16. M.B. Wilson and P.K. Nakane In *Immunofluorescence and Related Staining Techniques,* W. Knapp, K. Holubar, and G. Wick (ed.), Elsevier, Amsterdam, 1978.
17. K. Kato, Y. Hamaguchi, H. Fukui, and E. Ishikawa, *FEBS Lett* **56**:370, 1975.
18. K. Kato, Y. Hamaguchi, H. Fukui, and E. Ishikawa, *J Biochem* **78**:235
19. S. Avrameas and G. Lespinats, *C R Acad Sci* **265**:1149, 1967.

20. S.J. Singer and A. Schick, *J Biophys Biochem Cytol* **9**:519, 1961.
21. R.J. Smith, R.A. Capaldi, D. Muchmore, and F. Dahlquist, *Biochemistry* **17**:3719, 1978.
22. T. Kitagawa and T. Aikawa, *J Biochem* **79**:233, 1976.
23. J. Carlsson, H. Drevin, and R. Axén, *Biochem J* **173**:723, 1978.
24. G.I. Tesser and J.J.M. Lamberts, *Int J Pept Prot Res* **8**:559, 1976.
25. J.P. Kraehenbuhl, R.E. Galardy, and J.D. Jamieson, *J Exp Med* **139**:208, 1974.
26. C. Borrebaeck and B. Mattiason, *J Solid-Phase Biochem* **4**:57, 1979.
27. P.M. Hardy, G.J. Hughes, and H.M. Rydon, *J Chem Soc Perkin* **1**:2282, 1979.
28. P. Knight, *Biochem J* **179**:191, 1979.

Chapter 5

Recent Advances in Fluorescence Immunoassay Techniques

EDWIN F. ULLMAN

Fluorescence methods are frequently mentioned as the next logical generation of immunoassay techniques. In this chapter, I would like to try to place recent developments of fluorescence immunoassays into historical perspective and to discuss some of the advantages and disadvantages of these methods, which will play a role in their acceptance by the clinical chemistry community.

Fluorescence has played a particularly important role in the development of immunochemistry. One of the earliest immunochemical procedures that has survived practically unchanged is the fluorescence histochemical staining method first described by Coons et al. in 1941.[1] This procedure is still applied routinely for the immunochemical localization of tissue antigens. Tissue sections are first incubated with antibodies. After washing away the unbound antibody, they are then stained with fluorescer-labeled antibodies from another species directed against the bound IgG. The location of the specific tissue antigens can be visualized in a dark field microscope.

The Coons method was probably the first clinical procedure to employ a reporter group. Considering the wide acceptance of the procedure, it is rather surprising that the use of receptor groups in competitive immunoassays did not appear until 18 years later with the introduction of radioimmunoassay.[2] This important method provided the added ability to determine antigens in solution quantitatively and with exquisite

Syva Research Institute, Palo Alto, Calif. 94304

sensitivity. Despite its power, the technique was adopted slowly as a routine tool because of the difficulty of developing protocols that addressed the need for speed, simplicity, and easy automatability that are so necessary for routine determinations. Moreover, the method added problems of reagent stability, laboratory safety, waste disposal, and government regulations.

It occurred to us about 1970 that most of these problems could be overcome by using nonisotopic labels, provided procedures could be developed in which the separation of free from bound label was eliminated. Pursuit of this objective first led to the development of spin immunoassay (FRAT®), which employed a stable radical label,[3,4] and the later EMIT® enzyme immunoassay method.[5-7] Both of these methods employed a labeled antigen which produced a signal that was modified upon binding by antibody. Inhibition of binding caused by competitive binding to the analyte thus effected a change in the measured signal. We defined these assays as examples of "homogeneous" immunoassay.[5] This nomenclature was used to provide a distinction from heterogeneous methods such as RIA, which require separation of the bound and free labeled antigen prior to measurement.

Interestingly, fluorescence also played the leading role in the development of homogeneous immunoassays. Thus as early as 1964, Dandliker described the principles for a fluorescence polarization immunoassay.[8,9] This method was based on the fact that light absorption and emission has direction. The efficiency of light absorption by a chromophore is dependent on the angle between the electric dipole of the exciting light and the transition moment of the molecule. Thus a beam of polarized light will more efficiently excite molecules that are oriented so their transition moments are parallel to the plane of polarization. Conversely, oriented molecules will emit polarized light. Provided a fluorescent molecule absorbs and re-emits light within a time interval that is short relative to its rate of tumbling, the resulting fluorescence emission will be partially polarized. However, rapid tumbling would cause the initially oriented excited molecules to become randomized and the emitted light to be nonpolarized.

Dandliker took advantage of this phenomenon by studying the increase in polarized fluorescence when a small rapidly tumbling fluorescer-labeled hapten was allowed to bind to large slowly tumbling antibodies. The assay was applied to the detection of antipenicillin antibodies and more recently has been applied to an assay for gentamicin[10] and phenytoin,[11] in which the usual competitive immunoassay protocol was employed.

Unfortunately, fluorescence polarization immunoassays have serious problems that are unlikely to be readily resolved. The theoretical maximum polarization for fully oriented immobilized molecules is 0.5.

Thus only half of the fluorescence intensity can even theoretically be utilized. This figure is further reduced by incomplete immobilization of the labels in the immune complex due to flexing of their linking groups and to tumbling of the whole complex. The modulatable signal thus represents a small fraction of the total signal and the assay sensitivity is correspondingly limited. In addition, even weak interactions between the fluorescer-labeled hapten and macromolecules in the sample can affect the average tumbling rates and result in nonspecific serum interference.

A number of alternative fluorescence methods to be described below have much less serious problems with sample interference, and in addition avoid the relatively complex instrumentation required for fluorescence polarization measurements.

THE BACKGROUND FLUORESCENCE PROBLEM

In setting out to design fluorescence methods, one is struck by the concerns frequently expressed about reproducibility and background problems in fluorescence measurements. Experience shows that many of these difficulties can be traced to the use of cuvettes, which introduce errors due to dust particles, fingerprints, and positioning in the fluorometer. The use of a flow cell eliminates most of these variables. A remaining major source of error is the background fluorescence from endogeneous components in the sample, as well as light scattering from micellular or particulate material. These errors can be minimized by use of the proper combination of chemical and instrumental techniques. Serum fluorescence increases sharply at short wavelengths, and thus fluorescers that absorb at wavelengths greater than 500 nm where serum fluorescence is weak are particularly useful. To optimize the signal-to-background ratio, the fluorescent label should have a high extinction coefficient and high fluorescence quantum yield. Scattering problems can be reduced both by the use of highly monochromatic light sources and good filters and by using fluorescers having large Stokes shifts.

For many years fluorescein isothiocyanate has come closest to meeting these requirements. Conjugates of this compound to proteins have extinction coefficients near 80,000 $M^{-1}cm^{-1}$ and quantum yields near 0.5, although the quantum yields fall off with higher dye to protein ratios.[12] Unfortunately, the 520-nm emission maximum of conjugates of this dye is very close to the corresponding maximum of bound bilirubin. Longer wavelength dyes such as rhodamine derivatives are available, but their quantum yields in water are much lower. New fluorescein derivatives currently under development in our laboratory retain all of the desirable features of fluorescein but have absorption and emission maxima that are shifted to longer wavelengths by at least 30 nm and thus are much less susceptible to interference from serum constituents.

Several instrumental approaches to the elimination of serum background fluorescence and light scattering are also possible. One approach takes advantage of the possibility of designing an assay that is measured by determining the rate of change of a fluorescence signal. Since the background signal can be kept relatively static, rate measurements provide a simple means for subtracting the background signal. Reduction in background can also be obtained by simultaneous scanning of both the excitation and emission wavelengths while maintaining a constant difference between the two wavelengths equal to the Stokes shift of the fluorescent label. It is unlikely that any fluorescent constituent will have exactly the same absorption and emission maxima as the fluorescent label, and thus the double scanning approach tends to minimize, though not eliminate, contributions from these constituents.

Another instrumental method for the elimination of background fluorescence and light scattering is by the use of time-resolved fluorometry. In this technique a fluorescent label must be used that has an excited state lifetime that is relatively long compared to the lifetime of endogeneous fluorescence substances. Particularly attractive fluorescers for this purpose are rare earth chelates and polycyclic hydrocarbons such as pyrene. Fluorescence of these labels can be distinguished from background by using a pulsed light source and measuring the signal after the shorter lifetime background has decayed.[13] Alternatively, phase modulation spectroscopy can be employed, in which the phase shift between an intensity modulated exciting light source and the corresponding modulated fluorescence signal is measured.

Alternative approaches to the elimination of background depend on the chemical or physical removal of the interfering substances. Among the more effective chemical methods is pretreatment of the sample with peracids such as peracetic or persulfuric acid and quenching of the excess reagent with sulfite ion (J. Kam and R. Yoshida, unpublished results). Over 90% of serum background can be eliminated in this way, although not all analytes can survive this treatment. Charcoal can also be employed to eliminate background, the use of which will be discussed below.

HETEROGENEOUS FLUORESCENCE IMMUNOASSAYS

Most background problems can be directly avoided by separating the labeled reagents from the assay solution prior to measurement. Commercial methods have been worked out for heterogeneous fluorescence immunoassays that work in principle exactly like RIA.[14] By incubating a fluorescent-labeled antigen with antibodies attached to a solid phase, the immune complex can be separated. In one method employed by BioRad, antibody-labeled polyacrylamide beads are suspended in the assay medium, spun down, and then resuspended for measurement. In IDT's system, the antibody or antigen is fixed on a solid surface, which is incubated in the assay medium and washed prior to measurement. These systems have theoretical sensitivities limited only by the spectrometer design, the binding constants of the antibodies, and the intrinsic fluorescence of the support. Removal of nonspecifically bound label, however, is a problem and necessitates careful washing. This rather clumsy feature of these assays, which is shared by RIA, is counterbalanced in part by the absence of stringent requirements for purity of the labeled antigen. The latter requirement is a troublesome feature of some of the homogeneous methods.

HOMOGENEOUS FLUORESCENCE IMMUNOASSAYS

A particularly intriguing fluorescence immunoassay technique that involves two phases but is properly considered homogeneous, since no separation is required, was described by Kronick and Little.[15] The method employs antibody bound to an optically flat quartz slide. A beam of light is injected into the edge of the slide such that it travels through the quartz and undergoes total reflection off the surface. Fluorescer-labeled antigens that become bound to the surface antibodies couple to an evanescent wave, which extends for a fraction of a wavelength past the quartz surface. Since only surface fluorescers become excited, they fluoresce with little interfering fluorescence from the bulk solution, which is in contact with the surface of the slide. The method thus does not require formal separation and washing. However, it has so far not attained high sensitivity, and the handling and cost of the quartz slides seriously reduces the practical appeal of the method.

A variety of fluorescence methods have also been devised for detecting antigen-antibody interactions in solution without separating the bound and free components. In certain cases, antibody binding to hapten-fluorescer conjugates fortuitously affects the fluorescence quantum yield. Thus, for example, binding of antigentamicin[16] antibodies to the corresponding drug-fluorescein conjugates causes up to about 40% quenching, which may be inhibited by the presence of the free drug. Although this fluorescence quenching immunoassay procedure is attractive in its simplicity, unfortunately, the degree of quenching is dependent on the choice of hapten and is sometimes too small to provide a satisfactory signal response. Moreover, the method is not applicable to protein antigens. Probably, quenching is due to the presence of an amine or other electron donor group in the hypervariable region of the antibody, which lies in close proximity to the bound hapten.

It is interesting that with certain haptens such as thyroxine[17] and triiodothyronine, the effect can be turned around, in that antibody can produce up to an eight-fold enhancement of the fluorescence. The degree of enhancement in these fluorescence enhancement immunoassays depends on internal quenching caused by interaction of the heavy iodine atoms with the fluorescent probe. Conjugates in which the groups have the highest probability of being in contact are initially the most weakly fluorescent, and are more strongly enhanced when antibody binding interferes with the heavy atom–fluorescer interaction (P. Khanna and R. Yoshida, unpublished observations). However, like the fluorescence quenching immunoassays, fluorescence enhancement assays appear so far to have only limited practical utility. Nonspecific interactions with serum components, particularly albumin, partially relieve the heavy atom–fluorescer interaction and cause partial fluorescence enhancement. Since some portion of the labeled hapten in the assay solution will be free and available to bind to albumin, nonspecific sample-to-sample variations in signal intensity become unacceptably large. Inclusion of albumin in the assay mixtures decreases these variations, but it is still difficult to obtain acceptable reproducibility (T. A. Houk and R. Yoshida, unpublished observations).

Fluorescence Excitation Transfer Immunoassay

Dependence of the above fluorescence quenching immunoassay on the fortuitous presence of an electron donor near the binding site can be avoided by covalently attaching a quencher to the antibodies. In this way fluorescer-labeled antigen can be guaranteed of being quenched upon antibody binding.[18] The most effective quencher for this purpose is a dye that has intense absorption at the wavelengths of the fluorescence emission of the fluorophore. The rate of energy transfer from the excited fluorophore to such a quencher has been shown to be directly proportional to the rate constant for fluorescence emission of the fluorescer and inversely proportional to the sixth power of the distance between the two dyes.[19] When using fluorescein as the fluorescer and rhodamine as the quencher, the fluorescence intensity can be reduced by half when the two dyes are about 50 Å apart.[18] Thus by labeling antibodies with up to 15 rhodamines, greater than 90% quenching has been observed. This effect can be completely reversed by inhibiting binding to the fluorescein-labeled antigen with free antigen (Fig. 1).

Numerous assays have been constructed using this fluorescence excitation transfer immunoassay. These include assays for morphine,[18]

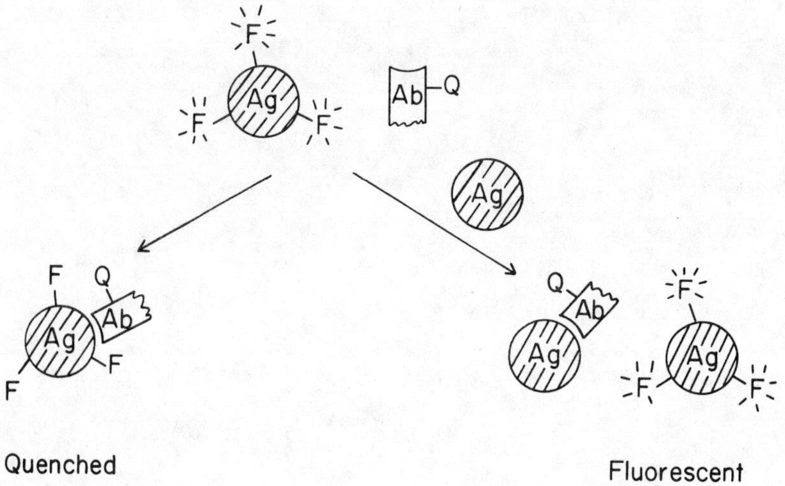

Fig. 1. Principle of fluorescence excitation transfer immunoassay. Antigen-antibody binding brings the quencher sufficiently near the fluorescer to permit energy transfer.

IgG,[18] IgA,[20] IgM[21] C3, C-reactive protein, α_1-antitrypsin, and transferrin. In each case, the analyte blocks antibody binding and thus causes an increase in the fluorescence intensity (Fig. 2). The method can also be applied to the determination of antibodies. Thus if fluorescer-labeled antigen and quencher-labeled antibody are employed, the analyte antibody can compete for sites on the antigen and decrease quenching by blocking binding by the labeled antibody. However, care must be taken to ensure that there is sufficient labeled antibody to saturate the antigenic sites when no analyte antibody is present. The presence of unbound sites permits the analyte antibody to crosslink the complexes of labeled antigen and labeled antibody with a resultant increase in quenching. This leads to a biphasic response, which can produce ambiguous readings (M. Schwarzberg, unpublished observations). Evidence that crosslinking is the source of the biphasic response was obtained by the elimination of this phenomenon when Fab fragments were used in place of intact analyte antibody (Fig. 3).

A practical limitation of the fluorescence excitation transfer immunoassay is the need to employ moderately purified fluorescer-labeled antigen in the assays. Purification of the antigen represents a significant limitation, since in some cases these materials may be scarce, difficult to characterize, or hazardous. Since these assays employ no separation step, any fluorescer-labeled impurities that are included with the labeled antigen add to unmodulated signal background. A large fluorescent background, even if it is nominally constant from sample to sample, lowers reproducibility and decreases instrumental sensitivity. For this

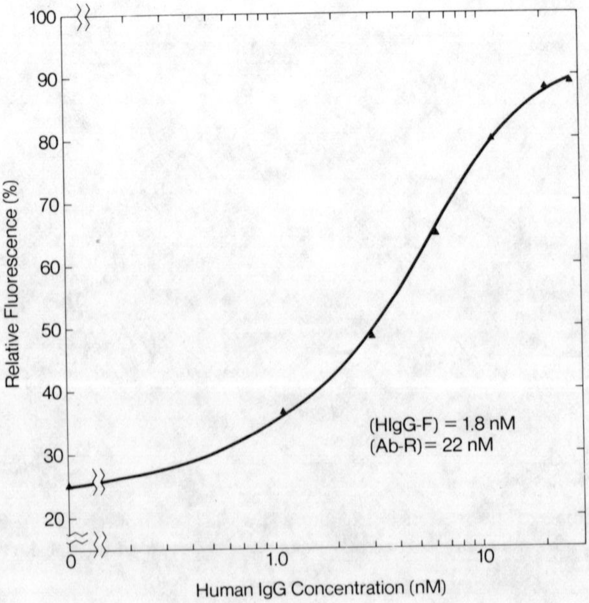

Fig. 2. Standard curve for human IgG by fluorescence excitation transfer immunoassay, using fluorescein (F) as fluorescer and rhodamine (R) as quencher.

reason, it is usually necessary to employ antigen preparations to at least 50% purity.

One way to avoid this limitation is to use an alternative protocol in which labeled antigen need not be used at all. Instead one portion of antibody is labeled with fluorescer and a second portion is labeled with quencher. Addition of analyte antigen, other than a hapten, to a mixture of thus labeled antibody causes separate molecules of antibody with each label to be brought into close spatial proximity at the antigen surface (Fig. 4).[18] Up to 60% quenching has been observed with this method, depending in part on the quenching efficiency of the fluorescer-quencher pair. Unfortunately, addition of excess antigen reverses the quenching by permitting the bound antibody to become spread over a large total antigen surface, which results in a biphasic standard curve (Fig. 5).

Although this antibody-labeled fluorescence excitation transfer immunoassay eliminates the need for labeled antigen in the assay, it requires that the fluorescer-labeled antibody be highly specific in order to avoid excessive unmodulatable background fluorescence. Since antibody purification usually requires tedious affinity chromatographic methods, this assay method is not currently a useful routine procedure. Nonetheless, the probable availability of monoclonal antibodies derived from hybridomas[22] may make this procedure particularly attractive in

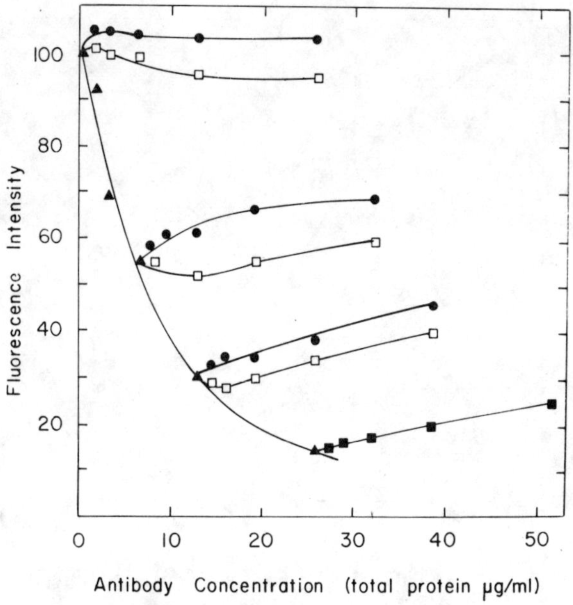

Fig. 3. Effect of unlabeled antibodies on the quenching of fluorescein-labeled human IgG (HIgG-F) by rhodamine-labeled antihuman IgG (Ab-R). One μg/ml solutions of HIgG-F were incubated with different amounts of Ab-R alone (▲) and in combination with unlabeled antibody (□) or unlabeled Fab fragments (●). With the largest volume of Ab-R, the responses due to unlabeled antibody and unlabeled Fab fragments were identical (■).

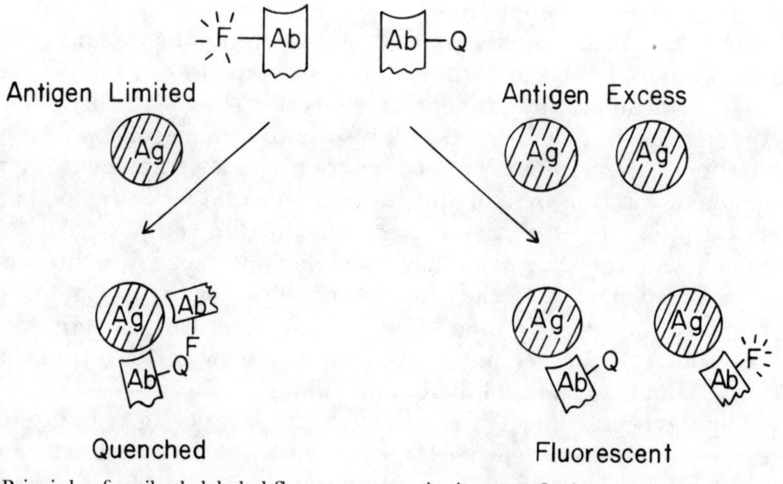

Fig. 4. Principle of antibody labeled fluorescence excitation transfer immunoassay showing origin of biphasic response.

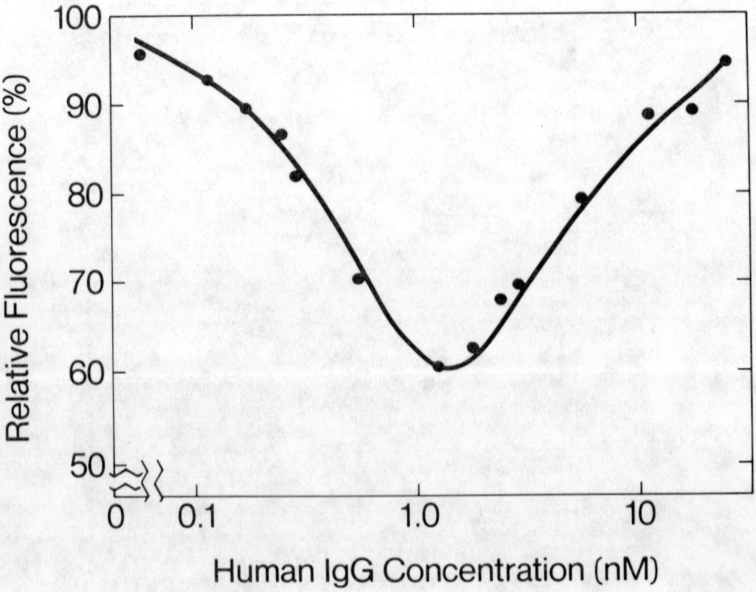

Fig. 5. Assay for human IgG with 1 : 5.4 mixture of fluorescein-labeled antibody and rhodamine-labeled antibody.

the future. The dependence of the method on the proximal binding of antibodies provides the opportunity to detect abnormal antigenic sites on otherwise normal proteins by letting specific fluorescer-labeled antibody bind to this site, while quencher-labeled antibody binds to adjacent normal antigenic determinants.

The antibody-labeled fluorescence excitation transfer method has been modified to simplify the isolation of pure antigen and antibody, and to eliminate the undesirable biphasic response. In this procedure, the IgG fraction of the antibodies is converted to Fab fragments, and the crude antigen is fractionated with respect to its molecular weight by gel filtration. After fluorescer labeling of the Fab fragments, they are combined with the partially purified antigen and again fractionated by gel filtration. In this second fractionation, the complexes of labeled antigen and Fab fragments have a higher molecular weight than any other component and can thus be readily separated (Fig. 6). These complexes can then be used in lieu of fluorescer-labeled antigen in the standard fluorescence excitation transfer immunoassay (M. Schwarzberg, unpublished observations).

This has been applied effectively to assays for IgG, IgA, and IgM. The respective impure quencher-labeled antibodies were found to quench fluorescer-labeled Fab-antigen complexes by up to 60, 75, and 70%, respectively, provided the Fab-to-antigen ratio was kept low; and

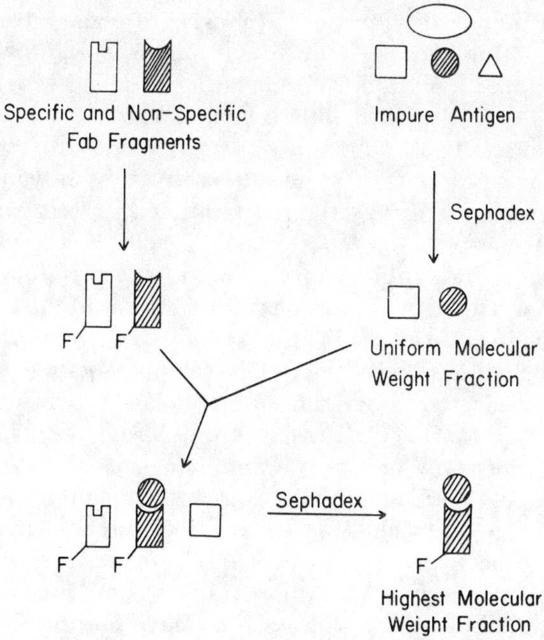

Fig. 6. General method for fluorescer (F) labeling and purification of labeled antigen.

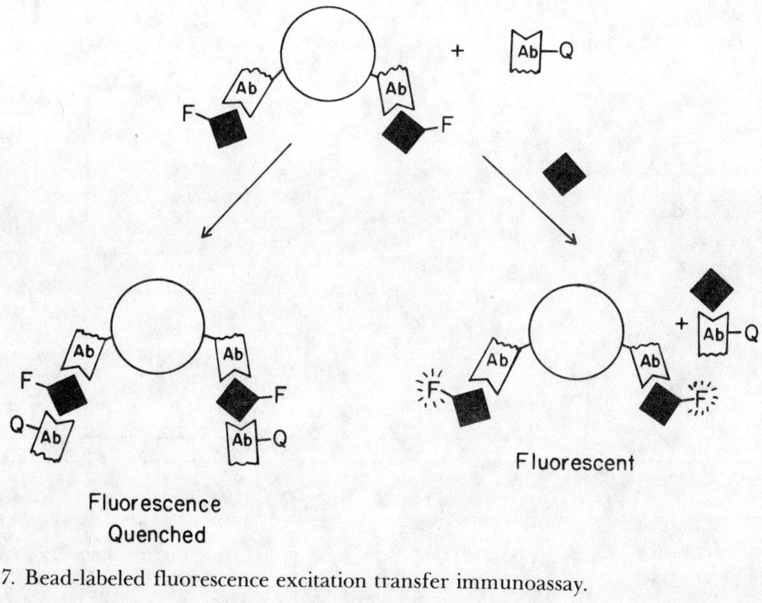

Fig. 7. Bead-labeled fluorescence excitation transfer immunoassay.

conventional monotonic response curves were obtained. Although the total change in fluorescence intensities is somewhat less than when using purified antigen, the simplification in antigen purification makes this an attractive technique for difficultly isolable antigens.

Another method of obtaining pure labeled antigen for use in fluorescence excitation transfer immunoassays takes advantage of phase separation techniques during the preparation of the reagents, while still avoiding a separation step in the assay itself. Polyacrylamide beads (BioRad) labeled with antibody are allowed to adsorb fluorescer-labeled antigen from a crude antigen preparation. After washing the beads, they are used as one reagent in the assay, the other reagent being quencher-labeled antibody (Fig. 7). After combining the antibody, sample, and beads, the fluorescence of the bead suspension is measured directly (R. Zuk and G.L. Rowley, unpublished work). Since the geometry permits only one of the antigenic sites of the antigen to be occupied by the antibody involved in attachment to the bead, the remaining sites are available for competition in the assay.

While this bead procedure in principle provides the simplest way of constructing fluorescence excitation transfer immunoassays, development of the method is not without difficulty. The principal problems concern nonspecific binding of fluorescer-labeled impurities and the need to leave sufficient space around each bound antigen to permit good

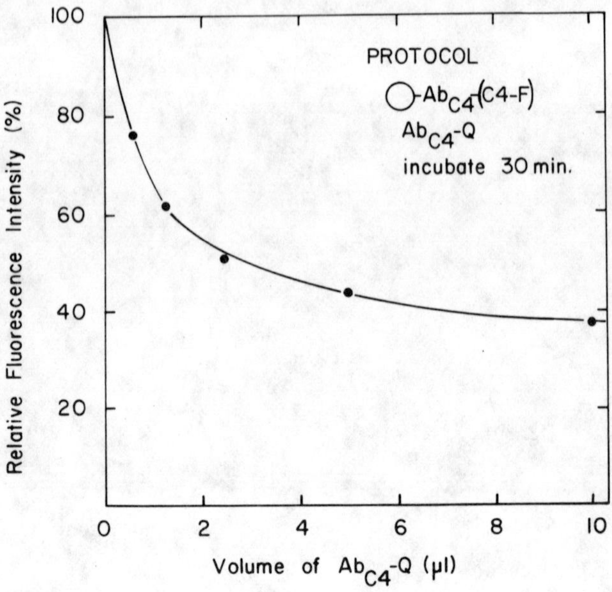

Fig. 8. Quenching of bead-bound fluorescer-labeled C4 (C4-F) by quencher-labeled anti-C4 (Ab_{C4}-Q).

quenching by quencher-labeled antibody. The magnitude of these problems varies with the antigen, although it is in principle solvable for all antigens. Thus after anti-IgG labeled beads had been treated with 1% pure IgG that had been fluorescer-labeled, they could be quenched up to 80% by quencher-labeled antibodies. However, beads similarly treated with 1% pure C4 were quenched only up to 60% (Fig. 8). Nevertheless, the fundamental simplicity of the method, which eliminates the need for characterizing the antigen at all, augurs well for the adoption of this technique as a standard immunoassay method.

Fluorescence Protection Immunoassay

An entirely different approach to fluorescence immunoassay has been employed that partially overcomes the antigen purification problem, permits a more direct determination of antibody as the analyte, and sometimes works where the fluorescence excitation transfer method breaks down. Fluorescence protection immunoassay was initially described for both haptens and proteins, specifically morphine and insulin,[23,24] and has more recently been demonstrated for albumin.[25] The method employs three reagents, an antigen-fluorescer conjugate, antibodies directed against the fluorescer, and antibodies directed against the antigen. Antigen from the sample is first allowed to complex with antibody. Upon addition of the conjugate, residual antibody binds to the conjugate. Since bound antibody directed against the antigen sterically interferes with antifluorescer binding, the degree to which it is bound can be determined by addition of the antifluorescer (Fig. 9). The inhibition of binding by the antifluorescer can be monitored directly, provided a fluorescer is employed that can be either quenched or

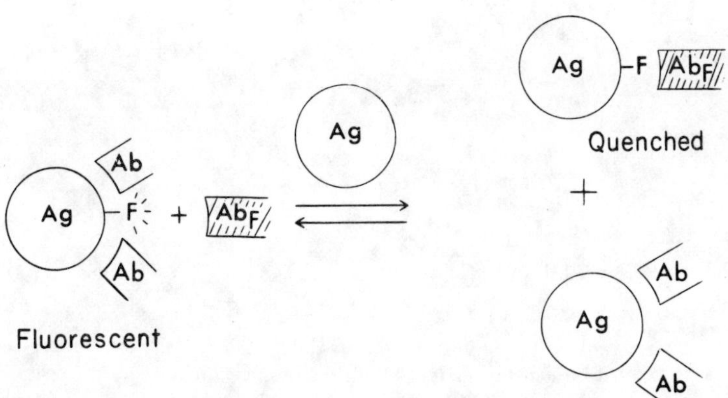

Fig. 9. Principle of fluorescence protection immunoassay.

activated upon antibody binding. When quenching antibodies are used that are very efficient, the method tolerates substantial quantities of fluorescent-labeled impurities, since they will be quenched prior to measurement.

A primary concern in developing fluorescence protection immunoassays is the efficiency by which antiantigen "protects" the fluorescer from binding by antifluorescer. Using a fluorescein isothiocyanate conjugate of human IgG as a model, the ability of antihuman IgG to protect the conjugate from quenching by antifluorescein was determined for antifluorescein preparations that varied in steric bulk.[26] In the absence of antihuman IgG, only 9% residual fluorescence remained after antifluorescein binding. When antihuman IgG was bound to the conjugate, the minimum residual fluorescence was increased to 28% using antifluorescein Fab fragments. This was further increased with increasing size of the antifluorescein up to 77% when antifluorescein bound to 500,000 dalton dextran was employed (Fig. 10).

While bulky antifluorescein preparations gave the largest modulation of the fluorescence intensity, they were only found useful if readings

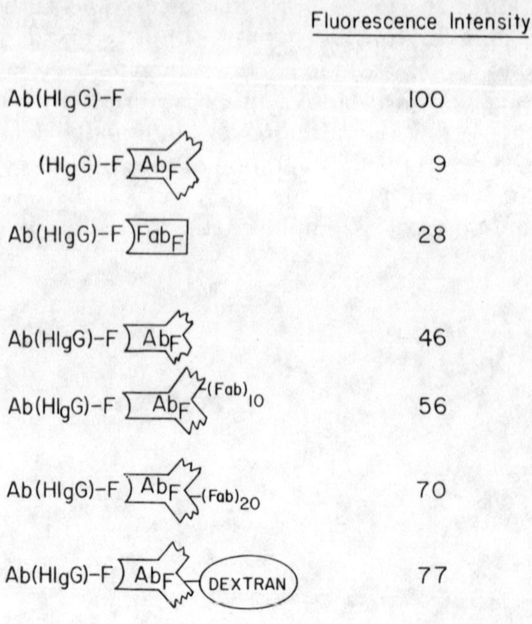

Fig. 10. Effect of various antifluorescein preparations on the fluorescence of fluorescein-labeled human IgG (HIgG-F) in the presence and absence of antihuman IgG (Ab). Intensities are given relative to antibody-bound HIgG-F. Modified rabbit antifluoresceins were prepared by incubation with 10- and 20-fold molar excess of sheep antirabbit Fab respectively, or by conjugation to 500,000 dalton dextran.

were made after equilibrium was approached. If the rate of quenching due to binding by antifluorescein is to be measured, absolute protection of the fluorescer must be avoided. Instead, in order to obtain a large signal modulation, the fluorescer should be fully quenchable even in the presence of antiantigen, and only the rates should be dependent on the degree of antiantigen binding.

There are two reasons why the rate protocol is to be preferred over the endpoint measurement. First, measurement immediately after addition of the antifluorescein obviates the need for two incubations. Second, the rate measurement automatically compensates for serum background fluorescence. Although Fab fragments of antifluorescein provided large modulation of rates, intact antibody was found to be even more effective and is therefore preferred.

Several applications for fluorescence protection immunoassay have been found in which this method appears to have advantages over fluorescence excitation transfer immunoassay. Using the endpoint method, a combination assay has been constructed that employs umbelliferone-labeled IgG, fluorescein-labeled IgM, antibodies to the two antigens, and antibodies to the two fluorophores (G. Rowley and T.A. Houk, unpublished work). Both fluorophore conjugates could be quenched by greater than 80% by the homologous antifluorophore. The antigens could each be determined independently in the same solution simply by exciting and measuring each dye separately at the appropriate wavelengths. The protocol entailed combining the sample, mixed antiantigen antibodies, and mixed labeled antigens. After incubation, the mixed antifluorescer antibodies were added, the mixture was incubated again, and then was measured. With appropriate instrumentation, it should be possible to simultaneously follow the rates of quenching, and thus the second incubation and a sample blank could be avoided. Construction of a similar combination assay employing the fluorescence excitation transfer method would be expected to be more complex because of the need to find four separate dyes that do not interfere with each other.

Perhaps the most generally useful application of fluorescence protection immunoassay is for the detection or quantitation of antibodies. In contrast to the fluorescence excitation transfer method, which is a competitive assay and requires both labeled antigen and labeled antibody, fluorescence protection immunoassays for antibodies are direct assays and employ only one labeled reagent, the antigen. One assay that is currently under study is for anticardiolipin in human serum. The method employs a fluorescein-cardiolipin conjugate, which represents 5% by weight of monolamellar phospholipid vesicles prepared from phosphatidyl choline and cholesterol by sonication in buffer. Incubation of this preparation with serum containing anticardiolipin is followed by addition of antifluorescein and measurement of the rate of quenching. Assays developed to date[27] are similar in sensitivity to the standard VDRL assay that employs cardiolipin-lecithin-cholesterol particles, which aggregate in the presence of antibody. Since the VDRL assays uses undiluted serum rather than the 2% serum used in the fluorescence protection assay, the intrinsic sensitivity of the latter method is about 50-fold more sensitive. It is expected that the use of other dyes that more effectively avoid serum interference will permit more serum to be used so that higher sensitivity to the serum concentration of the antibody can be achieved. In addition, longer wavelength dyes should eliminate the present need to determine a serum blank.

A similar fluorescent vesicle protection immunoassay has been applied to haptens. Thus phenobarbital has been covalently linked to phosphatidyl ethanolamine and incorporated into phospholipid vesicles containing fluorescein that was incorporated in a like fashion (Fig. 11). Although antibodies to phenobarbital caused a reduced rate of quenching by antifluorescein, there appeared to be no particular advantage of this over other methods of assaying this drug (J.M. Brinkley, unpublished work).

Fluorescence protection immunoassays have also been applied to the assay of thyroxine (G. Rowley and T.A. Houk, unpublished work). The sample was first incubated with antithyroxine and anilinonaphthalene

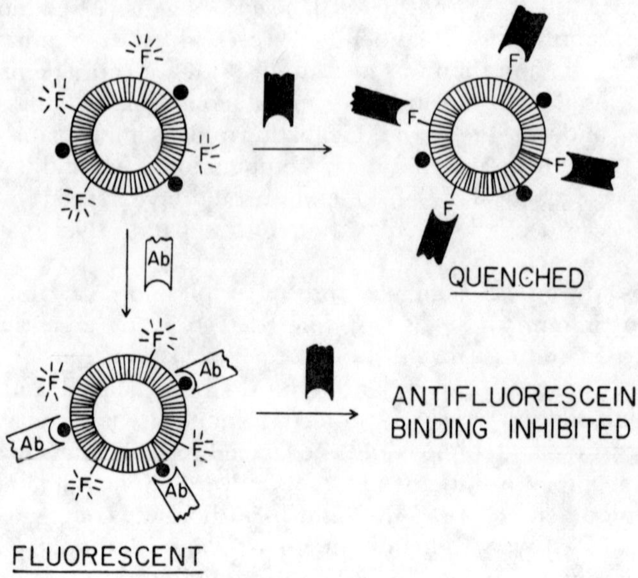

Fig. 11. Principle of fluorescent vesicle protection immunoassay.

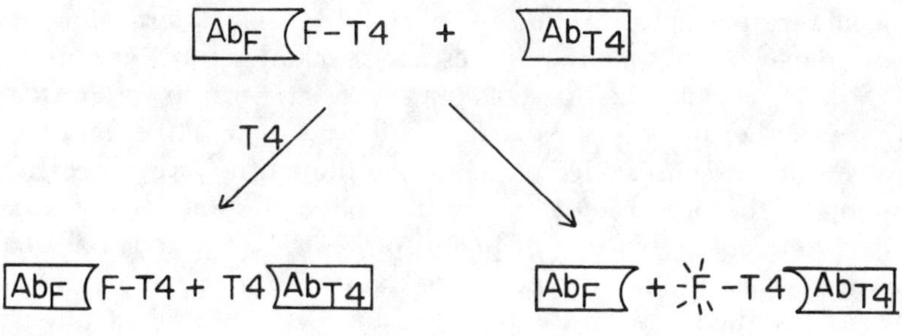

Fig. 12. Fluorescence protection immunoassay for thyroxine.

sulfonic acid (for release of thyroxine from thyroid binding globulin). A combined reagent consisting of antibodies to fluorescein and a fluorescein-thyroxine conjugate was then added and the rate of fluorescence enhancement measured (Fig. 12). The method differs from the fluorescence enhancement immunoassay,[17] where advantage is taken of the ability of antithyroxine to enhance the fluorescence of thyroxine-fluorescein conjugates. Unlike the fluorescence enhancement immunoassay, the conjugate is always bound to either antithyroxine or antifluorescein. As a result, enhancement due to nonspecific interaction of the conjugate with serum proteins is avoided.

One of the important theoretical advantages of fluorescence protection immunoassays is the opportunity to employ relatively impure antigen for labeling. In principle any labeled impurities will be quenched by antifluorescer antibodies and thus will not contribute to the background. In practice antifluorescein can only quench fluorescein fluorescence by about 90%. However, if rhodamine-labeled antifluorescein is used, the quenching efficiency increases to about 98%. With this labeled antibody, antigen with 90% impurity will have only 18% of its total fluorescence signal that cannot be modulated. Although this much background does not significantly affect the assay, when antigen with 95% impurity is used, the assay sensitivity is decreased.

Fluorescence Protection Immunoassay with Charcoal Scavenging

An important variation of the fluorescer protection assay utilizes a black particle in place of antifluorescer to cause quenching. In preliminary experiments it was demonstrated that fluorescein-labeled IgG could be almost completely quenched by common decolorizing charcoal. It is expected that any fluoresceins adsorbed directly to the charcoal surface would be quenched because of strong perturbation of the electronic states of the dye. However, fluoresceins attached to a portion of the bound protein that was not in contact with the particles must also have been quenched. Two mechanisms for quenching are probably responsible. First, dipole coupled energy transfer to the charcoal may occur, as in the fluorescence excitation transfer immunoassay. Second, the charcoal particle may act as an opaque screen that can intercept either or both the exciting light and the emitted light.

When fluorescein-labeled antibodies to human IgG were treated with charcoal in the presence of serum, the quenching was far less efficient due to competitive binding of serum proteins on the charcoal surface. However, when the same experiment was carried out with charcoal that was preadsorbed with antifluorescein antibodies, excellent quenching was obtained. Nearly complete fluorescence quenching was achieved with charcoal suspensions having an optical density of about 0.3 (1 mm pathlength) (Fig. 13). Most significantly, if the fluorescein-labeled antibodies were first allowed to bind to human IgG bound to Sepharose 4B, the resulting suspension was much less quenched by the charcoal (Fig. 14). Based on the fact that the antibodies were about 25% pure and the charcoal absorbed about half the light, it was calculated that binding of the fluorescein-labeled specific antibody to Sepharose protected over half of the bound fluoresceins from quenching by charcoal (R. Zuk, unpublished work).

These observations showed that an assay could be set up as illustrated in Figure 15. Fluorescein-labeled antihuman IgG antibody was first

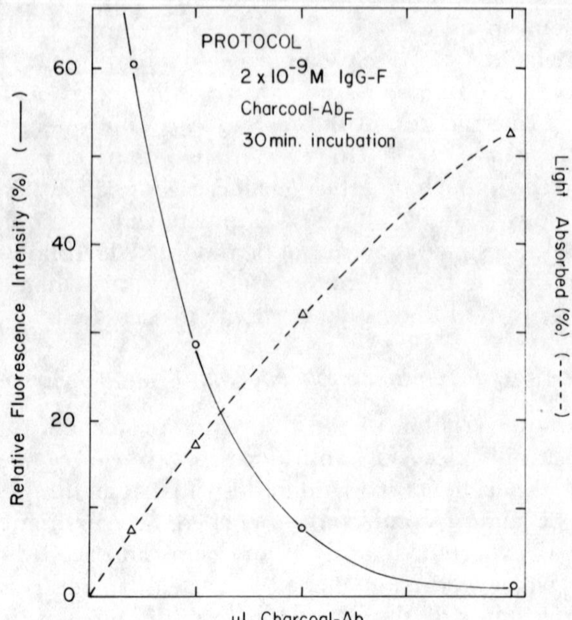

Fig. 13. Quenching of fluorescein-labeled IgG by charcoal labeled with antifluorescein.

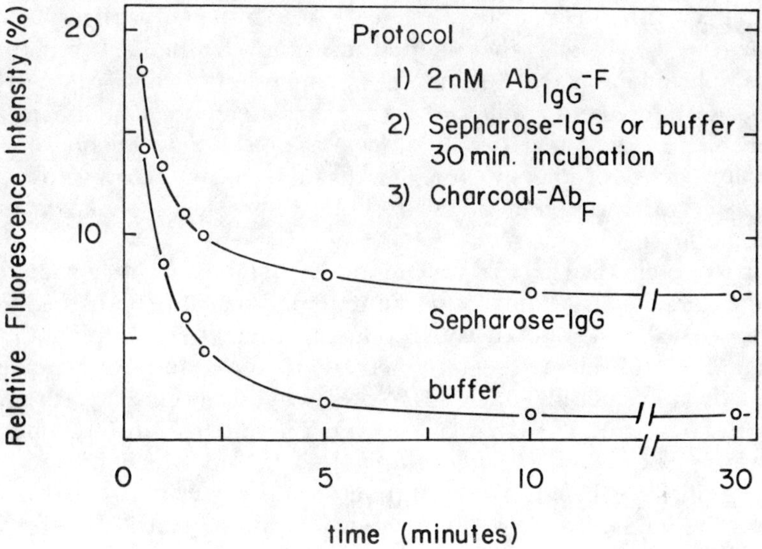

Fig. 14. Kinetics of quenching fluorescein-labeled antibodies to human IgG by charcoal labeled with antifluorescein.

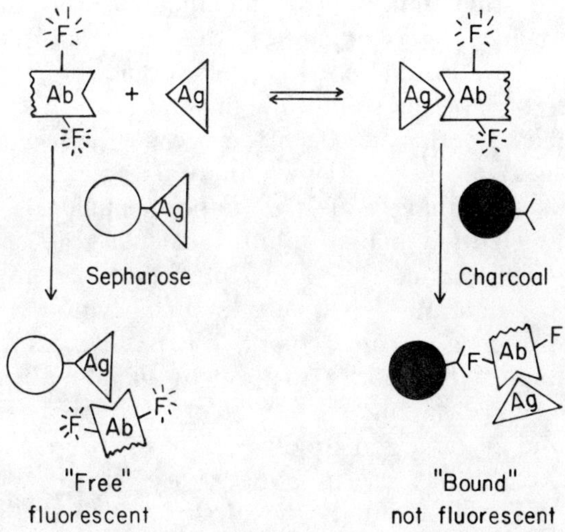

Fig. 15. Principle of fluorescence protection immunoassay with charcoal scavenging.

combined with the sample antigen. A suspension of antigen-labeled Sepharose beads was then added to cause binding of remaining uncomplexed antibody. Addition of a suspension of charcoal adsorbed with antifluorescein, followed by a half-hour incubation, caused quenching of the labeled protein that was not bound to Sepharose. In addition, most of the intrinsic background serum fluorescence was quenched. Measurement of the residual fluorescence then permitted quantitation of the antigen.

Up to a point the charcoal scavenging method is conceptually identical to heterogeneous fluorescence immunoassays. In both methods, fluorescer-labeled antibody is partitioned between free and immobilized antigen. In the heterogeneous method, the free and bound labeled antibody are physically separated to permit a fluorescence measurement of one fraction. The charcoal scavenging method differs only by providing a means of quenching the bound fraction and any nonspecifically labeled protein without requiring separation. Although only a preliminary study demonstrating a crude standard curve for IgG has so far been made, the technique should be just as adaptable to a variety of different situations as the heterogeneous method. Thus by suitable choice of reagents, the assay should be adaptable not only to the assay of antigens and antibodies, but by use of sandwich techniques, it should be possible to assay proteins with both a specific antigenic site and a specific receptor site, such as, for example, a specific IgM.

Other Methods

A variety of other immunoassay techniques employing fluorescence detection have been described. Most of these are not strictly fluorescence immunoassays because the labels are not simple fluorescent labels, and they will therefore be discussed only briefly.

Considerable attention has been focused on the use of phospholipid liposome labels in liposome lysis immunoassays.[28] Several of these methods take advantage of the impermeability of phospholipid membranes to charged or hydrophilic molecules. Liposomes filled with the fluorogenic enzyme substrate, umbelliferone phosphate, were caused to lyse when antibody against a surface antigen was allowed to bind in the presence of complement. Escape of the substrate into the external solution permitted its turnover by alkaline phosphatase with a concomitant increase in fluorescence.[29] Alternatively, a charged fluorescer and a charged quencher have been encapsulated in liposomes, and the increase in fluorescence produced upon lysis was monitored.[30] These methods have the advantage of substantial theoretical sensitivity because the binding of a few antibodies can in principle cause the release of a large number of fluorescent molecules. However, the calculated sensitivity based on the actual observations suggests a detection limit of 0.01–0.1 μg of antigen,[30] which at best is the same as fluorescence excitation transfer immunoassay. Moreover, the method is sensitive to the concentration of complement and the presence of inactive complement, factors that are difficult to control. The instability of complement represents a reagent problem and the appearance of active and inactive complement in varying amounts in serum is likely to contribute to significant serum interference.

A new method employing phospholipid vesicles, called vesicle fusion immunoassay, takes advantage of the ability of antibodies bound to the surface of unilamellar vesicles to inhibit calcium ion-induced fusion.[31] The fusion was monitored by incorporating rhodamine (quencher) into the phospholipid membrane of some vesicles and incorporating dansyl (fluorescer) into the membrane of other vesicles. Mixing of the dyes following fusion caused quenching. If hapten-labeled vesicles were used, the concentration of free hapten controlled the amount of antibody binding to the vesicles and thus the extent of quenching. However, the method was extremely sensitive to nonspecific binding by serum proteins and is therefore unlikely to have practical utility.

An interesting new application of fluorescence in homogeneous immunoassays is the use of fluorogenic enzyme substrates. These have been employed directly in an enzyme substrate inhibition assay in which the substrate is bound to an antigen.[32,33] Binding of antibody to the labeled antigen interferes with approach of enzyme and prevents turnover of the substrate. The theoretical sensitivity of the method is similar to the fluorescence excitation transfer and fluorescence protection immunoassays. It also shares the limitations of these methods in requiring that the antigen be partially purified. In its present state of development, serum background represents a serious limitation to the practical sensitivity of the method. The most attractive fluorogenic substrate so far described appears to be umbelliferyl β-galactoside, which is converted to the fluorescent umbelliferone by β-galactosidase. The relatively short wavelengths required to excite this dye also excite common endogeneous substances in serum, which fluoresce sufficiently strongly to reduce assay reliability despite the use of a rate measurement. Nevertheless, the method itself appears viable provided satisfactory substrates can be prepared.

An alternative use of fluorogenic enzyme substrates is in connection with homogeneous enzyme immunoassays. Recently, assays have been developed that are applicable to both haptens and macromolecular antigens.[34-36] These assays use bacterial β-galactosidase, which has the advantage of being active under conditions where the mammalian enzyme is inactive. A number of synthetic substrates have been devised for this enzyme, including fluorogenic substrates with longer wavelength absorption products than umbelliferone. However, the only substrate that has so far been studied is polymeric and gives rise to a nonfluorescent chromophore.

The potential amplification afforded by the use of an enzyme label coupled with fluorescence detection offers the possibility of exceptional sensitivity. These methods, which are still in an early stage of development, appear particularly promising. Provided practical fluorogenic substrates can be prepared, they will complement nicely direct fluorescence methods by providing the extra sensitivity required for the determination of low concentration antigens.

ADDENDUM

As the number of immunoassay methods proliferate, the nomenclature has become confused due to the use of arbitrary naming by several groups of investigators. In this review, I have employed a consistent nomenclature without regard to the assay names given by various authors. The naming was selected to conform as closely as possible to the most common usage and is outlined below.

Immunoassay methods can be divided into those that employ reporter groups (labels) and those that do not. Among the latter are *immunoelectrophoresis, immunoprecipitation,* and *immunodiffusion.* These methods all employ the prefix "immuno" and a suffix indicating the phenomenon being measured. Similar naming is also in common use where labels are employed, provided the objective of the procedure is to identify the location or distribution of an antigen (or antibody) on a slide or tissue section. Thus we speak of *immunofluorescence* or *immunoenzymatic* staining. Antigen localization using other labels should therefore be called by terms such as *immunoferritin* or *immunochemiluminescence* staining or *immunoradioautography.*

By contrast, methods that employ labels and are intended to establish the presence or quantity of an antigen (antibody) in a bulk sample are usually called *immunoassays*. Heterogeneous immunoassays, which require the separation of the free label from the bound label prior to measurement, can best be defined simply in terms of their label. Thus it is usually sufficient to introduce the name of the label before the word immunoassay as, for example, heterogeneous *enzyme* immunoassay,[37] *radio* (isotope) immunoassay,[2] *fluorescence* (label) immunoassay,[14] *chemiluminescence* (label) immunoassay,[38] etc. Where it is not obvious how the signal is measured, a descriptive word can be inserted after the label definition, e.g., metal *atomic absorption* immunoassay,[39] or surface *reflectance* immunoassay.[40]

Homogeneous immunoassays, which require no separation step, are most varied and may require both the name of the label and a word describing the effect of antibody-antigen binding on the signal. Thus a homogeneous enzyme immunoassay can be an enzyme *inactivation* immunoassay,[5] an enzyme *activation* immunoassay,[41] or an enzyme *channeling* immunoassay.[35] Other examples include fluorescence *polarization*,[8,9] fluorescence *protection*,[25-27] fluorescence *excitation transfer*,[18] spin *immobilization*,[3,4] fluorescence *total reflection*,[15] γ-ray emission *angular correlation*,[42] enzyme substrate *inactivation*,[32,33] liposome *lysis*,[28,29] vesicle *fusion inhibition*,[31] phage *inactivation*,[43] electrochemical *inactivation*,[44] etc.

Additional descriptive terms can of course be added to these basic names where required. Contractions such as enzymoimmunoassay or fluoroimmunoassay are to be avoided, since they are not sufficiently versatile to encompass the large range of possible labels. It is strongly urged that this frequently used but previously unformalized nomenclature be universally adopted to help facilitate communication in this rapidly growing field.

REFERENCES

1. A.H. Coons, H.J. Creech, and R.N. Jones, *Proc Soc Exp Biol Med* **47**:200, 1941.
2. S.A. Berson and R.S. Yalow, *J Clin Invest* **38**:1996, 1959.
3. R.K. Leute, E.F. Ullman, A. Goldstein, and L.A. Herzenberg, *Nature, New Biol* **236:**93, 1972.
4. R.K. Leute, E.F. Ullman, and A. Goldstein, *JAMA* **221**:1231 1972.
5. K.E. Rubenstein, R.S. Schneider, and E.F. Ullman, *Biochem Biophys Res Commun* **47**:846, 1972.
6. G.L. Rowley, K.E. Rubenstein, J. Huisjen, and E.F. Ullman, *J Biol Chem* **250**:3759, 1974.
7. R.S. Schneider, P. Lindquist, E. Tong-in Wong, K.E. Rubenstein, and E.F. Ullman, *Clin Chem* **19**:821, 1973.
8. W.B. Dandliker and G. Feigen, *Biochem Biophys Res Commun* **5**:299, 1961.
9. W.B. Dandliker, S.P. Halbert, M.C. Florin, R. Alonso, and H.C. Schapiro, *J Exp Med* **122**:1029, 1965.
10. R.A.A. Watson, J. Landon, E.J. Shaw, and D.S. Smith, *Clin Chim Acta* **73**:51, 1976.
11. A.R. McGregor, J.O. Crookall-Greening, J. Landon, and D.S. Smith, *Clin Chim Acta* **83**:161, 1978.
12. F. Sokol, A. Hulka, and P. Albrecht, *Folia Microbiol (Prague)* **7**:155, 1961.
13. I. Wieder, *In Immunofluorescence and Related Staining Techniques*, W. Knapp, H. Holubar, and G. Wick (eds.), Elsevier/North-Holland Biomedical Press, New York, 1978 p. 67.
14. A.J. Toussaint and R.I. Anderson, *Appl Microbiol* **13**:552, 1965.
15. M.N. Kronick and W.A. Little, *J Immunol Methods* **8**:235, 1975.
16. E.J. Shaw, R.A. Watson, J. Landon, and D.S. Smith, *J Clin Pathol* **30**:526, 1977.
17. D.S. Smith, *FEBS Lett* **77**:25, 1977.
18. E.F. Ullman, M. Schwarzberg, and K.E. Rubenstein, *J Biol Chem* **251**:4172, 1976.
19. T. Förster, *Z Naturforsch* **4a**:321, 1949.

20. R. Rodgers, M. Schwarzberg, P.L. Khanna, C.H. Chang, and E.F. Ullman, *Clin Chem* **24**:1033, 1978.

21. W.M. Eimstad, M. Schwarzberg, R. Rodgers, P.L. Khanna, C.H. Chang, and E.F. Ullman, *Clin Chem* **24**:1015, 1978.

22. G. Kohler and C. Milstein, *Nature* **256**:495, 1975.

23. E.F. Ullman, US Patent No. 3,998,943 (1976).

24. E.F. Ullman, *Clin Chem* **24**:973, 1978.

25. R.D. Nargessi, J. Landon, and D.S. Smith, *Clin Chim Acta* **89**:461, 1978.

26. R. Zuk, G.L. Rowley and E.F. Ullman, *Clin Chem* **25**:1554, 1979.

27. J.M. Brinkley, G.L. Rowley, P. Singh and E.F. Ullman, *Clin Chem* **25**:1077, 1979.

28. S.C. Kinsky, *In Methods in Enzymology*, Vol. 32, S. Fleischer and L. Packer (eds.), Academic, New York, 1974, p. 501.

29. H.R. Six, W.W. Young, Jr., K. Uemura, and S.C. Kinsky, *Biochemistry* **13**:4050, 1974.

30. M. Smolarsky, D. Teitelbaum, M. Sela, and C. Gittler, *J Immunol Methods* **15**:255, 1977.

31. P. VanDerWerf and E.F. Ullman, *Biochim Biophys Acta* **596**:302, 1980.

32. J.F. Burd, R.C. Wong, J.E Feeney, R.J. Carrico, and R.C. Boguslaski, *Clin Chem* **23**:1402, 1977.

33. R.C. Wong, J.F. Burd, R.J. Carrico, R.T. Buckler, J. Thoma, and R.C. Boguslaski, *Clin Chem* **25**:686, 1979.

34. I. Gibbons, C. Skold, G.L. Rowley, and E.F. Ullman, *Anal Biochem* **102**:167, 1980.

35. E.F. Ullman, *J Histochem Cytochem* **27**:717, 1979.

36. E.F. Ullman, *In Enzyme Immunoassay*, E. Maggio (ed.), CRC Press, West Palm Beach, Fla., 1980.

37. A.H.W.M. Schuurs and B.K. Van Weemen, *Clin Chim Acta* **81**:1, 1977.

38. L.S. Hersh, W.P. Vann, and S.A. Wilhelm, *Anal Biochem* **93**:267, 1979.

39. M. Cais, S. Dani, Y. Eden, O. Gandolfi, M. Horn, E.E. Isaacs, Y. Josephy, Y. Saar, E. Slovin, and L. Snarsky, *Nature* **270**:534, 1977.

40. A.L. Adams, M. Klings, G.C. Fischer, and L. Vroman, *J Immunol Methods* **3**:227, 1973.

41. E.F. Ullman, R.A. Yoshida, J.I. Blakemore, E. Maggio, and R. Leute, *Biochim Biophys Acta* **567**:66, 1979.

42. C.F. Meares, M.W. Sundberg, and J.D. Baldeschwieler, *Proc Natl Acad Aci (USA)* **69**:3718, 1972.

43. J. Haimovich, N. Novic, and M. Sela, *Israel J Med Sci* **5**:438, 1969.

44. W.R. Heineman, C.W. Anderson, and H.B. Halsall, *Science* **204**:865, 1979.

Chapter 6

The Development and Use of Immunoassays for Drugs

ALAN BROUGHTON, M.D.

INTRODUCTION

The increasing awareness of the general public to the dangers of the inappropriate use of many therapeutic agents, coupled with the scientific community's analysis that 6% of hospital admissions in 1977 were due to drug related illness, has led to a rapid increase in the development of assays to measure blood levels of drugs.

Although not the ideal measurement, the determination of blood levels affords some indication of drug efficacy and its probable therapeutic response. Assays for a few drugs have been available for some considerable time, but the recognition that a drug will behave as a hapten and produce an antibody response when injected into an animal, has allowed the development of sensitive, precise, and specific assays for many different drugs, both therapeutic and illicit. This chapter will outline the development of such assays and illustrate their use in health care.

Nichols Institute, 1300 S. Beacon Street, San Pedro, Calif. 90731.

ASSAY DEVELOPMENT: HAPTEN PROTEIN CONJUGATION

Most drugs are relatively small compounds with a molecular weight less than 1,000. Therefore, alone they are not good immunogens, but when conjugated to a macromolecule, they often produce high avidity, high titer antibodies. The choice of macromolecule often lies in personal preference, sometimes with availability and cost. I have used exclusively bovine serum albumin, because it is inexpensive, readily available, has high immunogenicity, resists denaturation, and is very soluble. The techniques of conjugation vary with the type of drugs being conjugated and the availability of functioning groups, either on the hapten or the protein carrier. These groups include free amine groups (the terminal amino group of lysine and the NH_2 terminal residues of the protein), free carboxyl groups (aspartic acid, glutamic acid, and the terminal carboxyl groups of the protein), imidazo groups (histidine), indolyl (tryptophan), sulfhydryl (cysteine), and guanidine (arginine) functions. When these groups are not available, the drug can often be derivitized to produce functional groups. Figure 1 illustrates some of these possibilities.

The methods used for conjugation must employ chemical conditions that do not cause significant structural alterations of the hapten and also do not denature the protein carrier so that it is rendered insoluble. A number of such methods have been described.[3,4,8,18,21] These methods have included the use of water soluble carbodiimides,[13] glutaraldehyde,[1] and a mixed anhydride.[11]

Landsteiner in 1945 showed,[17] and this was later confirmed by Erlanger,[12] that the incorporation of too many hapten molecules as well as too few in a hapten protein conjugate led to poor antibody response. Both these authors suggested that a ratio of 10:1 incorporation of hapten into the protein molecule seemed optimal when albumin was the choice of protein.

Therefore, it is recommended that the molar incorporation of the drug be determined prior to immunization. This can be done in several ways, for example, using the molar extinction coefficient[12] or by the incorporation of a radioactive tracer.[3]

IMMUNIZATION

There have been numerous regimens proposed for the immunization of animals. These regimens vary in animal choice, frequency, site of injection, and frequency of bleeds to evaluate the antisera. Usually, they are constant in the use of Freund adjuvant mixture or pertussis vaccine,[26] the latter being used when the amount of immunogen is

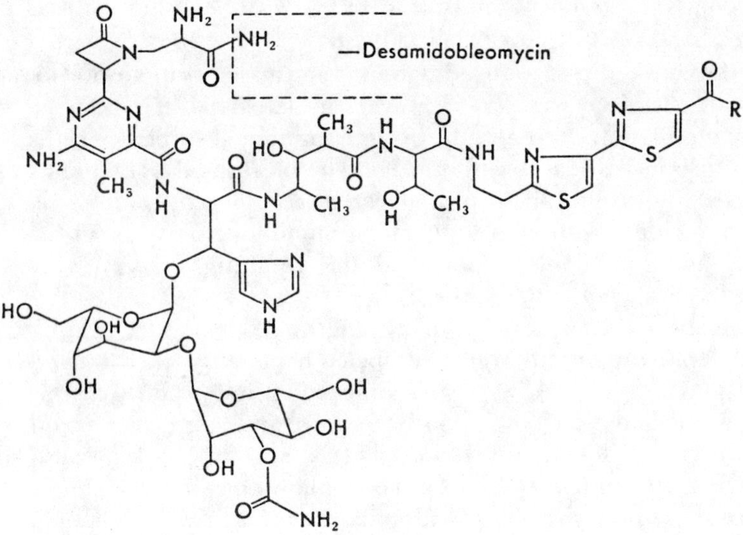

Fig. 1. The structural formulas of bleomycin and its analogs.

A_2: R = $NHCH_2CH_2CH_2S_+$ CH_3 / CH_3

B_2: R = $NHCH_2CH_2CH_2CH_2CH_2NHC$ NH / NH_2

B_1: R = NH_2

A_5: R = $NH\text{-}(CH_2)_3\text{-}NH\text{-}(CH_2)_4\text{-}NH_2$

Bleomycinic acid: R = OH

limited. The animal chosen most often is the rabbit or the guinea pig, although large animals such as the goat present an attractive alternative, particularly when large volumes of antisera are required. The practical problems associated with antibody production have been well reviewed by Hurn and Landon[14] and Hurn.[15]

EVALUATION OF ANTISERA

All antisera must be evaluated for specificity, avidity, and titer. Most animals immunized with a hapten protein conjugate will also produce antibodies against the carrier protein. Therefore, the method chosen for assessment of antisera must be one in which only the antibody specific for the hapten reacts. This is most conveniently done using a direct competitive reaction with the labeled hapten.

Usually, the antibodies produced against the carrier protein do not interfere with the assay system. However, if necessary, they can be removed by absorption onto an appropriate immunoabsorbent. If it is necessary to produce antisera without this type of antibody, the use of homologous albumin as a carrier protein can be considered. In this case, the hapten homologous albumin conjugate is immunogenic, whereas the homologous albumin alone is not, and the resulting antisera only contains antibodies against the hapten.

The specificity of the antisera is usually determined by demonstrating the displacement of an immunoreactive labeled hapten by closely related compounds and is expressed as a percentage. It is important that this percentage is calculated on a molar basis to insure an accurate reflection of the crossreactivity. The use of chemically related compounds has also afforded the opportunity to determine some interesting academic information regarding the immunodominance of certain functional groups. In my laboratory we were fortunate enough during the development of radioimmunoassays for bleomycin and its closely related drug tallysomycin to determine the effect of changes in functional groups on the crossreactivity of the various antisera.

The bleomycins (Fig. 1) differ from each other in their terminal amine moieties, and the results of our crossreactivity studies suggested that the presence and nature of this part of the molecule determined much of its immunoreactivity. Table 1 shows the percentage crossreactivity of

Table 1. Bleomycin Analog Immunoreactivity[a]

Drug	Mean concentration (pm)	Standard deviation (pm)	Percent crossreactivity (%)
Sulfate	3.45	±0.11	100
A_2	2.99	±0.22	115.4
B_2	4.63	±0.17	74.5
A_5	29.50	±5.14	11.7
Iso-A_2	13.70	±0.29	25.2
Acid	>100.00		<1.0
Bu2231B	>100.00		<1.0
Desamido A_2	8.26	0.51	44.6
B_1	214.2	15.9	1.6

[a]The indicated quantity of bleomycin analog was required to produce a 50% inhibition of iodine-125 labeled bleomycin sulfate bound to antibody. Results are expressed as the mean concentration, in picomoles, of the bleomycin analog determined in five separate analyses.

certain bleomycin analogs with the antisera developed against a bleomycin albumin conjugate. Bleomycins A2 and B2 compete more effectively than the other analogs, and although B2 has a somewhat different terminal moiety from A2, there is a structural resemblance between the two, as shown with molecular models. A5, which has a spermidine moiety as a terminal amine, competes only 11.7% as effectively against the antibody, and isobleomycin A2, which differs from A2 only in the translocation of the carbomoyl group in the amino sugar, competed with 25% the efficiency of bleomycin. Another compound, bleomycinic acid, which has no terminal amine moiety, failed to react with the antibody, and bleomycin B1, which has an amide group in lieu of a terminal amino acid, only reacted 1.6% as efficiently.

Desamidobleomycin, a metabolite of bleomycin produced by the inactivating enzyme described recently by Umezawa,[25a] has intact terminal amines, but the amine group on B aminalanamide has been removed. This compound crossreacted at 44% efficiency with the bleomycin antibody, whereas an antibody raised against desamido-bleomycin crossreacted 100% against bleomycin itself. Antisera raised against the tallysomycin gave further evidence to support the immunodominance of the terminal amines. These compounds, in addition to the existing disaccharide in bleomycin, contain a new amino sugar and a specific terminal amine moiety. The structure of these compounds is shown in Figure 2, and antibodies raised against them showed no crossreaction with bleomycin. For further information the reader is referred to Broughton.[5,6]

The relation of immunodominance to the site of conjugation is of more than theoretical interest. The drug methotrexate has biologically active sites in the pteroyl region of the molecule. Therefore, the amines in this region of the molecule should not be used for conjugation. Instead, the carboxyl moieties of the glutamic acid region should be used. A carbodiomide conjugation of methotrexate and methylated albumin produces such a conjugate, and antibodies specific for methotraxate can be produced in this manner.

PRODUCTION OF IMMUNOREACTIVE LABELED DRUGS

The development of any successful immunoassay requires the production of an immunoreactive label. These may be red cell indicators as in complement fixation tests or the classic radioactive labels for radioimmunoassay. The earlier immunoassays for drugs[13a,17a] used tritiated material. But the inherent technical difficulties involved with beta emitting isotopes make gamma emitters such as ^{125}I desirable for

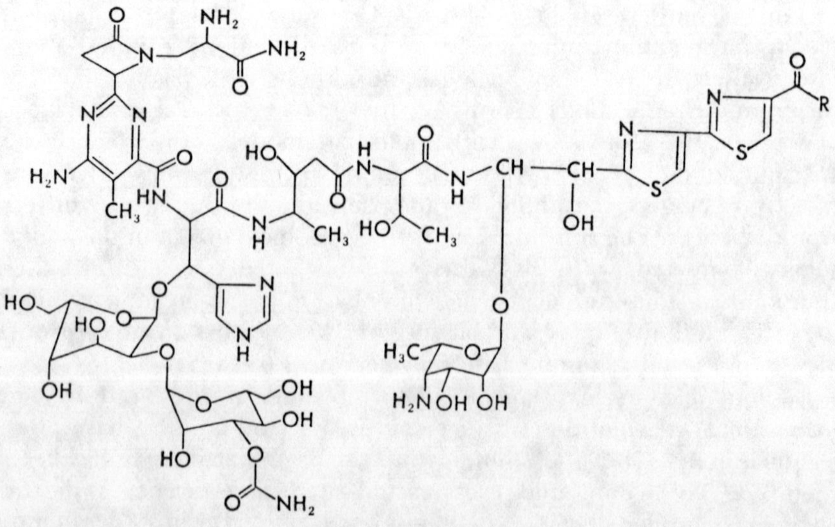

Fig. 2. The structural formulas of tallysomycin A and B.

Tallysomycin A: $R = -NH(CH_2)_3\text{-}\underset{NH_2}{CH}\text{-}CH_2\text{-}CO\text{-}NH\text{-}(CH_2)_3NH(CH_2)_4NH_2$

Tallysomycin B: $R = -NH(CH_2)_3NH(CH_2)_4NH_2$

any immunoassays. Most drugs lack suitable residues for iodination, and therefore the chemical manipulations similar to those used in the conjugation of the drugs to a carrier protein are used to form iodinatable derivates. This has been reviewed elsewhere.[2-4,5]

Once the derivative has been produced, it can be iodinated by any of the recognized techniques, for example, chloramine-T or lactoperoxidase. There are occasions when the drug can be directly iodinated by altering the conditions of iodination. An example of this is the iodination of bleomycin, the antineoplastic chemotherapeutic agent.[4]

The development of alternative tracers has been progressing rapidly. An enzyme-linked immunoassay for the antibiotic viomycin has been described using B galactosidase as the tracer,[16a] and the cardiac glycoside digoxin can be measured using a homogeneous enzyme immunoassay available through the Syva Corporation. More recently, the antimetabolite methotrexate and the anitbiotic gentamicin are also available on this system. The enzyme immunoassay of drugs is an attractive alternate to radioimmunoassay, allowing the small laboratory access to measurement of many compounds using existing spectrophotometric equipment. Additional advantages are the stability of reagents, no nuclear regulatory licenseship problems, and an ability to form stat tests when required.

Another approach to immunoassay makes use of fluorescence, either by polarization technique[27] or by the quenching of fluorescence.[7,25] In both of these techniques, the drug is conjugated to fluorescein isocyanate. This type of conjugate is stable, inexpensive, and easy to prepare. The former technique is based on the change of polarization when a small molecule such as fluorescein isocyanate/gentamicin binds to a large molecule such as its antibody. The competition between the unlabeled and labeled gentamicin for the antibody binding sites can be used to produce a dose response curve.

The latter technique depends upon the quenching of fluorescence when the fluorescein-labeled antigen reacts with its antibody. This competition between labeled and unlabeled antigen for the antibody reduces the amount of quenching, and again a dose response curve can be constructed. Principal advantages of these two techniques are that there is no separation phase required. A further modification of a fluoroimmunoassay has been recently reported by O'Donnell et al.,[20] where they use a heterologous system employing a solid phase second antibody. Recently Shaw et al.[24] have adapted the quenching fluoroimmunoassay of gentamicin to a continuous flow autoanalyzer system.

SEPARATION TECHNIQUES

The successful development of many immunoassays depends upon the use of an efficient agent to separate antibody bound material from free material. Many different techniques have been employed, and most workers in the field choose an agent suitable for their own needs. For most of our assays, we use dextran coated charcoal, although recent evidence suggests that with charcoal the incubation time is critical, and variations in this can result in imprecision.[22] The advantage of charcoal is wide applicability, in contrast to using rabbit antigammaglobulin, which introduces a second biological reagent with all its attendant problems. An alternative to charcoal is polyethyleneglycol (PEG), which has been used in a wide variety of assays,[10] and one which we are introducing into our laboratory.

The introduction by Catt[9] of solid phase antibodies for the assay of insulin introduced a new dimension into the separation of free from bound phases. He covalently linked antiinsulin onto polyethylene test tubes, thus obviating any need for specific separating agents. Since his report, many solid phases have been used (sephadex particles, glass beads, and cellulose). Most of these have been used in the determination of hormones, but a few have extended into the radioimmunoassay of drugs.

The advantage of some of the nonisotopic immunoassays is the lack of need for a separating agent. For example, polarizing and quenching fluorescence assays do not require separating agents, nor do the homogeneous enzyme immunoassays.

IMMUNOASSAY PROCEDURES

The reagents prepared and evaluated in the previous section have to be brought together into an assay system. The antibody is diluted in a suitable buffer to a titer that will displace 50% of the labeled material used in the assay. This titer varies for individual assays and antisera. The amount of labeled material used in the assay system is the minimum amount of material that will give an acceptable detection, depending upon whether it is an isotope, an enzyme, or a fluorescent-labeled compound. The sample size, of course, will depend again on the individual assay and varies according to the sensitivity and levels expected in the sample. It is customary to arrange dilutions of the samples to fall in the middle of the standard curve, which is prepared from appropriate dilutions of the drug under investigation.

The final volume is adjusted to one that is convenient to handle (approximately 0.5 ml). The order of addition of reagents is important. Zettner and Dooley[29] showed that the sensitivity of an assay can be increased by sequential addition of the label following preincubation of the unknown with the antisera; however, this technique is usually not necessary for hapten induced antisera. The usual order of addition is buffer, sample or standard, label material, and finally antisera.

The length of incubation and temperature are usually found by experiment. These assays are often equilibrium, not endpoint systems, and therefore incubation time can be critical. Following incubation, either a separation agent is added if required, or in the case of an enzyme immunoassay, the indicator system is added. If a second antibody is used as a separating agent, it has to be diluted to the appropriate dilution to precipitate all of the first antibody and its complexed antigen. This dilution will vary from batch to batch of antibody and may vary from analyte to analyte. Therefore, we prefer to use charcoal or PEG. The data generated either by radioimmunoassay and enzyme immunoassy or a fluorescence immunoassay can be handled several different ways; this has been reviewed recently by Shaw et al.[24] For convenience, we reduce our data by a log-logit transformation, both for the radioimmunoassays and the fluorescence immunoassays.

The last stage of development to any immunoassay system is to attempt to compare it with an existing assay, when one is available.

THE USE OF IMMUNOASSAYS

The development of these precise and sensitive systems has facilitated the investigation pharmacokinetics of many drugs and the monitoring of patients' blood levels to prevent the onset of toxicity. It is impossible in the space available to review all the drugs for which assays are now available, and I would like to illustrate the principles using two drugs as examples.

The chemotherapeutic agent bleomycin has been extensively studied in our laboratory. These investigations were first conducted on animals and then on patients receiving the drug as therapy for a variety of malignant disease.

Bleomycin Distribution

The animal chosen was the Wistar rat; the rats were divided into ten groups each containing five rats. The rats received an intraperitoneal injection of bleomycin (10 U/kg), and at a preselected time the animal was anesthetized with ether and heparinized blood was obtained using cardiac puncture. These samples were centrifuged and plasma separated. The red cells were washed with physiological saline and both the red cells and plasma were then frozen in dry ice and acetone and stored at −70°C until analyzed. The lungs, liver and a sample of skin were also frozen and immediately stored at −70°C.

The bleomycin was then extracted from the tissue using a dounce homogenizer attached to a drill press, its concentration was determined in the extract and expressed per gram of wet tissue. A group of control rats was also treated the same as the experimental rats, except saline injections were administered without bleomycin. Aqueous extracts from the control rats' tissues were used to detect interference with the bleomycin assay.

The results of these experiments showed that the plasma level reached a peak within one hour of injection and fell rapidly with an initial halflife of 15 min. The terminal elimination halflife was approximately seven hours and reflected the elimination of bleomycin from the tissues. The tissue levels were initially lower than the plasma levels, however. Four hours following the injection, tissue levels were greater than plasma levels, clearly demonstrating a multicompartmental distribution of the drug.

PHARMACOKINETICS IN HUMAN SUBJECTS

The patients included in these studies all gave informed consent and had a variety of neoplastic disorders. The patients received multiple day, intravenous infusions or short-term 10-min infusions during the course of the study. Blood specimens were collected in heparin containing tubes, centrifuged, and the serum was stored frozen (−70°C) until analyzed. Urine samples were obtained by 24-h urinary collections and the samples frozen for later analysis. The patients were arranged into three groups for data analysis.

Group I consisted of four patients receiving long-term (4–5 days) continuous infusion of 30 u of the drug for 24 h, for whom serum concentrations were available during onset, study state, and postinfusion. Group II consisted of seven patients receiving a 10-min infusion, for whom postinfusion specimens were available. Group III was composed of patients receiving long-term infusion (4–5 days), but for whom serum samples were only available postinfusion. For each group, serum samples were analyzed by a weighted nonlinear least squares regression computer program.[19]

Initial analysis of the results obtained in patients receiving the 10-min infusion showed multiple compartmental characteristics, as did analysis of those patients receiving bleomycin by continuous intravenous infusion. These patients had reached their steady state 12–24 h following initiation of infusion, and their decay curve showed an initial halflife of 2.98 h, which corresponded to the terminal halflife of those patients receiving 15 u by 10-min infusion. However, the terminal halflife of patients receiving the multiple-day continuous infusion was 14.8 h, and this was not observed in patients receiving the 10-min infusion. Further analysis of this data was made using the nonlin program,[19] and the summary of these findings is listed in Table 2. Two sets of data were generated for both groups I and III in this investigation. One set is all the data points included in the computer analysis, while the other set excluded data points less than 10 μU/ml. This was done in an attempt to explain the long terminal elimination phase seen in the multiple-day infusion, but not in the 10-min infusion. This phase is approximately 12 h after the termination of the long infusion, when concentrations of the drug were less than 10 μU/ml. The average estimated for the three groups depicted in Table 2 revealed that the pharmacokinetic parameters obtained for groups I and III agreed more closely with group II when bleomycin levels less than 10 μU/ml were excluded.

The results of this investigation raised questions concerning pharmacokinetics of bleomycin. According to pharmacokinetic models, the time necessary to reach 95% steady state concentration of the drug should be four elimination halflives. But the time necessary to reach 95%, steady state concentrations for many patients was around 12–24 h. This was less than the time predicted by the terminal elimination for patients receiving the continuous infusion when all data points were

Table 2. Averaged Estimates[a]

	k_{12} (h^{-1})	k_{21} (h^{-1})	k_{10} (h^{-1})	V_1 (liters/kg)	B (h^{-1})	$t_{1/2}$ (h)	$V_{d\beta}$ (liters/kg)
Group 1 (all data points used)	0.104	0.0979	0.519	0.251	0.0768	14.5	3.83
Group 1 (points less than 10 μU/ml excluded)	1.58	0.747	0.980	0.145	0.243	2.98	0.458
Group 2	1.31	1.18	0.981	0.142	0.371	2.03	0.354
Group 3 (all data points used)	0.0872	0.117	0.469	0.260	0.0832	9.53	1.74
Group 3 (points less than 10 μU/ml excluded)	0.369	0.431	0.676	0.200	0.236	3.90	0.608

[a]The following abbreviations were used: k_{12}, rate constant for drug transfer, central to peripheral compartment; k_{21}, rate constant for drug transfer, peripheral to central compartment; k_{10}, rate constant for elimination of drug from central compartment; V_1, volume of distribution for central compartment; B, slope of the terminal elimination phase; $t_{1/2}$, halflife of the terminal elimination phase; $V_{d\beta}$, volume of distribution for the drug.

included. However, when concentrations less than 10 μU/ml were excluded, the time to reach steady state was approximately four times the average elimination halflife. This suggests that metabolites are present to a greater degree in the plasma following multiple day infusions, and their concentration becomes significant at low levels of the parent compound. The metabolism of bleomycin has been studied, and an inactivating enzyme has been purified.[25a] Additionally, Umezawa's pharmacokinetic analysis of bleomycin distribution indicates a significant nonrenal pathway for drug elimination that could include metabolism.[5] It's unclear whether the radioimmunoassay recognizes inactive metabolites, since little is known about metabolism of bleomycin and few metabolites have been isolated. However, one of the metabolites of bleomycin, desomidobleomycin, does react in the radioimmunoassay, and it is possible that after a five-day continuous infusion, concentration of desomidobleomycin is significant. Thus the pharmacology of bleomycin using the immunoassay has to be interpreted with caution. This illustrates a problem that is not unique to radioimmunoassay when studying the metabolism of the pharmacology of drugs.

The group of antibiotics called the aminoglycosides are nephrotoxic and autotoxic.[16] The use of radioimmunoassay has allowed the measurement of blood levels of the aminoglycosides much lower than originally anticipated. The published halflife for all the aminoglycosides is 120 min, with a one-compartmental type of distribution. However, when one follows patients who have received therapy with tobramycin by collecting samples for many hours after the infusion, one can still detect tobramycin at levels of 0.1 μg/ml after 18 h and show that the excretion halflife of the drug can be anything from 18–36 h. This model suggests that the drug has more than the accepted compartments and is bound to some deeper tissues for a varying length of time. This phenomenon could explain some of the hitherto complex problems regarding the incidence of nephrotoxicity and autotoxicity.

CONCLUSIONS

The development of the use of immunoassays for drugs presents an exciting opportunity for the clinical pathologist and the clinical pharmacologist to get together and investigate drugs using analytical methods previously unavailable. The results of these investigations should prove fruitful in designing therapeutic regimes to meet individual patients' needs and decrease the steadily increasing number of patients admitted to hospitals for drug related illnesses.

REFERENCES

1. S. Avrameas and T. Ternynek, *Immunochemistry,* **6**:53, 1969.

2. A. Broughton and J.E. Strong, *Clin Chem* **22**:726, 1976.

3. A. Broughton and J.E. Strong, *Clin Chem Acta* **66**:125, 1976.

4. A. Broughton and J.E. Strong, *Cancer Res* **36**:1418, 1976.

5. A. Broughton *In Bleomycin Current Status and New Developments,* S.K. Carter, S.T. Crooke, and H. Umezawa (eds.), Academic, New York, 1978, p. 107.

6. A. Broughton, *In Clinical Immunochemistry,* eds. S. Natelson, A.J. Pesce, and A.A. Dietz (eds.), AACC, Washington D.C., 1978, p. 445.

7. A. Broughton and M. Frazier, *Clin Chem* **24**:1033, 1978.

8. V.P. Butler Jr. and S.M. Beiser, *Advan Immunol* **17**:255, 1972.

9. K.J. Catt, *Acta Endocrinol* **142**(Suppl):222, 1970.

10. B. Desbuquois and G.D. Aurback, *J Clin Endrocrinol Metab* **33**:732, 1971.

11. B.F. Erlanger, F. Borek, S.M. Beiser, and S. Lieberman, *J Biol Chem* **228**:713, 1957.

12. B.F. Erlanger, *Pharmacol Rev* **25**:271, 1973.

13. T.L. Goodfriend, L. Levine, and G.D. Fasman *Science* **144**:1344, 1964.

13a. T.W. Smith, V.P. Butler Jr., and E. Haber, *New England J Med* **281**:1212, 1969.

14. B.A.L. Hurn and J. Landon, *In Radioimmunoassay Methods,* K.E. Kirkham and W.M. Hunter (eds.), Churchill, Livingston, Edinburgh, 1971, p. 21.

15. B.A.L. Hurn, *Br Med Bull* **30**:26, 1974.

16. G.G. Jackson and G. Arcieri, *J Infect Dis* **124**(Suppl):130, 1971.

16a. T. Vitagawa, T. Fujitake, and H. Taniyamia, *J Antibiot* **29**:1343, 1976.

17. K. Landsteiner, *The Specificity of Serological Reactions,* Harvard University Press, Cambridge, Mass., 1945.

17a. J.E. Lewis, J.C. Nelson, and H.A. Elder, *Nature* **204**:214, 1972.

18. V. Marks, B.A. Morris, and J.D. Teale, *Br Med Bull* **30**:80, 1974.

19. C.M. Metzler, NONLIN a Computer Program for Parameter Estimation in Non Linear Situations, The Upjohn Company, Kalamazoo, Mich., 1969.

20. M. O'Donnell, S. Suffin, J. McBride, and A. Broughton, *Clin Chem* **25**:1077, 1979.

21. C.W. Parker, *Progr Clin Pathol* **4**:103, 1972.

22. C.W. Parker, *In Radioimmunoassay of Biologically Active Compounds,* C.W. Parker (ed.), Prentice-Hall Foundations of Immunology Series. Prentice-Hall, Englewood Cliffs, N.J., 1976, p. 156.

23. E.J. Shaw, R.A.A. Watson, and J. Landon, *J Clin Pathol* **13**:526, 1977.

24. W. Shaw, J. Smith, F.W. Spierto, and S.T. Agnese, *Clin Chem Acta* **76**:15, 1977.

25. E.J. Smith, R.A.A. Watson, and D.S. Smith, *Clin Chem* **25**:322, 1979.

25a. H. Umezawa, S. Hori, T. Sawa, T. Yoshiovat, and T. Takenchi, *J. Antibiot* **27**:419–424, 1974.

26. J. Vaitukaitis, J.B. Robbins, E. Nieschlag, and G.T. Ross, *J Clin Endocrinol Metab* **33**:988, 1971.

27. R.A.A. Watson, J. Landon, and E.J. Shaw, *Clin Chem Acta* **73**:51, 1976.

28. J.H. Wilfert, J.P. Burke, and H.A. Bloomer, *J Infect Dis* **124**(Suppl):S130, 1971.

29. A. Zettner and R.E. Duly, *Clin Chem* **20**:5, 1974.

Chapter 7

Recent Advances in Homogeneous Enzyme Immunoassay

RICHARD S. SCHNEIDER, Ph.D.

INTRODUCTION

The development of homogeneous enzyme immunoassay techniques for the quantitative detection of drugs and hormones in biological fluids provides clinical chemists and physicians with powerful new tools in the management of disease. Assays have been developed to detect drugs of abuse, antiepileptic agents, cardioactive drugs, antiasthmatic drugs, antimicrobial drugs, and to measure thyroid function.

Using the principles of competitive protein binding, the EMIT® enzyme immunoassay system provides an immunochemical technique free of the problems of shelf life, stability, health hazards, and a separation step common to radioimmunoassays. An enzyme is used as a ligand label in place of a radioisotope. Such labeled enzyme conjugates are able to bind drug specific antibodies with a concomitant change of enzymatic activity caused by antibody binding. This change in activity is reversed by the presence of the free drug or hormone.

A primary feature of a homogeneous assay system is that assays can be performed without a separation step to bring about a partition of bound and free drug. Assays can be performed on spectrophotometric equipment. The method combines the features of sensitivity, specificity, and quantification with rapid measurement and ease of sample manipulations.

Syva Company, 3181 Porter Drive, Palo Alto, Calif. 94304

During the preceding five years, there has been a veritable explosion of new analytical techniques that have found application in the field of clinical diagnostics. This growth has been fueled in part by the need for additional biomedical information on the part of physicians and by the rapid accumulation of knowledge in the fields of biochemistry and pharmacology. Scientific knowledge about antibodies, their preparation, specificity, and other characteristics have contributed to the general field of analytical biochemistry. These developments, coupled with progress in radioimmunoassay (RIA), particularly since 1969, share responsibility for the development of other more advanced immunochemical concepts that have led to wide-scale improvements in RIA and, in some cases, to completely new analytical systems.[1-13]

This chapter has been designed as a review of recent developments in the field of homogeneous enzyme immunoassay for drugs. Some emphasis will also be placed on the pharmacology of certain drugs as they may serve as examples to establish a rationale for measuring the concentration of the drug in serum. This bioanalytical technique does not use radioisotopes as biochemical markers and, therefore, is free from problems associated with reagent stability, licensing, disposal, and separation techniques. The method utilizes an enzyme as a label in place of the radiochemical marker used in RIA. Since the assay system employs only one phase and no separation step is needed, the term homogeneous enzyme immunoassay has been used to differentiate this technique from others that also use enzymes as labels but require separation procedures.[13] The EMIT® system is a commercial application of homogeneous enzyme immunoassay developed by Syva Company, Palo Alto, Calif.[1]

There are many different immunochemical techniques described in the literature for both qualitative and quantitative determinations of antigens (Table 1). Some techniques employ no labeled reactants at all; however, these techniques are generally qualitative in nature. An example of a technique utilizing no chemically labeled reactant is the hemagglutination assay used, for example, to determine pregnancy.

Table 1. A Classification of Available Immunoassay Techniques for Antigens

1. Employing no labeled reactant
2. Employing labeled antigen
   a. With separation
   b. Without separation
3. Employing labeled antibody
   a. Sandwich technique
   b. Labeled second antibody
   c. Direct label

time takes advantage of the catalytic nature of the enzyme system. Thus increased sensitivity can often be obtained simply by allowing the reaction mixture to incubate for a longer period of time. Use of absorption spectrometers, rather than gamma or scintillation counters, and gas liquid or high pressure liquid chromatographs greatly simplifies the sample and the data handling required to perform an assay. Spectrophotometric equipment, both manual and automated, has already found a secure home in clinical laboratories. Now it is possible to perform many heretofore esoteric and difficult assays on one type of equipment with simplicity and ease.

The technical manipulations used for all EMIT enzyme immunoassays for haptens are similar. Fifty microliters (50 μl) of sample (urine, serum, or plasma) are mixed with the antibody reagent containing antibodies to the particular drug and the substrate(s) for the enzyme. Binding occurs to the drug(s) in the sample that is (are) recognized by the antibody. Next a drug labeled with the enzyme is added. The labeled drug combines with any remaining unfilled antibody binding sites, and the enzyme activity is measured.

DRUGS OF ABUSE

The first commercial application of the EMIT assay principle was in the development of assays for the detection of drugs of abuse in urine.[16] Assays have been developed to detect the compounds listed in Table 3. These assays, with the exception of the assays for phencyclidine and THC, utilize the enzyme lysozyme. The lysozyme based assays have been limited to tests for drugs and/or their metabolites in urine, since the presence of endogenous lysozyme in serum and saliva makes background interference from these fluids unacceptable. A recent report[17] of the application of these assays to fluids other than urine describes an extraction step prior to the analysis to eliminate endogenous enzyme interference. The assay for phencyclidine (PCP) employs glucose-6-phosphate dehydrogenase (G6PDH), while the THC assay uses malate dehydrogenase (MDH). Recent experiences with phencyclidine abuse warrant a somewhat more detailed description of this new test. A discussion of the THC metabolite assay[20,21] will be reported elsewhere.

Phencyclidine (PCP) was originally synthesized and tested as a potential analgesic-anesthetic.[42,43] The drug was found to produce serious and prolonged postanesthetic confusion and delirium and in 1967 was abandoned for use in humans. As one of the most commonly encountered drugs of abuse, PCP was initially favored for its

Table 3. EMIT Assays for Drugs and Hormones

Drug abuse urine assays
Opiates
Barbiturates
Amphetamines
Methadone
Cocaine metabolite
Benzodiazepines
Propoxyphene
Phencyclidine (PCP)[18,19]
Cannabinoids (THC)[20,21]
Antiepileptic drug assay
Phenytoin
Phenobarbital
Carbamazepine
Primidone
Ethosuximide
Valproic acid[23]
Antiasthmatic drugs
Theophylline[22]
Cardioactive drugs
Digoxin[24,25]
Lidocaine[26,27]
Procainamide[28]
N-acetylprocainamide[29]
Quinidine[30]
Propranolol[31]
Disopyramide
Chemotherapeutic agents
Methotrexate[33]
Antimicrobial drugs
Gentamicin[34]
Tobramycin[32]
Amikacin; under development
Endogenous hormone assays
Thyroxine (T-4)[35-37]
T-3 uptake[38,39]
Cortisol[40]
Estriol; under development
Toxicology assays
Benzodiazepines[41] (serum)
Barbiturates[41] (serum)

Technique employing labeled antigens can be divided into two general classifications, those with and those without a separation step. Examples of separation-type assays utilizing a labeled antigen are radioimmunoassays. Recent advances in fluorometric immunoassays also employing a separation step have been reported.[14,15] Separation-type assays using an enzyme label have generally come to be known as enzyme-linked immunoabsorbent assays (ELISA) for antigens. This elegant work, performed largely by groups in Japan, the United Kingdom, and Scandinavia, has done much to broaden the concepts on non-radiolabeled immunoassay techniques.

The third type of immunoassy technique employs a labeled antibody. The antibody can be labeled directly with a radioligand or an enzyme, or a labeled second antibody can be used. Another variation is the so-called "sandwich" technique.

All immunochemical techniques require the preparation of specific antibodies. The key to immunoassays is the fact that antibodies will bind tightly only to a specific compound or very closely related compounds. Antibodies can be prepared for nearly any medically interesting compound.

The total immunoassay system is composed of three parts: (1) a specific antibody, (2) a labeled compound, and (3) a sample or compound to be analyzed. The specific antibody and labeled compound are added to a solution containing the compound to be assayed. Since an insufficient number of antibody binding sites are provided, the labeled and unlabeled compounds compete for the limited number of available sites. The more unlabeled compound present in the unknown solution, the less labeled compound will be bound to the antibody. In radioimmunoassay, the bound and free radiochemically labeled compounds are both present in the solution. In order to determine the concentration of the drug in the patient sample, separation of the bound and free labeled antigen must take place. This can be accomplished by adsorbing the free antigen using dextran-coated charcoal, or by employing antibodies immobilized on a solid support. Regardless of the degree of sophistication employed to perform this step, the separation procedure remains one of the major potential sources for error associated with the test. It is largely these considerations that have led researchers to design immunochemical systems free both from separation steps and radiochemical labels.

Homogeneous enzyme immunoassay[1] permits determination of amounts of free and bound labeled compounds without the necessity of a physical separation step. Elimination of this step greatly simplifies the assay procedure and offers a way to improve overall precision and accuracy. This technique is called "homogeneous" immunoassay because only one phase is employed.

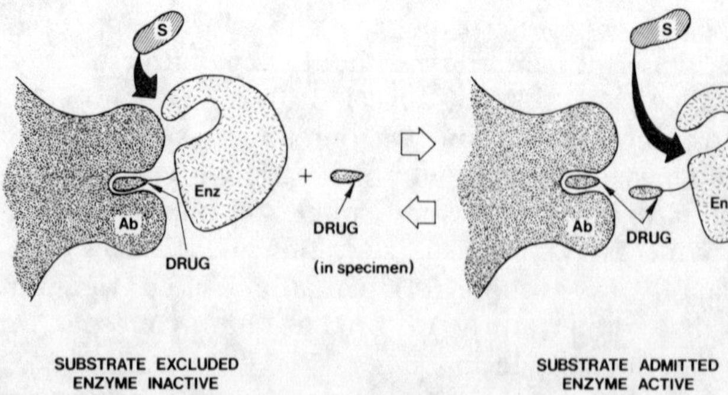

Fig. 1. Schematic representation of homogeneous enzyme immunoassay.

EMIT assays are homogeneous immunoassays that can be used for the microanalysis of specific compounds in biological fluids. In this technique, the drug is labeled by an enzyme instead of by a radiochemical marker. When the enzyme-labeled drug becomes bound to an antibody against the drug, the activity of the enzyme is modified. Free drug in a sample competes with the enzyme-labeled drug for the antibody and thereby decreases the antibody induced modulation of enzyme activity (Fig. 1). Enzyme activity correlates with the concentration of drug introduced in the sample and is measured spectrophotometrically. Two enzymes that have found broad utility for EMIT assays are lysozyme and glucose-6-phosphate dehydrogenase (Table 2).

Sensitivity is related to the specific activity of the enzyme used. It is also related to the measurement period, since increased measurement

Table 2. EMIT Assays: General Information

General data	Lysozyme	Glucose-6-phosphate dehydrogenase (G6PDH)
Substrate	*M. lysodeikticus*	glucose-6-phosphate
Cofactor	None	NAD
Sample volume	50 λ	8.3 λ
Preparation required	None	None
pH	6.0 ± 0.2	8.1 ± 0.1
Temperature (±0.1°C)	37°C	30°C
Wavelength	436 nm	340 nm
Timing		
Delay time	10 s	15 s[a]
Measure time	40 s	30 s[a]

[a]Due to increased sensitivity requirements, the digoxin assay is not performed with this protocol.

sample-to-sample variation between 50 samples is small compared to the difference observed due to the presence of drug. The assay is specific for phencyclidine and is not affected by other drugs of abuse.

Detailed discussion for each of the EMIT assays for drugs is beyond the scope of this presentation. A summary of the available assays is given in Table 3. Details can be obtained from the cited references. Assays for a few compounds have been selected as recent examples of new applications for homogeneous enzyme immunoassay.

ANTICONVULSANT ASSAYS

The initial application of the EMIT system to the detection and quantitation of drugs in serum was in the development of assays for antiepileptic drugs.[62] The compounds listed in Table 3 represent the most common alternatives to physicians for treatment of patients with epilepsy. During the past decade the value of routine monitoring of serum antiepileptic drug levels as an adjunct to better patient care has been repeatedly demonstrated. Clinical studies have shown a strong correlation between serum antiepileptic drug concentrations and seizure control. All these assays are performed in an identical manner, utilizing the same sample/reagent handling, the same enzyme and other assay variables. The enzyme utilized is glucose-6-phosphate dehydrogenase (G6PDH) isolated from the bacterium *Leuconostoc mesonteroides.* Interference from human G6PDH activity is minimized by use of NAD, the preferred coenzyme for the bacterial enzyme.

The sample volume used per test is less than 10 μl. Therefore, from 50 μl of a sample, it is possible to perform up to five assays, making this technique ideal for pediatric applications. Accurate temperature control to $\pm 0.1°C$ is essential for good reproducibility and hence, good performance. Equally important to performance is a precise pipetter/diluter. Reagent stability of the lyophilized agent is at least one year when stored at 2–8°C. These reagents, reconstituted with distilled water, are stable for a period of 3–4 months if kept refrigerated when not in use.

Figure 4 shows a standard curve obtained in the assay for phenytoin. Special graph paper that provides a straight line calibration curve is prepared for each assay and is included in each reagent kit. The logarithmic concentration of the drug (in μg/ml) is plotted on the horizontal axis; the vertical axis is a refined logit function of the enzyme rate. The typically sigmoidal immunoassay standard curve is transformed into a straight line, thus allowing improved, more precise data interpretation.

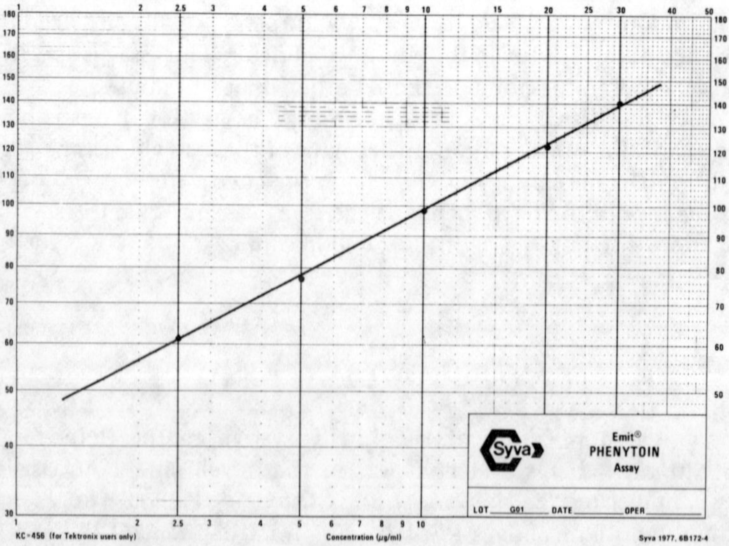

Fig. 4. Typical phenytoin standard curve.

Serum-based calibrators and controls are provided for each assay to define the subtherapeutic, therapeutic, and toxic ranges for the drug. The specificity provided by each antibody permits the combination of all five drugs in the calibrators and control. The calibrator/reagent system is sufficiently stable to permit samples to be analyzed without the need of frequent calibration. A standard curve can be used for at least a working day and often for longer if adequate controls are employed. Performance data for the EMIT antiepileptic drug assays have been reported elsewhere.[63,64]

CARDIOACTIVE DRUGS

EMIT assays have been developed for many cardioactive drugs.[65,69] This group of compounds (see Table 3) is important in the treatment of cardiac disease. Assays for all of these compounds are now available.

THEOPHYLLINE ASSAY

Recent developments in the clinical pharmacology of theophylline have resulted in a renewed emphasis and improved use of this drug in the treatment of asthma.[70,72] Today, theophylline is considered the most useful and primary drug of choice in the treatment and prevention of psychomimetic effects. Potent and unwanted side effects, however, caused a rapid decline in its popularity as a recreational drug.[44,45] Phencyclidine has subsequently reappeared in preparations misrepresented as containing LSD, mescaline, cocaine, or tetrahydrocannabinol (THC). Most recently, PCP has regained its position as an intended drug of abuse.[46] Controlled under the Drug Abuse Prevention and Control Act of 1970,[47] phencyclidine continues to gain popularity on the illicit drug market. It has been identified in street samples sold under as many as 46 different names appearing as powders, tablets, leaf mixtures, and "rock" crystals with variations in purity ranging from 10 to 100%. PCP can be taken orally, by inhalation (smoking), insufflation (snorting), and, rarely, by an intravenous method.[44,48]

PCP is an arylcyclohexylamine compound closely related to an anesthetic agent, ketamine (Fig. 2). The drug acts on the central nervous system either as a stimulant or a depressant and its effects are considered to be dose-dependent.[49,50] Although the presenting picture most often resembles a mixture of paranoid schizophrenia and catatonic excitement,[51] cases involving ingestion of high doses, which present as undiagnosed coma, may be difficult to differentiate from other causes.[47] It has been reported that the concentration of PCP in urine bears little or no quantitative relationship to the degree of impairment.[52] Fatal cases have been reported in which the urinary concentration ranged from 0.6 to 330 μg/ml, while samples from living chronic users and nonfatal overdoses have produced concentrations from 0.3 to 92 μg/ml.[53] One investigator reported that urine samples from 41 known PCP users were in the range of 0.5 μg/ml to 23 μg/ml, with the majority falling in the range of 2–5 μg/ml PCP.[52]

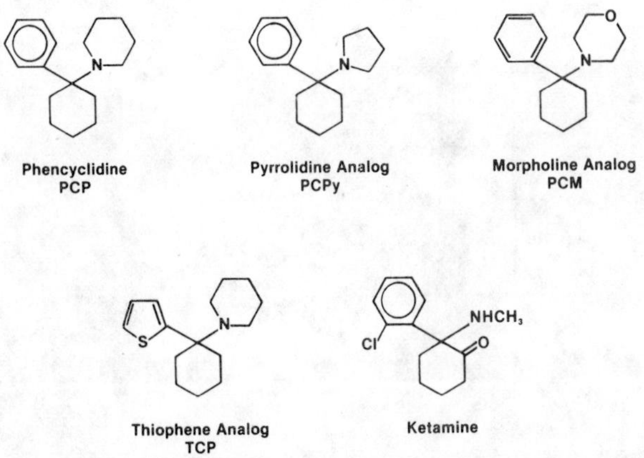

Fig. 2. Structures of phencyclidine and related compounds.

Two conjugated hydroxylated metabolites of PCP, 1-(1-phenyl-cyclohexyl)-4-hydroxypiperidine and 4-phenyl-4-piperidinecyclohexanol, have been identified; however, the biotransformation of phencyclidine in humans is not yet clear.[55,57] The exact clinical picture after ingestion of PCP is variable and depends on dose, time since ingestion, presence or absence of concurrent psychiatric or organic disease and hypoxia.[54] In many cases, administration of sympathomimetic drugs is cautioned due to the stimulant as well as depressant effects of phencyclidine. Specific diagnosis and therapy, therefore, depend upon identification of the drug before initiation of treatment.

Both quantitative and qualitative analytical techniques for measuring PCP in urine are available, including gas chromatography (GC), either alone or followed by mass spectrophotometry (GC/MS), thin layer chromatography (TLC), ultraviolet (UV) spectrophotometry and radioimmunoassay (RIA).[58,61] Limited by either costly equipment, special handling requirements, or lengthy turnaround times, the utility of these methods as rapid screening procedures can be problematic.

The EMIT® Phencyclidine Assay is designed as a primary screening system to detect positive samples in a largely negative population. Negative immunoassay results can be interpreted as evidence that the drug in question is not present in excess of the detection limit of the assay. The EMIT homogeneous enzyme immunoassay for phencyclidine makes it possible to obtain a semiquantitative result within minutes of receipt of the sample.

The facile differentiation between drug-free samples and those containing 150 ng/ml phencyclidine is shown in Figure 3. The

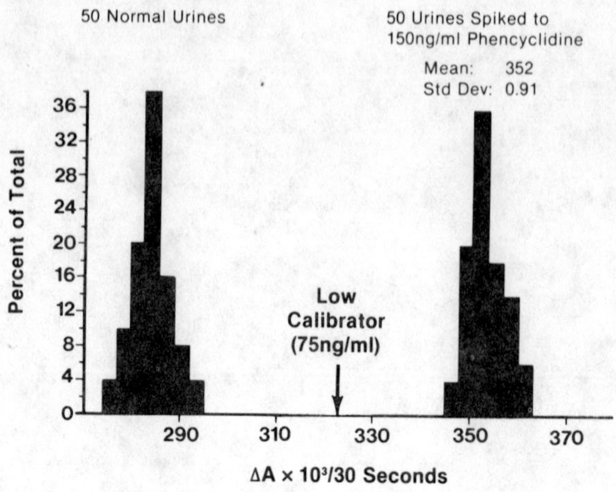

Fig. 3. EMIT® phencyclidine assay performance summary.

Table 4. Summary of Clinical Investigations Using the EMIT® Theophylline Assay

A. Accuracy: analysis of ten serum samples containing known concentrations of theophylline

Method	Correlation coefficient	Slope	Intercept (μg/ml)	Mean EMIT (μg/ml)	Spike (μg/ml)	Standard error of the estimate (μg/ml)
EMIT	0.999	0.95	0.45	13.4	13.6	0.36
HPLC	0.999	1.00	0.65	14.2	13.6	0.51
UV	0.992	0.56	0.51	8.1	13.6	0.74

B. Comparative analysis: an analysis of clinical samples with the EMIT® theophylline assay and an alternate methodology

Correlation statistics: comparative analysis of theophylline patient samples

	Lab 1	Lab 2	Lab 3	Lab 4	Lab 5	Lab 6	Lab 7
Number of samples	101	90	112	100	102	85	96
Correlation coefficient	0.98	0.97	0.95	0.95	0.87	0.86	0.97
Mean (μg/ml)							
EMIT	12.16	14.69	13.22	8.01	9.25	15.23	13.30
HPLC or UV	11.45	15.80	12.67	7.75	8.45	16.02	11.37

which was not obtainable with lower doses. High-dose therapy has been used successfully in the management of acute leukemia, non-Hodgkin's lymphoma, osteogenic sarcoma, and primary cancer of the lung. Its effectiveness in the treatment of other types of malignancies is under clinical investigation. The structures of methotrexate and some related analogues are shown in Figure 7.

Methotrexate (MTX), by interfering with the biochemical process of DNA synthesis, arrests cells as they undergo division. Inside the cell, MTX binds irreversibly to dihydrofolate reductase, the enzyme responsible for converting folic acid to the reduced folate cofactors essential to DNA synthesis. When the MTX-saturated cell enters the S-phase (DNA synthesis) of its life cycle, it lacks the reduced folates necessary for replication and thus dies. MTX, however, is toxic not only to neoplastic cells, but also to normal cells, such as those comprising the skin and bone marrow. Because these tissues continually renew themselves, DNA synthesis occurs frequently and is fatal to those cells saturated with MTX. To prevent MTX-induced toxicity to normal cells, leucovorin "rescue" is administered as an adjunct to high-dose MTX therapy.

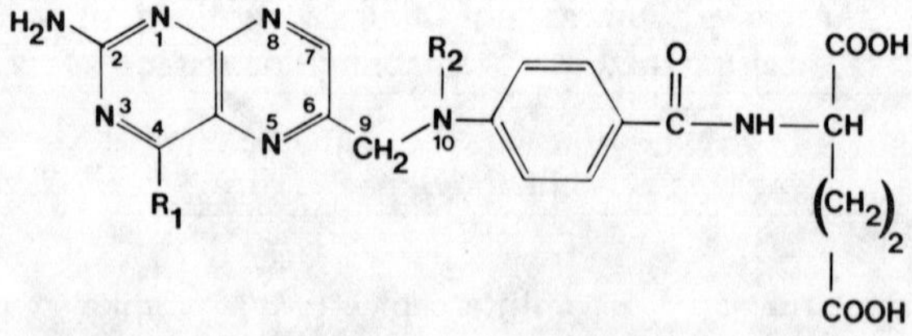

Substance	R_1	R_2
Methotrexate (Amethopterin)	$-NH_2$	$-CH_3$
Aminopterin	$-NH_2$	$-H$
Methopterin	$-OH$	$-CH_3$
Folic Acid (Pteroylglutamic Acid)	$-OH$	$-H$

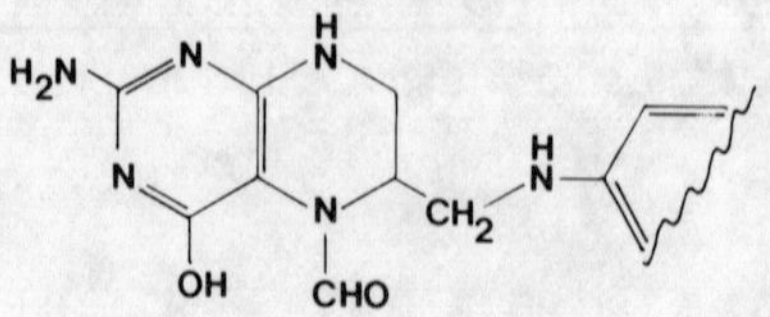

Folinic Acid-SF, (5-Formyl-5,6,7,8-tetrahydrofolic Acid) Citrovorum Factor, Leucovorin

Fig. 7. Structures, methotrexate and analogs.

Massive doses of MTX have produced successful responses in neoplastic diseases previously found to be resistant to lower doses.[75] The rationale of the high-dose approach is to drive a sufficient number of MTX molecules into the neoplastic cell to irreversibly bind all of the cell's dihydrofolate reductase.[75] Maximal suppression of DNA synthesis is achieved when the intracellular MTX level exceeds that required to bind all of the cell's dihydrofolate reductase.[76]

Two basic types of high-dose regimens are in use. The first consists of a 4–6 h bolus infusion of >20 mg/kg of MTX; the goal of this approach is to maximize the intracellular MTX concentration.[77] Blood levels reach 10^{-2}–10^{-4} mol/liter during such regimens, with an exponential decline thereafter. The second type of protocol calls for a 20–42 h high-dose infusion, in which blood levels remain in the range 10^{-4}–10^{-6} during infusion and then decline exponentially. The rationale of the latter regimen is to encompass more of the cell cycle of neoplastic cells.[77] An interval of 2–6 weeks is generally allowed between administrations of high-dose MTX under either type of protocol to permit the recovery of normal cells.

Both methods of high-dose MTX administration place normal cells in jeopardy and, therefore, require the use of leucovorin (folinic acid, citrovorum factor) "rescue" to replenish the reduced folates depleted by MTX. Leucovorin may be administered i.v., i.m., or orally, and is

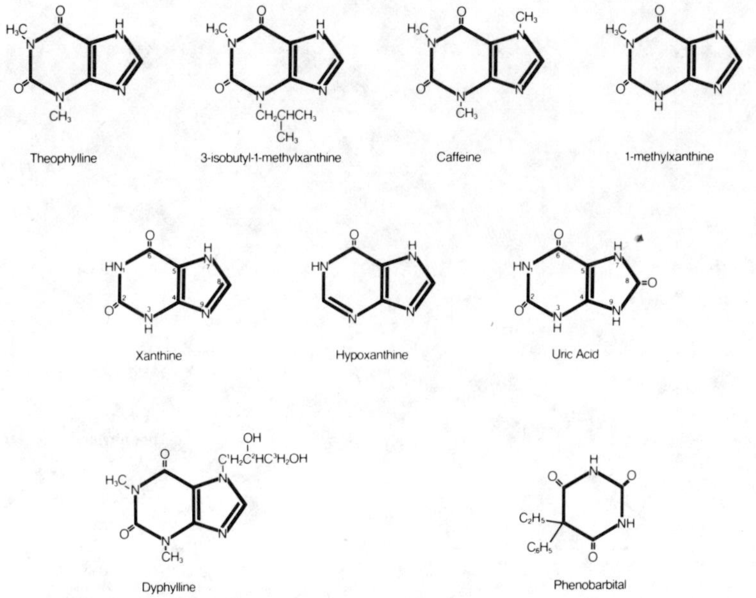

Fig. 5. Theophylline and related structures.

asthmatic symptoms in children and adults. The relationship between theophylline dosage and the likelihood of achieving both therapeutic effect and toxicity has been reported. However, because there are remarkable variations in the rate of individual metabolism of theophylline in both children and adults, large percentages of patients in any population receiving the useful dosage will either not achieve a therapeutic effect or be at risk of toxicity. This is particularly true in the case of young infants, as they are very susceptible to seizure, while other adverse side effects are usually difficult to recognize. Current data suggest that safe, effective use of theophylline in adults and children requires careful dosage adjustment based on theophylline serum measurements. Theophylline dosages that achieve the serum concentration range of 10–20 μg/ml are usually effective in suppressing chronic asthmatic symptoms. The development of a homogeneous enzyme immunoassay for theophylline should be important in the treatment of this disease.

Figure 5 is a diagram indicating the variety of structurally related substances that are important in an assay for theophylline. Variations in the alkyl substituents on the nitrogen atoms provide a dazzling array of substituted xanthines and hypoxanthines for consideration. In order for an assay to be widely useful, the antisera must differentiate theophylline from caffeine, theobromine, and other common xanthine derivatives.

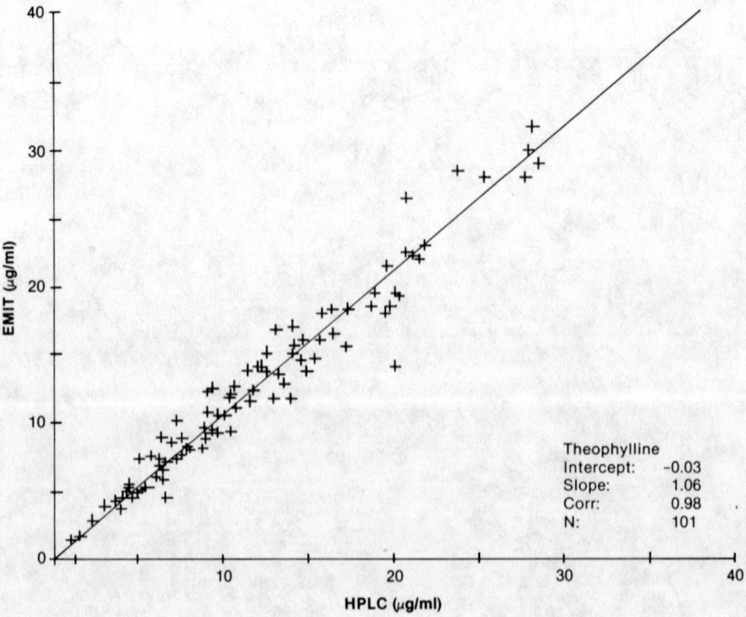

Fig. 6. Comparative analysis of patient samples for theophylline.

While laboratory data obtained by artificially challenging the assay with an array of theophylline metabolites and related compounds indicated no substantial interference,[73] it remained for a thorough study[22] of actual patient samples to validate the clinical specificity of the test. The data in Figure 6 and Table 4 are from field studies of patient samples. Data from both the EMIT assay and reference methods (HPLC, UV) were analyzed. No significant difference between the results has been observed, thereby giving credence to the postulate that metabolites or drugs with similar structure do not interfere with the EMIT theophylline assay.

METHOTREXATE ASSAY

Methotrexate (amethopterin), a folic acid antagonist, has been in clinical use for over 20 years.[33,74] Prior to 1967, it was used in comparatively small doses in the treatment of acute leukemia and diseases such as severe psoriasis, sarcoidosis, and Wegener's granulomatosis. Considerable clinical experience with high-dose methotrexate regimens in treating a variety of neoplastic diseases has been gained during the past decade, supporting the hypothesis that saturation of certain neoplastic cells with the drug could elicit an effect

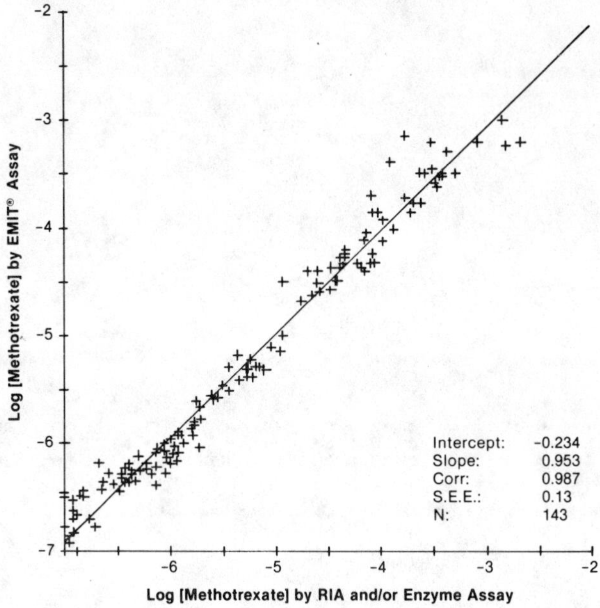

Fig. 8. Comparative analysis of patient samples for methotrexate.

minimally absorbed when given orally, therapeutic levels are obtained only when the drug is administered by the intramuscular or intravenous route. The drug, which is not bound to plasma proteins, is distributed in a volume similar to that of the extracellular fluid, and its serum halflife in patients with normal renal function is approximately two hours.[87] Gentamicin is not metabolized and is excreted by the kidney. The structures of gentamicin and related aminoglycoside antibiotics are shown in Figure 9.

Gentamicin is highly effective against a variety of organisms; it is used primarily in the treatment of serious gram-negative bacterial infections. Peak serum gentamicin levels in the range of 5–10 μg/ml are necessary for maximum therapeutic efficacy in treating gram-negative infections.[89] No evidence has been found that peak concentrations greater than 10 μg/ml are more effective than lower levels. Subtherapeutic doses are not only ineffective in treating serious infections, but may also encourage the development of antibiotic resistance in the infecting organism.[90] Overdosing may result in renal impairment.[87,88,91-94] Serum levels of <2 μg/ml may indicate tissue accumulation of gentamicin[94] and have been correlated with the emergence of symptoms of nephrotoxicity.[88,91-94]

Individual patients exhibit a high degree of variability in response to a given dose of gentamicin both in terms of peak plasma levels

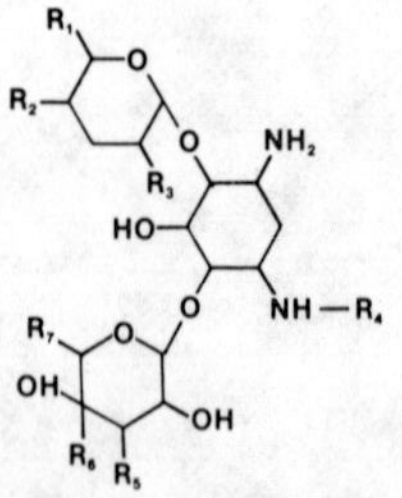

		R_1	R_2	R_3	R_4	R_5	R_6	R_7
	C_1	$CH(CH_3)$-$NHCH_3$						
Gentamicin	C_1A	CH_2NH_2	H	NH_2	H	$NHCH_3$	CH_3	H
	C_2	$CH(CH_3)$-NH_2						
Sisomicin*		CH_2NH_2	H	NH_2	H	$NHCH_3$	CH_3	H
Tobramycin		CH_2NH_2	OH	NH_2	H	NH_2	H	CH_2OH
Kanamycin A		CH_2NH_2	OH	OH	H	NH_2	H	CH_2OH
Amikacin		CH_2NH_2	OH	OH	$NHCOCOH$-$CH_2CH_2NH_2$	NH_2	H	CH_2OH

*Sisomicin contains a double bond between the two ring carbon atoms containing R_1 and R_2.

Fig. 9. Structures of aminoglycoside antibiotics.

attained[89,90,92,93,96-100] and in rates of elimination from plasma.[89,94,97-99] Peak levels vary according to body weight, body surface area, and other factors that affect the volume in which the drug is distributed. Because gentamicin is eliminated almost entirely by renal excretion, its plasma elimination halflife is dependent upon the rate of renal clearance.[89,94,97--100,102] Thus serum gentamicin concentrations cannot reliably be predicted from an administered dose at the outset of therapy. It is well established that monitoring serum gentamicin levels is the most effective means of ensuring adequate therapy.[89-95,96-102]

Until the development of more rapid and accurate techniques, serum gentamicin assays were performed almost exclusively by microbiological methods. The original agar plate diffusion technique[103] is impractical for routine monitoring because of its lengthy turnaround time (18–24 h) and its susceptibility to interference from penicillins and cephalosporins, which may be administered concurrently with gentamicin. Improved agar plate diffusion assays require shorter incubation periods (2–4 h) and are less subject to interference from beta-lactam antibiotics.[104-106] The urease method,[107] a three-hour microbiological assay, is relatively complicated to perform and has been found to be less accurate than plate diffusion assays.[108]

Radioimmunoassays[109-111] and radioenzymatic assays,[112-116] which offer better sensitivity and specificity than the microbiological methods, have been widely used in the routine monitoring of serum gentamicin levels. Although these methods require the use of radiochemicals and specialized instrumentation, they provide results within several hours of generally begun within several hours of the start of MTX infusion. Leucovorin is rapidly metabolized to 5-methyl-tetrahydrofolate, the predominant reduced folate in humans; this compound in turn is converted to 5,10-methylene-tetrahydrofolate, which enters the cell cycle beyond the MTX-induced block. It has been hypothesized that leucovorin brings about the resumption of DNA synthesis in normal cells to a greater extent than in neoplastic cells, although the mechanism for selectivity has not been established.[78] Leucovorin administration is generally continued until MTX blood levels drop to concentrations at which normal DNA synthesis can resume or until there is evidence that the final phase of MTX clearance is proceeding at a normal rate.

Each organ system and tissue has a particular time and concentration threshold for suppression of DNA synthesis by MTX.[77] Thresholds have not yet been determined for many organs and tissues; it is known, however, that when MTX blood levels exceed 10^{-8} M for over 42 h, DNA synthesis in the bone marrow and intestinal epithelium is suppressed.[79] Leucovorin rescue is designed to minimize the effects of MTX on these tissues during and immediately after high-dose MTX administration. Standard leucovorin rescue is not always successful in preventing serious toxicity to the bone marrow and intestinal epithelium. Patients with renal dysfunction, a frequent side effect of high-dose MTX therapy, may retain high levels of MTX for periods exceeding the protection capability of the standard leucovorin regimen. Early recognition of delayed MTX clearance is important so that supplemental rescue doses and efforts to increase renal clearance can be initiated before bone marrow and gastrointestinal toxicity ensue. Some oncologists monitor serum MTX levels throughout the course of high-dose therapy and discontinue leucovorin rescue when MTX blood levels of 10^{-7} or 10^{-8} M are reached.[77] Others have begun to use their knowledge of the drug's pharmacokinetics to determine time and concentration thresholds that, when exceeded, indicate the need for supplemental leucovorin rescue. Wang et al.,[80] Stoller et al.[81] and Nirenberg et al.[82] have successfully predicted toxicity on the basis of blood levels measured 48 h after the start of high-dose MTX infusions. These investigators have correlated 48-h blood levels exceeding approximately 10^{-6} M with impending toxicity and the need for supplemental rescue efforts. Forty-eight hour levels less than 10^{-6} M were correlated with a satisfactory rate of clearance and no subsequent toxicity.

Many of the techniques previously reported for the measurement of plasma methotrexate have somewhat limited utility in routine monitoring due to the length of time required to carry out the assays. Among the numerous assay methods reported (for example, RIA,[83] CPB,[84] HPLC[85] enzymatic inhibition[86]), only two, a radioimmunoassay technique and a competitive protein binding (CPB) method, have been commercially available in kit form. Both of these methods require batch assaying of multiple dilutions of every sample. The speed and simplicity of the EMIT assay make it the method of choice for "stat" determinations used in predicting impending toxicity. The greater sensitivity of the RIA and CPB methods, however, may be desirable in cases in which the oncologist chooses to monitor serum MTX levels until they decline to very low concentrations or in monitoring patients receiving MTX for dermatologic disorders.

The EMIT® Methotrexate Assay[33] has been designed for routine use in monitoring blood levels during and following the administration of high-dose MTX. Because it provides results within one to five minutes of a sample's receipt, the assay permits immediate identification of patients in need of supplemental leucovorin rescue. The assay can also be used to monitor serum MTX levels throughout the course of therapy as the concentration declines to the 10^{-7} *M* region. The assay's range of quantitation, 0.3–2.0 μM (3×10^{-7} to 2×10^{-6} *M*), encompasses levels typically observed at 48 h. Samples containing up to 2,600 μM are easily analyzed by preparing serial dilutions to bring them into the range of quantitation.

The specificity of the EMIT® Methotrexate Assay is comparable to that of the enzymatic (dihydrofolate reductase inhibition) method and greater than that of the RIA technique. Endogenous folates, dihydrofolic acid, and leucovorin do not interfere with the assay. Metabolites and contaminants of the high-dose MTX preparation may produce a 30% quantitation error in samples containing 1.0 μM of MTX at concentrations above the following minimum levels:

7-hydroxymethotrexate	$> 1.00\ \mu M$
4-amino-4-deoxy-N^{10}-methylpteroic acid (APA)	$\sim 0.3\ \mu M$
Methopterin	$> 1.0\ \mu M$
Trimethoprim	$> 100.0\ \mu M$
Aminopterin	$\sim 0.3\ \mu M$

Analysis of samples obtained from patients on methotrexate therapy is shown in Figure 8. This figure is a comparison of results obtained to the EMIT® Methotrexate Assay and those obtained by a radioimmunoassay and an enzymatic assay for methotrexate. Since the drug concentration of interest spans four orders of magnitude, logarithmic axes are used in Figure 8.

GENTAMICIN ASSAY[34]

Gentamicin is an aminoglycoside antibiotic that acts by inhibiting normal protein synthesis in susceptible bacteria. Since gentamicin is

THYROID FUNCTION ASSAYS

The thyroid hormones are important regulators of body metabolism. Their presence is critical to growth, development, and maintenance of good health. So important are these hormones that abnormal levels at any age can produce mental and physical disabilities. In newborns, for example, undetected thyroid deficiency can cause irreparable mental retardation and physical deformity. With the recognition of the importance of thyroid hormones to good health and the difficulty in differentiating thyroid disease from other illnesses, tests to confirm or rule out this endocrine problem are usually included in an initial diagnostic workup. Today, clinicians consider blood level measurements of these hormones important diagnostic tools. As thyroid testing methods become easier and less expensive, many laboratories will no doubt add thyroid tests to traditional biochemical screens or organ profiles.

A progression of methodologies have been used to monitor thyroid functions by measurements of thyroxine. Historically, the most important procedures begin with the measurement of protein-bound iodine. This analysis was performed in the clinical chemistry lab due to the procedural requirements of the test. This initial method was replaced by the more sensitive radioassays involving competitive protein binding. The procedure described by Murphy and Patee[130] allowed the relatively specific measurement of thyroxine. Interestingly, the radiolabel employed in the method resulted in the migration of the test from the clinical chemistry laboratory to the nuclear medicine area. The movement was enhanced by the introduction of sensitive radioimmunoassays using specific antithyroxine antibodies.

Recently, EMIT thyroxine assays have been introduced to accommodate existing single and multichannel enzyme analyzers. With this innovation, thyroxine assays can once again be performed in the clinical chemistry laboratory. More important, existing automated analyzers can be employed to perform T-4 determinations by the same technicians who currently carry out enzyme and blood chemistry tests.[35,126,127]

A variety of EMIT thyroxine assay systems are listed in Table 6 with various performance characteristics. All systems result in coefficients of variation less than 10% with equivalent quantitation and normal range values. Correlation between the EMIT ABA thyroxine and a commercial RIA thyroxine kit is presented in Figure 12.

The manual T-4 assay is performed in batches containing up to 60 samples. A sample throughput of 40–60 samples per hour makes this test useful for smaller hospitals and clinics that do not have a high workload, and, therefore, do not require faster throughput and less technician involvement. The ABA-100 or Centrifugal Analyzer T-4

Table 6. EMIT Thyroxine Assays

	ABA-100[23]	Centrifichem®[32]	Manual	Autochemist[31]
Sample volume (μl)	20	25	50	75
Total assay time (min)[a]	45	30	45	
Technician time (min)[a]	20	15	20	
Potential throughput, assay/h	80–100	100–150	50	180
Reagent stability				
Lyophilized	1 year	1 year	1 year	
Reconstituted	4 months	4 months	4 months	6 months

[a]Batch of 28–30 assays. Precision: less than 8% coefficient of variation (μg/dl). Accuracy: comparison of RIA methods gives correlation coefficients of 0.92–0.96. Specificity: no known clinically significant. Crossreactants: minimal interference from grossly abnormal serum specimens (hemolysis, lipemia, icterus).

a sample's receipt. Additional assay techniques that have been reported for the quantitation of serum gentamicin are high-pressure liquid chromatographic methods,[117-119] a gas-liquid chromatographic (GLC) assay,[120] fluorimmunoassays,[121-123] and enzyme immunoassays.[124,125]

The EMIT assay[34] for gentamicin utilizes gentamicin specific antibodies and a gentamicin-G6PDH conjugate. As with the AED assays, a single determination requires only 50 μl of serum and is completed in one minute. Both within-day and day-to-day precision of the assay at 2 and 8 μg/ml levels are <10%, with recoveries of 102% and 100%, respectively. The related antibiotics sisomicin and netilmicin are also recognized by the gentamicin antibodies and therefore could potentially interfere with the gentamicin assay. However, since these drugs are not administered concomitantly with gentamicin in clinical practice, no clinically significant specificity problem exists. Other aminoglycosides such as tobramycin and amikacin, as well as all other common antibiotics, do not interfere in the assay.

Serum based calibrators are provided that contain gentamicin in the range of 0–16 μg/ml. A typical standard curve is shown in Figure 10.

Accuracy of the EMIT® Gentamicin Assay was assessed by comparison of patient sample quantitation with several currently employed assay methodologies: microbiological assay (BIO), radioenzymatic assay

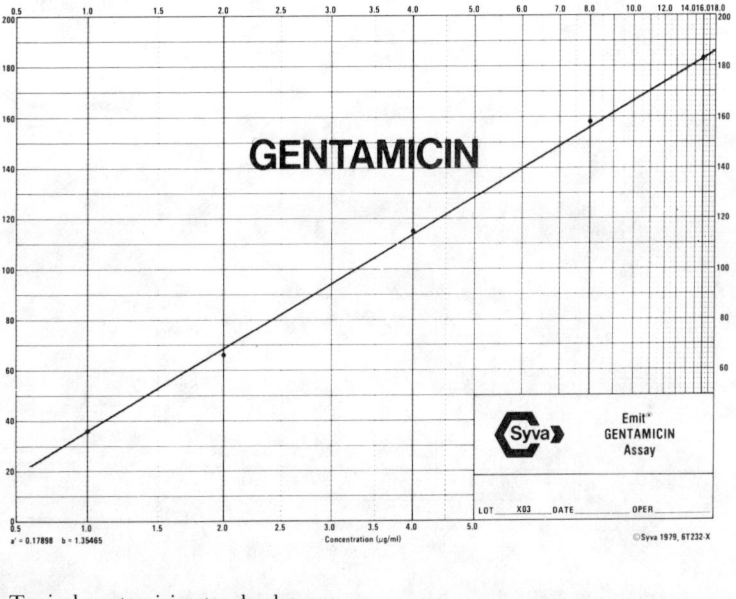

Fig. 10. Typical gentamicin standard curve.

Table 5. Correlation Statistics: EMIT Assay Versus Reference Analysis for Gentamicin

	Lab 1	Lab 2	Lab 3		Lab 4
Correlation coefficient	0.90	0.97	0.94	0.94	0.98
Slope	0.83	0.98	1.22	1.04	1.02
Mean EMIT (μg/ml)	4.68	3.82	2.47	2.47	2.96
Reference (μg/ml)	5.12	3.80	2.42	2.56	3.39
Number	82	82	100	100	98
Method	RIA	RIA	RIA	BIO	ENZ

(ENZ), and radioimmunoassay (RIA). Table 5 lists the statistical results of the comparative analyses. The data from a representative laboratory (Lab 2) is shown in Figure 11. These results indicate a relatively high correlation between the EMIT® Gentamicin Assay and the most common reference techniques. The enzyme immunoassay procedure should find use where speed of results is important or where automation is required.

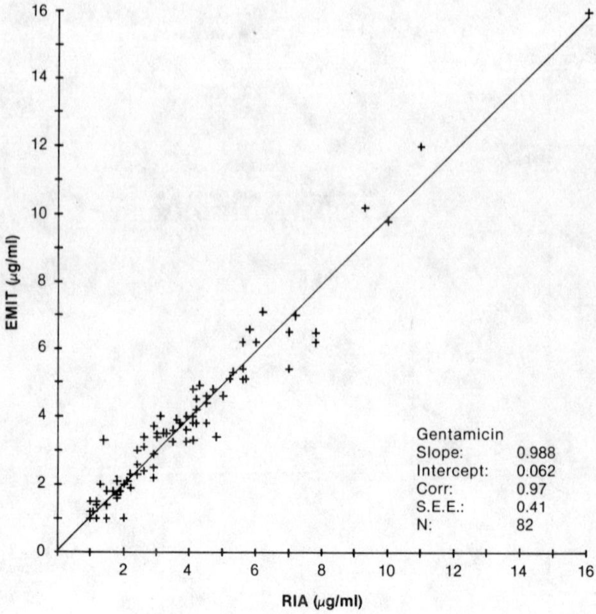

Fig. 11. Comparison of RIA and EMIT® assays for gentamicin.

their consistent efforts over the past years to provide the technical background, documentation, and imagination that has been responsible for bringing homogeneous enzyme immunoassay to its current stage of development and application.

REFERENCES

1. K.E. Rubenstein, R.S. Schneider, and E.F. Ullman, "Homogeneous" enzyme immunoassay. A new immunochemical technique. *Biochem Biophys Res Comm* **47**:846–851, 1972.
2. R.K. Leute, E.F. Ullman, A. Goldstein, and L.A. Herzenberg, Spin immunoassay technique for determination of morphine. *Nature* **236**:253, 1971.
3. M. Goldman, *Fluorescent Antibody Methods,* Academic, New York, 1968.
4. W.B. Dandliker, R.J. Kelly, J. Dandliker, J. Farguhar, and J. Levin, Fluorescence polarization immunoassay. Theory and experimental method. *Immunochemistry* **10**:219, 1973.
5. R.A.A. Watson, J. Landon, E.J. Shaw, and D.S. Smith, Polarisation fluorimmunoassay of gentamicin. *Clin Chim Acta* **73**:51–55, 1976.
6. A.R. McGregor, J.O. Crookall-Greening, J. Landon, and D.S. Smith, Polarisation fluoroimmunoassay of phenytoin. *Clin Chim Acta* **83**:161–166, 1978.
7. E.J. Shaw, R.A.A. Watson, J. Landon, and D.S. Smith, Estimation of serum gentamicin by quenching fluoroimmunoassay. *J Clin Pathol* **30**:526–531, 1977.
8. D.S. Smith, Enhancement fluoroimmunoassay of thyroxine, *FEBS Lett* **77**:25–27, 1977.
9. E.F. Ullman, M. Schwarzberg, and K.E. Rubenstein, Fluorescent excitation transfer immunoassay. *J Biol Chem* **251**:4172–4178, 1976.
10. J.F. Burd, R.C. Wong, J.E. Feeney, R.J. Carrico, and R.C. Boguslaska, Homogeneous reactant-labeled fluorescent immunoassay for therapeutic drugs exemplified by gentamicin determination in human serum. *Clin Chem* **23**:1402–1408, 1977.
11. H.R. Schroeder, F.M. Yeager, R.C. Boguslaski, E.O. Snoke, and R.T. Buckler, Immunoassay for thyroxine monitored by chemiluminescence. *Clin Chem* **23**:1123, 1977.
12. R.J. Carrico, J.E. Christner, R.C. Boguslaski, and K.K. Yeung, A method for monitoring specific binding reactions with cofactor labeled ligands. *Anal Biochem* **72**:283–292, 1976.
13. A.H.W.M. Schuurs and B.K. Van Weemen, Enzyme-immunoassay. *Clin Chem Acta* **81**:1–40, 1977.
14. C.M. O'Donnell and S.C. Suffin, Fluorescence immunoassays. *Anal Chem* **51**:33A–40A, 1979.
15. E. Soini and I. Hemmila, Fluoroimmunoassay: present status and key problems. *Clin Chem* **25**:353–361, 1979.
16. R.S. Schneider, P. Lindquist, E.T. Wong, K.E. Rubenstein, and E.F. Ullman, Homogeneous enzyme immunoassay for opiates in urine. *Clin Chem* **19**:821–825, 1973.
17. E.L. Slightom, The analysis of drugs in blood, bile and tissue with an indirect homogeneous enzyme immunoassay. *Forensic Sci* **23**(2), 1978.
18. H. Tom, D.S. Kabakoff, C.I. Lin, P. Singh, M. White, P. Westkamper, C. McReynolds, K. dePorceri-Morton, Homogeneous enzyme immunoassay for PCP in urine. *Clin Chem* **25**(6):1144, 1979.

19. C. Walberg and R. Gupta, Quantitative estimation of phencyclidine in urine by homogeneous enzyme immunoassay (EMIT®). *Clin Chem* **25**(6):1144, 1979.

20. A.J. Mann, C. Crowl, and R. Rodgers, An EMIT® assay for cannabinoid metabolites, Abstr. Amer. Acad. of Forensic Sciences, 31st Annual Meeting, Abstr. K-3, February 1979.

21. R. Rodgers, C.P. Crowl, W.M. Eimstad, M.W. Hu, J.K. Kam, R.C. Ronald, G.L. Rowley, E.F. Ullman, Homogeneous enzyme immunoassay for cannabinoids in urine. *Clin Chem* **24**:95–100, 1978.

22. J.Y. Chang and R.J. Bastiani, Clinical study no. 41, summary report: performance evaluation of the EMIT® theophylline assay, Syva Co., Palo Alto, Calif., 1977.

23. A. Izutsu, D. Leung, C. Araps, P. Singh, A. Jaklitsch, D.S. Kabakoff, Homogeneous enzyme immunoassay for valproic acid in serum. *Clin Chem* **25**(6):1093, 1979.

24. D. Scoggin, J. Petrehn, and D. Besemer, Homogeneous enzyme immunoassay for digoxin on the ABA-100 and CentrifiChem® 400. *Clin Chem* **24**:1055, 1978.

25. J.J. Chang, C.P. Crowl, and R.S. Schneider, Homogeneous enzyme immunoassay for digoxin, *Clin Chem* **21**:967, 1975.

26. M.E. Cobb, N. Buckley, M.W. Hu, J.G. Miller, P. Singh, and R.S. Schneider, Homogeneous enzyme immunoassay for lidocaine in serum. *Clin Chem* **21**:967, 1975.

27. B.E. Pape, R. Whiting, K.M. Parkey, and R. Mitra, Enzyme immunoassay and gas liquid chromatography compared for determination of lidocaine in serum. *Clin Chem* **24**:2020–2022, 1978.

28. R.A. Fanciullo, N. Huber, A. Izutsu, M.R. Pirio, N. Buckley, P. Singh, J.B. Gushaw, J.G. Miller, and R.S. Schneider, Homogeneous enzyme immunoassay for procainamide in serum. *Clin Chem* **24**:1056, 1978.

29. A. Izutsu, M.R. Pirio, N. Buckley, P. Singh, J.B. Gushaw, J.G. Miller, and R.S. Schneider, Homogeneous enzyme immunoassay for N-acetylprocainamide in serum. *Clin Chem* **24**:1055, 1978.

30. C. Collins, M. Hu, C.P. Crowl, D.S. Kabakoff, and P. Singh, A homogeneous enzyme immunoassay for quinidine in serum. *Clin Chem* **25**(6):1093, 1979.

31. K. Chegwidden, M.R. Pirio, P. Singh, J.B. Gushaw, J.G. Miller, and R.S. Schneider, Homogeneous enzyme immunoassay for propranolol in serum. *Clin Chem* **24**:1056, 1978.

32. D. Leung, Y. Tsay, P. Singh, A. Jaklitsch, and D.S. Kabakoff, Homogeneous enzyme immunoassay for tobramycin in serum. *Clin Chem* **25**:1094, 1979.

33. J.B. Gushaw and J.G. Miller, Homogeneous enzyme immunoassay for methotrexate in serum. *Clin Chem* **24**:1032, 1978.

34. D.S. Kabakoff, D. Leung, and P. Singh, An EMIT® assay for gentamicin. *Clin Chem* **24**:1055, 1978.

35. A.P. Jaklitsch, R.S. Schneider, R.J. Johannes, J.E. Levine, and G.L. Rosenberg, Homogeneous enzyme immunoassay for T-4 in serum. *Clin Chem* **22**:1185, 1976.

36. R.S. Galen and D.W. Forman, Enzyme immunoassay of serum thyroxine with the "Auto Chemist" multichannel analyzer. *Clin Chem* **23**:119, 1977.

37. D.M. Besemer and J.R. Chandler, Application of homogeneous enzyme immunoassay for thyroxine on a centrifugal analyzer. *Clin Chem* **23**:1083, 1977.

38. R.A. Fanciullo, A.C. Brown, L.J. Winfrey, H.M. Greenwood, and K.E. Rubenstein, Homogeneous enzyme immunoassay for serum T-3 uptake on the ABA-100. *Clin Chem* **25**:1103, 1979.

39. A.P. Jaklitsch, H.M. Greenwood, A.C. Peterson-Brown, J.E. Lavine, and D.K. Leung, Serum T-3 uptake by homogeneous enzyme immunoassay. *Clin Chem* **23**:1123, 1977.

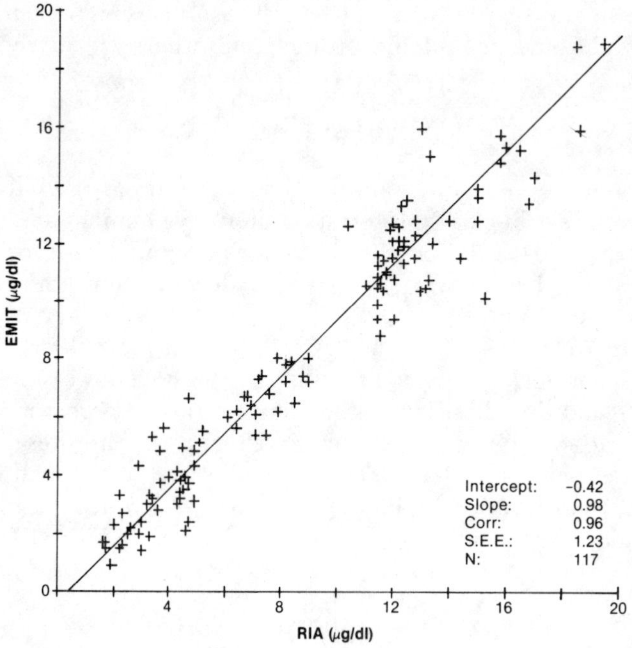

Fig. 12. Comparison of RIA and EMIT® ABA thyroxine assay.

assays allow hundreds of samples to be analyzed per day, making these systems applicable for larger clinical laboratories or for screening applications. Of course, incorporation of the T-4 test into the domain of multichannel analyzers makes the possibility of screening patients for thyroid abnormality quite intriguing.

Measurement of thyroid binding capacity (TBG) is provided by the EMIT® T-3 Uptake Assay.[128] The results from this assay, coupled with that for serum T-4, provide the free thyroxine index (FTI). The incorporation of the EMIT T-3 Uptake Assay onto manual and automated instrumentation will provide a valuable tool for the diagnosis and treatment of thyroid disease.

PROTEIN ASSAYS

Recent developments into the understanding of the mechanism of homogeneous enzyme immunoassay have led Ullman and coworkers to expand the scope of these assays to include assays for proteins.[129] Thus using β-galactosidase and a macromolecular substrate of O-phenyl-β-galactoside attached to dextran, these investigators have been able to demonstrate a competitive inhibition of the protein labeled enzyme in the presence of protein antibody. Clinically useful assays for human IgG, IgA, and IgM have been demonstrated, and others will surely follow.

ONGOING PROJECTS

Applications of enzyme immunoassay have progressed to include many other areas of clinical interest. Under development are assays for cortisol and estriol. Also, the widespread clinical use of tricyclic antidepressants has caused us to begin development for assays for compounds in this group.

The application of EMIT assays to toxicology problems is readily apparent, considering the need for almost instantaneous results in order to properly aid the physician in the identification of a potentially lethal drug overdose. Therefore, serum assays for barbiturates and benzodiazepines have been developed. Working with the National Institutes of Health, Syva has developed an assay for Δ9-tetrahydrocannabinoic acid, a major urinary metabolite from marijuana.

SUMMARY

Clearly, the application of homogeneous enzyme immunoassay has progressed much further than our original attempts at the detection of drugs of abuse in urine. The application of this technology to a wide variety of clinical problems is evident from the data presented thus far. Homogeneous enzyme immunoassay appears to be a general, broadly based analytical technique for the assay of haptens and proteins, which will greatly aid physicians in the clinical diagnosis and therapeutic monitoring of patients. In addition, adoption of this technique provides a clinical laboratory with a single analytical technique that can perform a great variety of test services day or night with minimal technician training. The EMIT system is a core technology for the clinical laboratory. This technique should find a place in laboratories devoted to optimized patient care with a minimum of capital investment, training, and time utilized to provide accurate, precise, and economical results.

ACKNOWLEDGMENTS

The author wishes to express his gratitude to Ms. Wendy Thole, Mary Specker, and Signe Gotcher for their superb help in documentation of the numerous articles cited in the bibliography and for their considerable literary skills. Also, the entire research and development scientific staff of the Syva Company deserves special consideration for

79. B.A. Chabner and R.C. Young, Threshold methotrexate concentration for in vivo inhibition of DNA synthesis in normal and tumorous target tissues. *J Clin Invest* **52**:1804–1811, 1973.

80. Y. Wang, E. Lantin, and W.W. Sutow, Methotrexate in blood, urine and cerebrospinal fluid of children receiving high doses by infusion, *Clin Chem* **22**:1053–1056, 1976.

81. R.G. Stoller, K.R. Hande, S.A. Jacobs, S.A. Rosenberg, and B.A. Chabner, Use of plasma pharmacokinetics to predict and prevent methotrexate toxicity, *N Engl J Med* **297**:630–634, 1977.

82. A. Nirenberg, C. Mosende, B.M. Mehta, A.L. Gisolfi, and G. Rosen, High-dose methotrexate with citrovorum factor rescue: predictive value of serum methotrexate concentrations and corrective measures to avert toxicity. *Cancer Treat Rep* **61**:779–783, 1977.

83. Methotrexate Radioimmunoassay Kit Instruction Manual, Diagnostic Biochemistry Inc., San Diego, Calif., June, 1978.

84. C.E. Myers, M.E. Lippman, H.M. Eliot, and B.A. Chabner, Competitive protein binding assay for methotrexate, *Proc Natl Acad Sci USA* **72**:3683–3686, 1975.

85. E. Watson, J.L. Cohen, and K.K. Chan, High-pressure liquid chromatography determination of methotrexate and its major metabolite, 7-hydroxymethotrexate, in human plasma, *Cancer Treat Rep* **62**:381–387, 1978.

86. L.C. Falk, D.R. Clark, S.M. Kalman, and T.F. Long, Enzymatic assay for methotrexate in serum and cerebrospinal fluid. *Clin Chem* **22**:785–788, 1976.

87. G.B. Appel and H.C. Neu, Gentamicin in 1978, *Ann Intern Med* **89**:528–538, 1978.

88. M. Barza and R.T. Scheife, Drug therapy reviews: anti-microbial spectrum, pharmacology and therapeutic use of antibiotics — Part 4: aminoglycosides *Am J Hosp Pharm* **34**:723–737, 1977.

89. M. Barza and M. Lauermann, Why monitor serum levels of gentamicin?, *Clin Pharmacokinet* **3**:202–215, 1978.

90. P. Noone, T.M.C. Parsons, J.R. Pattison, R.C.B. Slack, D. Garfield-Davies, and K. Hughes, Experience in monitoring gentamicin therapy during treatment of serious gram-negative sepsis. *Br Med J* **1**:477–481, 1974.

91. W.L. Hewitt, Gentamicin: toxicity in perspective, *Post-grad Med J* **50**(Suppl. 7):55–59, 1974.

92. J.G. Dahlgren, E.T. Anderson, and W.L. Hewitt, Gentamicin blood levels: a guide to nephrotoxicity. *Antimicrob Agents Chemother* **8**:58–62, 1975.

93. E.L. Goodman, J. VanGelder, R. Holmes, A.R. Hull, and J.P. Sanford, Prospective comparative study of variable dosage and variable frequency regimens for administration of gentamicin, *Antimicrob Agents Chemother* **8**:434–438, 1975.

94. J.J. Schentag, T.J. Cumbo, W.J. Jusko, and M.E. Plaut, Gentamicin tissue accumulation and nephrotoxic reactions, *JAMA* **240**:2067–2069, 1978.

95. G.G. Jackson and G. Arcieri, Ototoxicity of gentamicin in man: a survey and controlled analysis of clinical experience in the United States. *J Infect Dis* **124**(Suppl.):S130–S137, 1971.

96. G.G. Jackson and L.J. Riff, Pseudomonas bacteremia: pharmacologic and other bases for failure of treatment with gentamicin. *J Infect Dis* **124**(Suppl.):S185–S191, 1971.

97. L.R. Riff and G.G. Jackson, Pharmacology of gentamicin in man, *J Infect Dis* **124**(Suppl.):S98–S105, 1971.

98. D. Kaye, M.E. Levison, and E.D. Labovitz, The unpredictability of serum concentrations of gentamicin: pharmacokinetics of gentamicin in patients with normal and abnormal renal function. *J Infect Dis* **130**:150–154, 1974.

99. M. Barza, R.B. Brown, D. Shen, M. Gibaldi, and L. Weinstein, Predictability of blood levels of gentamicin in man. *J Infect Dis* **132**:165–174, 1975.

100. G.R. Siber, P. Echeverria, A.L. Smith, J.W. Paisley, and D.H. Smith, Pharmacokinetics of gentamicin in children and adults, *J Infect Dis* **132**:637–651, 1975.

101. J.E. Pennington, D.C. Dale, H.Y. Reynolds, and J.D. MacLowry, Gentamicin sulfate pharmacokinetics: lower levels of gentamicin in blood during fever. *J Infect Dis* **132**:270–275, 1975.

102. R.J. Sawchuck, D.E. Zaske, R.J. Cipolle, W.A. Wargin, and R.G. Strate, Kinetic model for gentamicin dosing with the use of individual patient parameters. *Clin Pharmacol Ther* **21**:362–369, 1977.

103. E.M. Oden, H. Stander, and M.J. Weinstein, Microbiological assay of gentamicin, *Antimicrob Agents Chemother,* 8–13, 1963.

104. L.D. Sabath, J.I. Casey, P.A. Ruch, L.L. Stumpf, and M. Finland, Rapid microassay of gentamicin, kanamycin, neomycin, streptomycin, and vancomycin in serum or plasma. *J Lab Clin Med* **78**:457–463, 1971.

105. M.E. Lund, D.J. Blazevic, and J.M. Matsen, Rapid gentamicin bioassay using a multiple-antibiotic-resistant strain of *Klebsiella pneumoniae. Antimicrob Agents Chemother* **4**:569–573, 1973.

106. D.C. Shanson, A two-hour plate assay for gentamicin, *J Antimicrob Chemother* **1**:247–249, 1975.

107. P. Noone, J.R. Pattison, and D. Samson, Simple, rapid method for assay of aminoglycoside antibiotics. *Lancet,* 16–19, July 3, 1971.

108. I. Phillips, C. Warren, and S.E. Smith, Serum gentamicin assay: a comparison and assessment of different methods. *J Clin Pathol* **27**:447–451, 1974.

109. R.A.A. Watson, E.J. Shaw, and C.R.W. Edwards, A ^{125}I-based radioimmunoassay for serum gentamicin. *Int. Congr Chemother,* J.D. William (ed.), Plenum, NY, 1976, Vol. 2, pp. 107–110.

110. A. Broughton and J.E. Strong, Radioimmunoassay of iodinated gentamicin. *Clin Chim Acta* **66**:125–129, 1976.

111. D.J. Casley, An improved radioimmunoassay for serum gentamicin levels using ^{125}I-labeled gentamicin. *Clin Exp Pharmacol Phys* **4**:525–532, 1977.

112. D.H. Smith, B. Van Otto, A.L. Smith, A rapid chemical assay for gentamicin, *N Engl J Med* **286**:583–586, 1972.

113. R.K. Holmes and J.P. Sanford, Enzymatic assay for gentamicin and related aminoglycoside antibiotics. *J Infect Dis* **129**:519–527, 1974.

114. J.M. Broughall and D.S. Reeves, The acetyltransferase enzyme method for the assay of serum gentamicin concentrations and a comparison with other methods. *J Clin Pathol* **28**:104–145, 1975.

115. P. Stevens, L.S. Young, and W.L. Hewitt, Radioimmunoassay, acetylating radioenzymatic assay, and microbioassay of gentamicin: a comparative study. *J Lab Clin Med* **86**:349–359, 1975.

116. K.P. Shannon and I. Phillips, The use of aminoglycoside 2′-N-acetyltransferase for the assay of gentamicin in serum, plasma, and urine. *J Antimicrob Chemother* **3**:25–33, 1977.

117. J.P. Anhalt, Assay of gentamicin in serum by high-pressure liquid chromatography. *Antimicrob Agents Chemother* **11**:651–655, 1977.

118. G.W. Peng, M.A.F. Gadalla, A. Peng, V. Smith, and W.L. Chiou, High-pressure liquid chromatography method for determination of gentamicin in plasma. *Clin Chem* **23**:1838–1844, 1977.

40. L.J. Winfrey, L. Johns-Stephens, and H.M. Greenwood, Development of an automated homogeneous enzyme immunoassay for serum cortisol on the ABA-100 bichromatic analyzer. *Clin Chem* **25**:1151, 1979.

41. H. Tom, R.S. Schneider, R. Ernst, W. Khan, P. Singh, and D.S. Kabakoff, Homogeneous enzyme immunoassays for barbiturates and benzodiazepines in serum. *Clin Chem* **25**:1094, 1979.

42. F.E. Greifenstein, M. DeVault, V. Yoshitaki, and J.E. Gajewski, A study of 1-arylcyclo-aexylamine for anesthesia, *Anesth Analgesia* **37**:283–294, 1958.

43. E.F. Domino, Neurobiology of PCP (Sernyl), a drug with an unusual spectrum of pharmacological activity, *Int Rev Neurobiol* **6**:303–347, 1964.

44. S.E. Lerner, Testimony before U.S. Senate Subcommittee on Juvenile Deliquency and U.S. Senate Subcommittee on Alcoholism and Drug Abuse, Washington, D.C., June 7, 1978.

45. National Clearinghouse for Drug Abuse, Information on Phencyclidine (PCP), Series 14/1, 1–11, 1973.

46. R. Aronow and A.K. Done, Phencyclidine overdose: an emerging concept of management. *JACEP* **7**(2):56–59, February, 1978.

47. S.R. Burns, S.E. Lerner, R. Corrado, S.H. James, and S.H. Schnoll, Phencyclidine — status of acute intoxication and fatalities, *West J Med* **123**(5):345–349, November, 1975.

48. S.D. Lundberg, R.C. Gupta, and S.H. Montgomery, Phencyclidine: patterns seen in street drug analysis. *Clin Toxicol* **9**(4):503–511, 1976.

49. R. Aronow and A.K. Done, Phencyclidine overdose: an emerging concept of management, *JACEP* **7**(2):57, 1978.

50. J.W. Eastman and S.N. Colen, Hypertensive crisis and death associated with phencyclidine poisoning, *JAMA* **231**(12): March 24, 1975.

51. P.U. Luisada and B.I. Brown, Clinical management of the phencyclidine psychosis. *Clin Toxicol* **9**(4):539–545, 1976.

52. P.C. Reynolds, Clinical and forensic experiences with phencyclidine, *Clin Toxicol* **9**(4):547–552, 1976.

53. S.R. Burns and S.E. Lerner, Street PCP use: clinical studies of the acute and chronic intoxicated state. Presented at Calif. Assoc. of Toxicologists Quarterly Meeting, San Jose, Calif., August, 1975.

54. J.A. Marshman, M.P. Ramsay, and E.M. Sellers, Quantitation of phencyclidine in biological fluids and application to human overdose, *Toxicol Appl Pharmacol* **35**:129–136, 1976.

55. E.F. Domino, Neurobiology of phencyclidine — an update. *In Phencyclidine (PCP) Abuse: An Appraisal.* National Institute on Drug Abuse (NIDA) Monograph, series 21, August, 1978.

56. D.C. Lin, A.F. Fentiman, R.L. Foltz, R.D. Forney, and I. Sunshine, Quantification of phencyclidine in body fluids by gas chromatography-chemical ionization mass spectrometry and identification of two metabolites, *Biomed Mass Spectrometry* **2**:204–205, 1975.

57. L.K. Wong and K. Biemann, Metabolites of phencyclidine in humans, *Biomed Mass Spectrometry* **2**:204–205, 1975.

58. H.I. Finkle, Phencyclidine identification by thin-layer chromatography. A rapid screening procedure for emergency toxicology. *Am Soc Clin Pathol,* 287–290, August, 1978.

59. P.E. Froelich and G. Ross, Separation and detection of phencyclidine in urine by gas chromatography. *J Chromatogr* **137**:135–143, 1977.

60. W.D. MacLeod, D.E. Green, and E. Seet, Automated analysis of phencyclidine in urine by probability based matching GC/MS. *Clin Toxicol* **9**(4):561–572, 1976.

61. R.C. Gupta, I. Lee, O. Goat-Lee, and G. Lundberg, Determination of phencyclidine in urine and illicit street drug samples, *Clin Toxicol* **8**(6):611–621, 1975.

62. C.E. Pippenger, R.J. Bastiani, and R.S. Schneider, Evaluation of experimental homogeneous immunoassay for quantitation of phenytoin and phenobarbitone in serum or plasma. *In Clinical Pharmacology of Antiepileptic Drugs,* H. Schneider, D. Janz, C. Gardner-Thorpe, H. Meinardi, and A.L. Sherwin (eds.), Springer-Verlag, New York, 1975, pp. 331–336.

63. D.D. Schottelius, Homogeneous immunoassay system (EMIT®) for quantitation of antiepileptic drugs in biological fluids. *In Antiepileptic Drugs: Quantitative Analysis and Interpretation,* C.E. Pippenger, J.K. Penry, and H. Kutt (eds.), Raven Press, New York, 1978.

64. R. Bastiani and J. Chang, Performance evaluation of the EMIT® antiepileptic drug assays, Summary Report, Syva Co., Palo Alto, Calif., 1978.

65. C.B. Walberg, Immunoassay of cardioactive drugs in serum. *In Enzyme Labelled Immunoassay of Hormones and Drugs,* S.B. Pal (ed.), Walter de Gruyter, New York, 1978, pp. 429–436.

66. C.B. Walberg and S.H. Wan, Clinical evaluation of the EMIT® procainamide and N-acetylprocainamide assay, *In Therapeutic Drug Monitoring,* Vol. 1, Raven Press, New York, 1979.

67. D.P. Lehane, P.J. Wissert, P. Menyharth, A.C. Levy, and M.A. Kukucka, Enzyme immunoassay for serum lidocaine in antiarrhythmic therapy. *Clin Chem* **25**:614–616, 1979.

68. C.B. Walberg, Lidocaine by enzyme immunoassay, *J Anal Toxicol* **2**: July/August, 1978.

69. L.J. Haywood, K. Claiborne, and C.B. Walberg, Lidocaine: clinical use of rapid method for determining serum levels. *Clin Res* **27**: February, 1979.

70. J.B. Gushaw, M.W. Hu, P. Singh, J.G. Miller, and R.S. Schneider, Homogeneous enzyme immunoassay for theophylline in serum, *Clin Chem* **23**:1144, 1977.

71. M.L. Eppel, J.S. Oliver, H. Smith, A. Mackay, and L.E. Ramsay, Determination of theophylline in plasma: comparison of high-performance liquid chromatography and an enzyme multiplied immunoassay technique. *Analyst* **103**:1060–1065, October 1978.

72. Comparison of homogeneous enzyme immunoassay and high-pressure liquid chromatography for the determination of theophylline concentration in serum, *Rev Resp Dis,* 117 (1978).

73. J.B. Gushaw, M.W. Hu, P. Singh, J.G. Miller, and R.S. Schneider, Homogeneous enzyme immunoassay for theophylline in serum, *Clin Chem* **23**:1144, 1977.

74. C. dePorceri-Morton, J. Chang, M. Specker, and R. Bastiani, Performance evaluation of the EMIT® Methotrexate Assay, Syva Co., November, 1978.

75. I. Djerassi, J.S. Kim, N.P. Nayak, H. Ohanissian, and S. Adler, High-dose methotrexate with citrovorum factor rescue: a new approach to cancer chemotherapy. *In Recent Advances in Cancer Treatment,* H.J. Tagnon and M.J. Staquet (eds.), Raven Press, New York, 1977, pp. 201–225.

76. D. Goldman, Analysis of the cytotoxic determinants for methotrexate (NSC-740): a role for "free" intracellular drug, *Cancer Chemother Rep* **6**:51–61, 1975.

77. W.A. Bleyer, The clinical pharmacology of methotrexate. New applications of an old drug. *Cancer* **41**:36–51, 1978.

78. E. Frei III, N. Jaffe, M.H.N. Tattersall, S. Pitman, and L. Parker, New approaches to cancer chemotherapy with methotrexate. *N Engl J Med* **292**:846–851, 1975.

Chapter 8

ELISA

F.R. BISHAI, Ph.D.

INTRODUCTION

Enzyme-linked immunosorbent assay (ELISA) is a combination of enzymology and immunology disciplines. This reflects that ELISA is potentially a sensitive and specific test. In addition, the technique is normally completed within a short time; therefore, it can be considered as a special candidate for use for rapid diagnosis. Several articles have described the application of ELISA for the detection of drugs, hormones, polypeptides, steroids, plasma proteins, antibodies to pathogens, and antigens from pathogens.

ELISA has been established for the detection of some drugs and hormones such as cortisone,[10] procainamide,[37] thyroxin,[31] thyroid stimulating hormones,[25] human chorionic gonadotropin,[32,33] insulin,[19,21] and progesterone.[11] ELISA has been established for the detection of plasma proteins such as IgG,[12] IgE,[17] and alpha-fetoprotein.[2] Bile acids in serum were also detected by ELISA.[23]

Again, ELISA has been used for the detection of antibodies against pathogens like *E. granulosus*,[8] syphilis,[34] salmonella 0-antigens,[9] and *E. coli*,[20] antibodies against diseases such as malaria[35] and cholera,[18] and antibodies against viruses such as rubella virus,[8,14,36] herpes virus,[15] and influenza and parainfluenza viruses.[5] ELISA could be used for the detection of viral pathogens such as herpes simplex virus,[24] influenza virus A and B,[4] and rotavirus,[38] and to differentiate between different types of human rotavirus in patients' specimens.[4a,7]

Laboratory Services Branch, Ontario Ministry of Health, Box 9000, Terminal A, Toronto, Ontario M5W 1R5

ELISA, particularly, has been a promising technique for use in the detection of viral infection, because laboratory diagnosis for viral infections is based on the isolation of the virus in an experimental host, on the one hand, and the demonstration of specific antigens and antibodies, on the other. Virus isolation techniques are often difficult, time consuming, and expensive. In case of antibody determination, tests widely spaced in time have to be carried out on serum specimens in order to demonstrate a specific sero-conversion. The time required to arrive at useful results is often too long, and while the results may be useful to the epidemiologist, they will be of little practical value in patient's care.

Rapid techniques such as immunofluorescence (IF) and electron microscopy (EM) for the detection of the viral antigens are available. However, they have to be performed by highly trained personnel, and the necessary pieces of equipment for these techniques are not always available in every diagnostic laboratory. These techniques also have their own limitations. Electron microscopy is not sensitive; normally, it can only detect virus particles when their concentration reaches at least 10^8 particles per ml. The immunofluorescence technique is more sensitive than the EM technique. However, it is a tedious technique and, in many instances, it is troubled with nonspecific results, and the results are always subjective.

The radioimmunoassay (RIA) and enzyme-linked immunosorbent assay (ELISA) are the most sensitive techniques. RIA has recently been introduced to the field of virology for the detection of hepatitis B antigens and their antibodies; however, it is not yet universally accepted because of the handling of radioactive materials and the expense of the necessary equipment. ELISA is also highly sensitive, the shelf life of reagents is long, reading of the results is objective, inexpensive (colorimeter) equipment is satisfactory for registering the results, and the procedure can be automated for mass screening. ELISA appears to be superior to other existing sensitive techniques, yet it has not been widely accepted in the field of virology because the technique has not been rigidly standardized. Our laboratory, therefore, started a few years ago to develop ELISA techniques, with adequate standardization for the detection of different viruses and their antibodies, that could be used in routine diagnosis.

Viruses can be divided into two main categories: the first category includes viruses that can propagate efficiently in cell culture systems, such as influenza and adenoviruses; while the second category includes viruses that do not propagate efficiently in cell culture systems, such as human rota- and hepatitis viruses. Therefore, two main systems of ELISA have been developed in our laboratory for the detection of viruses, their antigens and antibodies. The first system is called the

119. S.K. Maitra, T.T. Yoshikawa, J.L. Hansen, I. Nillson-Ehle, W.J. Palin, M.C. Shotz, and L.B. Guze, Serum gentamicin assay by high-performance liquid chromatography. *Clin Chem* **23**:2275–2278, 1977.

120. J.W. Mayhew and S.L. Gorbach, Gas-liquid chromatographic method for the assay of aminoglycoside antibiotics in serum, *J Chromatogr* **151**:133–146, 1978.

121. R.A.A. Watson, J. Landon, E.J. Shaw, and D.S. Smith, Polarization fluoroimmunoassay of gentamicin *Clin Chim Acta* **73**:51–55, 1976.

122. E.J. Shaw, R.A.A. Watson, J. Landon, and D.S. Smith, Estimation of serum gentamicin by quenching fluoroimmunoassay, *J Clin Pathol* **30**:526–531, 1977.

123. J.F. Burd, R.C. Wong, J.E. Feeney, R.J. Carrico, and R.C. Boguslaski, Homogeneous reactant-labeled fluorescent immunoassay for therapeutic drugs exemplified by gentamicin determination in human serum. *Clin Chem* **23**:1402–1408, 1977.

124. B. Mattiasson, K. Svensson, C. Borrebaeck, S. Jonsson, and G. Kronvall, Non-equilibrium enzyme immunoassay of gentamicin, *Clin Chem* **24**:1770–1773, 1978.

125. J.C. Standefer and G.C. Saunders, Enzyme immunoassay for gentamicin. *Clin Chem* **24**:1903–1907, 1978.

126. G.L. Rowley, K.E. Rubenstein, J. Huisjen, and E.F. Ullman, Mechanism by which antibodies inhibit hapten-malate dehydrogenase conjugates. *J Biol Chem* **250**:2759–3766, 1975.

127. G.L. Rowley, K.E. Rubenstein, S.T. Weber, and E.F. Ullman, Mechanism by which antibodies inhibit hapten-glucose-6-phosphate dehydrogenase. In Abstracts of the 172nd American Chemical Society National Meeting, San Francisco, August 29, 1976, Biological Chemistry Section, abstract no. 151.

128. R.A. Fanciullo, A.C. Brown, L.J. Winfrey, H.M. Greenwood, and K.E. Rubenstein, Homogeneous enzyme immunoassay for serum T-3 uptake on the ABA-100. *Clin Chem* **25**(6):1103, 1979.

129. I. Gibbons, C. Skold, G.L. Rowley, and E.F. Ullman, *Clin Chem* **25**:1078, 1979 (Abstract).

130. B.E.P. Murphy and C.J. Pattee, *J Clin Endocrinol* **24**:187, 1964.

solid-phase "amplified" ELISA procedure, which has been established for detection of influenza viruses. The other is called the *solid-phase "sandwich" ELISA* procedure, which has been established for detection of human rotavirus.

MATERIALS AND METHODS

Solid-Phase "Amplified" ELISA

This test is a combination of tissue culture and immunoassay techniques. It has been established in our laboratory to detect and to identify viruses that can be propagated efficiently in tissue culture, such as influenza viruses.

Antigen Preparations

Seed viruses of influenza A/Victoria/3/75, influenza A/Hong Kong/1/68, influenza A/Texas/1/77, influenza A/Singapore/1/57, influenza A/USSR/90/77, influenza B/Hong Kong/5/72, and parainfluenza type 1 were obtained from the National Reference Centre (LCDC) in Ottawa, Ontario.

Stock Virus

Each virus was propagated in a monolayer of African green monkey tissue culture and/or in allantoic fluid of embryonated eggs. After 3–5 days incubation, the total fluid containing the virus was collected as the crude harvest of the virus. The harvest was then partially purified by low-speed centrifugation (3,000 × *g* for 20 min). The supernatant fluid was then collected and centrifuged again for 5 h at 100,000 × *g* at 40°C in a Beckman L2-65B ultracentrifuge. The supernatant fluid was removed, and the pellet was then suspended in sterile phosphate-buffered saline solution (PBS) (pH 7.3) to 1/200 of the original volume.

Purified Virus for Antibody Production

The stock partially purified virus prepared from the allantoic fluid was further purified by the adsorption-elution method[1] or by a two-step centrifugation method using a sucrose gradient as described by Arora et al.[3]

Preparation of Antisera

Each purified virus was used for the production of its specific antibodies in rabbits and in guinea pigs as described by Bishai et al.[7]

Preparation of Solid-Phase Coupled Antigen

Cell Cultures. One ml of African green monkey kidney cell suspension (purchased from Connaught Laboratories Ltd., Toronto) was planted in wells of the plastic Linbro tissue culture multiwell plates (24 flat-bottom wells per plate, Linbro Scientific Co., Inc.). The plates were sealed and incubated for 6 days at 37°C. The fluid was replaced with maintenance medium containing 2% fetal calf serum. The plates were then incubated for another 24 h until they were inoculated with virus.

Inoculation Procedure. The monolayer cell cultures in 16 wells of each plate were inoculated with 200 median tissue culture infective dose ($TCID_{50}$) of influenza virus, either A, B, or parainfluenza type 1 virus. The remaining eight wells were kept uninfected for use as negative controls.

Fixation Procedure. When heavy infection was demonstrated in the monolayer cells by cytopathic effect (CPE) or hemadsorption (HAd), a mixture of cold (−20°C) absolute ethyl alcohol and acetone (4:1) was added to each well. After 20 min the alcohol-acetone mixture was aspirated, and the plates were air-dried in a sterile cabinet. The plates were then stored at −70°C until used. In the present report, the fixed infected cells are referred to as solid-phase coupled antigen, whereas the fixed uninfected cells are referred to as solid-phase coupled no antigen. The latter were used as controls to detect nonspecific reactions.

BSA Treatment. Bovine serum albumin (BSA) treatment was performed to eliminate nonspecific reaction to the solid support after the plates had been treated with the fixative. The fixed plates were brought to room temperature. A 1-ml portion of 1% BSA solution (1 g of BSA fraction V dissolved in 100 ml of PBS, pH 7.3) was added to each well. After 30 min, the BSA solution was aspirated and the plate was air-dried.

Serum Diluent

The test sera were diluted with 0.5% BSA solution containing 0.05% Tween-20.

Enzyme Conjugate

Horseradish peroxidase conjugated antihuman immunoglobulin G (antihuman IgG) or antirabbit IgG prepared in goat serum was used. These conjugates were supplied by Miles Laboratories. This preparation was diluted 1:100 with 1% BSA solution containing 0.01% Tween-20. Also, specific antibodies to the different strains of influenza A were conjugated with horseradish peroxidase after Nakane and Kawaoi's method[26] with slight modification as described later.

Substrate Solution

A 20-mg portion of *O*-dianisidine dihydrochloride (Sigma Chemical Co.) and 37.2 mg of ethylenediaminetetraacetic acid disodium salt was dissolved in 80 ml of acetate buffer (pH 3.8). A 50-μl portion of purified Triton X-100 and 5 μl of 30% H_2O_2 were added; then the final volume of the solution was adjusted to 100 ml with acetate buffer.

Washing Solution

Washing was done with 0.1 M PBS (pH 7.3) containing 0.05% Tween-20.

Negative and Positive Controls

The following three assays were performed. (1) The serum diluent was assayed as a negative control to determine the background nonspecific reactivity. (2) Negative sera: preimmune rabbit sera, and human sera negative to influenza A, B, and parainfluenza type 1 by complement fixation (CF) and by hemagglutination inhibition (HAI) were also assayed by ELISA. Only those sera which gave identical low optical density (OD), when tested on solid-phase coupled antigen and on solid-phase coupled no antigen, were used as negative controls in the ELISA test. (3) Positive control sera: immune rabbit and human sera positive to influenza A/Hong Kong/1/68 or influenza A/Victoria/3/75, influenza B/Hong Kong/5/72, and parainfluenza type 1 by CF and/or HAI were used as positive controls in the ELISA test.

Test Procedure

BSA solution (0.2 ml) was inoculated into each of four wells, two wells containing solid-phase coupled antigen and two wells containing solid-phase coupled no antigen. This step was repeated in triplicate for negative and positive control sera and in duplicate for the unknown sera. The plates were then covered and incubated at room temperature for one hour, after which the wells were washed 10 times with the washing solution using an automatic washer. Either peroxidase conjugated antihuman or antirabbit IgG prepared in goat (0.2 ml) was added to each well and incubated for another hour. The type of the conjugate used depended on the test sera, whether from human or rabbit origin. The wells were then washed 15 times. Enzyme substrate solution (2 ml) was added to each well. The enzyme reaction was allowed to proceed for 20 min at room temperature before it was stopped by adding 0.1 ml of 1 N NaOH. The intensity of the color developed as the result of the enzymatic reaction was measured at 450 nm by a Brinkmann colorimeter 600/D with a stainless steel probe. All readings were registered within 15 min after the addition of the NaOH solution.

Confirmatory Test

Positive sera were confirmed by blocking the antibodies with their homotypic antigen by the following procedure. One hundred μl of the serum were added to 100 μl of the partially purified, concentrated homotypic virus. A negative control sample was prepared by adding 100 μl of test serum to 100 μl of diluent. Both samples were incubated for 18 h at 4°C, then centrifuged at 3,000 $\times$ *g* for 15 min. An aliquot from the supernatant was then diluted with the serum diluent to a final dilution of 1:40. These sera were then assayed for antibodies by ELISA. The optical densities of the color developed were compared between the untreated serum and serum treated with the virus. The specimen was considered positive if the optical density (OD) of the specimen was reduced by 60% or more after it had been treated with the homotypic virus.

Interpretation of ELISA Results for the Detection of Influenza Antibodies

The results were interpreted on the following basis.

1. Serum diluent, when used as inoculum, should yield negligible optical density values. The values obtained reflect the nonspecific color, developed as a result of the nonspecific attachment of the conjugate to the solid phase.

2. The negative and positive sera, when tested on solid-phase coupled no antigen, should also yield no or very low optical density values. The intensity of the color developed reflects the amount of the nonspecific antibodies attached to the solid phase.

3. The negative and positive sera, when tested on solid-phase coupled antigen, should yield a significant difference between the optical density values. The difference between the values of positive and negative reflected the amount of antibodies in the positive specimen and was defined as *ELISA specific activity* for antibody. In order to determine the positivity of an unknown specimen for specific antibodies to influenza A, B, or parainfluenza type 1, the following equation was used:

$$\text{Ratio} = \frac{\text{OD of the unknown specimen} - \text{OD of BSA}}{\text{OD of the negative control} - \text{OD of BSA}}$$

If the ratio was two or more, the specimen was considered to be positive for the antibody in question. If the ratio was less than two, the specimen was considered to be negative.

Detection and Identification of Influenza Viruses in Patients' Throat Washings

Each throat washing was inoculated into eight wells of Linbro plastic plate containing a monolayer of African green monkey cells; 100 μl of the test specimen was added to each well. The specimens were adsorbed to the cells for 1 h at 37°C. One ml of tissue culture media containing antibiotics was then added to each well. The wells were sealed and incubated at 37°C for 24–48 h. If the patient's specimen contained virus, it would replicate in the cell culture. At the end of the incubation period, the wells were fixed with a mixture of cold ethyl alcohol and acetone (4:1) as described previously. This step produced (1) a solid-phase coupled antigen in wells that were inoculated with patients' specimens containing virus; or (2) a solid-phase coupled no antigen in the wells that were inoculated with patients' throat washings containing no virus. Negative and positive controls were included in each plate. Each well was then treated with 1 ml of BSA solution for ½ hour. One hundred μl of a mixture of antibodies produced in rabbit against the different strains of influenza A, influenza B, and parainfluenza type 1 were added to two wells of the eight that were inoculated by the same specimen. Every two wells of the remaining six wells received 100 μl of specific antibodies to either influenza type A, influenza type B, or parainfluenza type 1. The plates were then incubated for 1 h at room temperature, after which the wells were washed 10 times. Peroxidase-labeled antirabbit IgG (100 μl) was then added to each well and incubated for another 1 h at room temperature. The wells were washed 15 times with washing solutions, then 2 ml of the enzyme-substrate were added. No color was formed in the wells that were inoculated with the negative control and with the patients' specimens free from the virus. However, brownish-yellow color was produced in wells inoculated with the positive control as well as with specimens containing influenza viruses.

For example, if the patient's specimen contained influenza A virus, four wells out of the eight that were inoculated with the same specimens should be positive: the two wells to which a mixture of the antibodies to influenza A, B, and parainfluenza type 1 was added, and the other two wells to which the specific antibodies to infuenza A were added. This test not only detected the presence of the virus in the specimens, but also identified the virus, whether it was A, B, or parainfluenza type 1.

Solid-Phase "Sandwich" ELISA

The solid-phase "sandwich" ELISA procedure has been used for the detection of viruses that do not propagate efficiently in tissue culture, such as human rotaviruses. Human rotaviruses were found to be antigenically similar to Nebraska calf diarrhea virus (NCDV) and simian (SA11) rotaviruses, which could easily be propagated in tissue culture. Therefore, NCDV and SA11 were used for the production of their specific antibodies in animals for use in this test.

Preparation of Rotaviruses

NCDV or SA11 rotaviruses were propagated in monolayers of BS-C-1 cell culture. Each virus was harvested and purified by the cesium chloride ultracentrifugation method described by Fauvel et al.[13] The purified, complete virus particles, which were banded at a density of 1.355 g per ml, were used for the preparation of anti-NCDV and anti-SA11 in rabbits or guinea pigs.

Antisera Preparation

Antisera against each virus were prepared in both rabbits and guinea pigs as described above.

Enzyme Conjugate

The method used was similar to that used by Nakane and Kawaoi[26] with a minor modification. The modification consisted of the elimination of the addition of sodium borohydrite, $NaBH_4$, to the mixture of immune gamma globulin and horseradish peroxidase aldehyde solution. Separation of the horseradish peroxidase-labeled antibody from the free enzyme by Sephadex G-200 was also unnecessary.

Detection of Rotaviruses by the Solid-Phase "Sandwich" ELISA Procedure

Falcon polystyrene tubes* (style 2054) were coated with immune gamma globulin (IgG) containing antibodies to NCDV or SA11 rotavirus prepared in rabbits. The tubes were previously treated with 1% glutaraldehyde solution in order to produce a satisfactory solid-phase coupled antibody.[4a] The coated tubes were stored at 4°C until used. Each specimen was tested in duplicate. Three positive and three negative control specimens were included in every test. Two hundred μl of the test material were added to either anti-NCDV coated or anti-SA11 rotavirus coated tubes. The tubes were then placed in a slightly slanted rotating tissue culture roller drum for 2 h at 37°C. Following this incubation period, the tubes were washed again and 200 μl of peroxidase-labeled anti-NCDV or anti-SA11 were added to each tube.

*Supplied by Falcon Plastics, U.S.A.

The conjugate was incubated as before for 1 h at 37°C, then the tubes were washed. One ml of the substrate solution, prepared as described above, was added, and the reaction proceeded for 20 min at room temperature. The optical density of the color was measured at 450-nm wavelength using a Brinkmann colorimeter 600/D with a stainless steel probe.

BLOCKING TEST (CONFIRMATORY TEST)

Test material was mixed with an equal volume of immune guinea pig anti-NCDV or anti-SA11 serum and incubated at 4°C for 18 h followed by 2 h at 37°C. Equal amounts of test material and preimmunization guinea pig sera were mixed and processed in the same manner as the control. The mixtures were then centrifuged and the supernatant was tested by ELISA as described above.

Other Tests Used for Comparison with ELISA

COMPLEMENT FIXATION (CF)

The CF procedure used was the microtiter technique described by Sever.[28] Usually, sera were tested at a starting dilution of 1:8.

HEMAGGLUTINATION INHIBITION (HAI)

The HAI procedure used was that described by Hierholzer et al.[16] Sera were tested at a starting dilution of 1:10.

HEMADSORPTION METHOD (HAd)

The rate of infection was tested by the hemadsorption described by Shelokov et al.[29]

ELECTRON MICROSCOPY (EM) AND COUNTERIMMUNOELECTROPHORESIS (CIEP)

These tests were carried out by the methods that were described previously by Spence et al.[30]

VIRUS ISOLATION PROCEDURE (VI)

This test involved the use of tissue cell culture for the isolation of the virus as described by Lennette and Schmidt.[22]

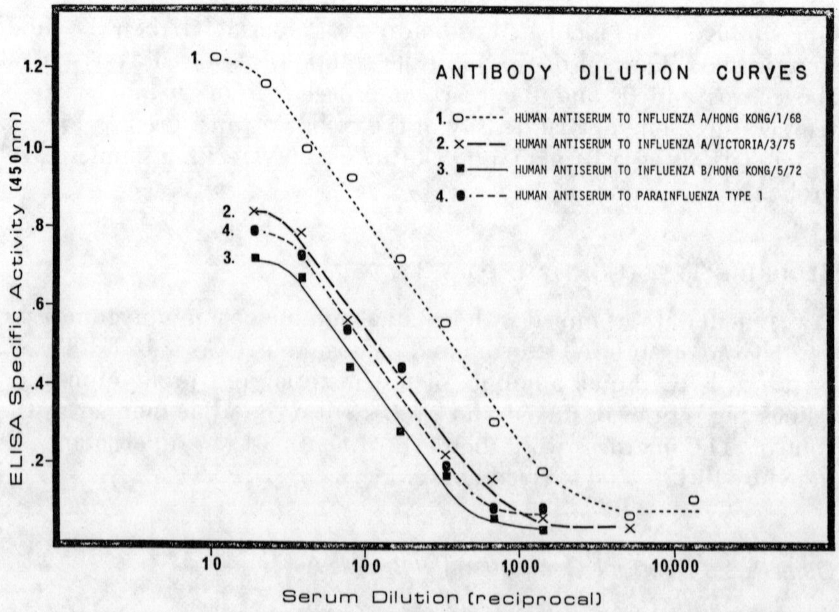

Fig. 1. Titration of four human antisera to (1) influenza A/Hong Kong/1/68, HAI titer 1:80; (2) influenza A/Victoria/3/75, HAI titer 1:40; (3) influenza B/Hong Kong/5/72, HAI titer 1:40; (4) parainfluenza type 1, CF titer 1:16. These sera were tested against their homotypic viruses.

RESULTS

Solid-Phase "Amplified" ELISA

Detection of Antibodies to Influenza Viruses

A dose response test was performed in duplicate in serial twofold dilutions on four different positive reference human sera (influenza A/Hong Kong/1/68, A/Victoria/3/75, B/Hong Kong/5/72, and parainfluenza type 1). Each sera was tested against its homotypic antigen. A typical sigmoid shaped curve was obtained in all cases (Fig. 1).

Specificity and Sensitivity of Amplified ELISA

Reference rabbit and human sera containing antibodies to either influenza A, B, or parainfluenza type 1 viruses were titrated by ELISA, HAI, and CF tests. The results obtained (Table 1) showed that there was

Table 1. Antibody Titers[a] to Influenza Type A, Type B, and Parainfluenza Type I by Complement Fixation (CF), Hemagglutination Inhibition (HAI), and Enzyme-Linked Immunosorbent Assay (ELISA) Techniques

Antisera	Influenza type A									
	Victoria strain			Hong Kong strain		Influenza type B			Parainfluenza type I	
	CF	HAI	ELISA	HAI	ELISA	CF	HAI	ELISA	CF	ELISA
Antiinfluenza A Victoria strain Rabbit	32	320	1280	20	80	<16[b]	10	40	<16[b]	40
Antiinfluenza A Hong Kong strain Rabbit	256	20	320	640	5120	<16[b]	<10	<40	<8	<40
Antiinfluenza B Hong Kong strain Rabbit	<10	10	≤40	<10	<40	40	80	2560	<10	<40
Antiparainfluenza type I Rabbit	<40[b]	10	40	10	40	<40[b]	10	<40	80	640
Antiinfluenza A Human	128	320	≥5120	40	160	<16[b]	<10	40	<16[b]	80
Antiinfluenza B Human	8	10	<40	10	<40	512	320	1600	8	<40
Antiparainfluenza type I Human	8		40		40	<8		<40	16	160

[a]Reciprocal of serum dilution.
[b]Anticomplementary at lower dilutions.

no crossreaction between antibodies to influenza A and/or B and/or parainfluenza type 1 when the ELISA method was used. The ELISA antibody titers for all the sera tested were 8–64 times higher than those obtained by CF or HAI methods.

Comparison Between ELISA and HAI Techniques for the Detection of Antibodies to Influenza A and B in Acute and Convalescent Clinical Specimens

Several clinical specimens were tested by ELISA and HAI. ELISA titers were always higher. The rise in titer in the convalescent sera was always demonstrated by ELISA as well as by HAI. As an example, Table 2 shows the results obtained by ELISA and HAI for acute and

Table 2. ELISA and HAI Titers of Antibodies to Influenza A and B in Clinical Specimens

	Reciprocal of antibody titers			
	Influenza A/Victoria 3/75		Influenza B/Hong Kong/ 5/72	
	HAI	ELISA	HAI	ELISA
Case I				
Acute	<10	10	<10	<40
Convalescent	80	2,560	<10	<40
Case II				
Acute	160	2,560	10	80
Convalescent	320	>10,240	20	80
Case III				
Acute	<10	10	20	80
Convalescent	80	640	20	160
Case IV				
Acute	>10	40	<10	<40
Convalescent	40	2,560	<10	<40
Case V				
Acute	<10	<40	<10	<40
Convalescent	<10	<40	40	640
Case VI				
Acute	40	40	10	<40
Convalescent	40	40	80	1,280
Case VII				
Acute	<10	<40	10	<40
Convalescent	<10	<40	80	640
Case VIII				
Acute	10	40	<10	40
Convalescent	10	40	40	320

convalescent sera obtained from eight patients. Four patients were infected with influenza A virus while the other four were infected with influenza B virus.

Comparison Between ELISA and HAI Techniques for the Detection of Antibodies to Influenza A in Unknown Sera

Seventy-four unknown sera were tested by ELISA and HAI methods for the presence of antibodies to influenza A. As seen from Table 3, 19% of the total specimens tested were only positive by ELISA. These specimens were confirmed to be positive by the blocking test. These results indicated that because ELISA is more sensitive than HAI, the weakly positive sera that could not be detected by HAI were easily detected by ELISA.

Table 3. Comparison Between ELISA and HAI Techniques for the Detection of Antibodies to Influenza A/Victoria/3/75 in Unknown Patients' Sera

	HAI	
ELISA	Pos.	Neg.
Pos.	43	14
Neg.	0	17

Detection of Influenza Virus by Amplified ELISA

Influenza viruses are usually found in patients' throat washings in low quantities and are usually coated by patients' cell debris, mucus, or IgA secretion. Therefore, it became necessary to inoculate the throat washing specimens in tissue culture. This process not only increased the amount of original virus present in the sample by allowing the virus to replicate in the cells for 24–48 h, but it also purified the virus from biological material excreted along with the virus.

To determine the sensitivity of this method for the detection of influenza viruses in patients' throat washings, we simulated the test by adding a known amount of influenza A/Victoria/3/75 to throat washings known to be free from live viruses. Throat washings negative for virus were used as a negative control. An aliquot of 100 μl of throat washings containing different amounts of virus particles were inoculated in each well of four Linbro tissue culture plates containing a monolayer of African green monkey cells. Four wells in each plate were inoculated with throat washings containing no virus as control. After the adsorption was completed, each well received 1 ml of tissue culture medium; then it was sealed. After every 24 h, one plate was examined by aspirating the tissue culture media; then the monolayer was fixed with ethyl alcohol-acetone mixture to produce solid-phase coupled antigen or solid-phase coupled no antigen as described above. The plate was treated with BSA and then tested for the presence of the virus as described above. The results in Table 4 show that one median tissue culture dose ($TCID_{50}$) could be detected after 24 h by ELISA, while it could be detected only after 3–4 days by the hemadsorption technique. Similar results were obtained when influenza type B or parainfluenza type 1 viruses were tested by this method.

Table 4. Detection of Influenza A/Victoria/3/75 in Throat Washings by Enzyme-Linked Immunosorbent Assay and Hemadsorption Methods at Different Intervals After Inoculation

Units of $TCID_{50}$	Ratio of OD of positive / OD of negative				Hemadsorption test			
	24 h	48 h	72 h	96 h	24 h	48 h	72 h	96 h
500	8	8	7	7	+	+	+	+
100	5	9	8	8	+	+	+	+
10	3.5	8	9	8	−	+	+	+
1	2	4	8	7	−	−	±	+
0.1	1.6	1.4	1.4	1.0	−	−	−	−
0.01	1.7	1.4	1.4	1.0	−	−	−	−
0.001	1.7	1.4	1.4	1.0	−	−	−	−

Detection of the Presence of Influenza A/Texas/1/77 in Patients' Specimens

Throat washings that were collected from 31 patients with respiratory diseases were supplied to our laboratory under code numbers. The specimens were then tested by the amplified ELISA technique in our laboratory as well as by the conventional isolation methods in another laboratory. By the amplified ELISA technique, six specimens were found to be positive within 24–48 h for influenza A/Texas/1/77. Twenty-five specimens were negative for influenza A (Table 5). All specimens that were negative by the ELISA test were also negative by the virus isolation technique. The same six positive specimens detected by ELISA were also detected as positive by the isolation technique. The final results for the amplified ELISA were obtained within 48 h. However, the final results for the virus isolations were obtained after two weeks.

Table 5. Detection of Influenza A/Texas/1/77 in Patients' Throat Washings by Amplified ELISA and Virus Isolation Techniques

Amplified ELISA (Results obtained within 24–48 h)	Virus isolation technique (Results obtained within 5–15 days)	
	Pos.	Neg.
Pos.	6	0
Neg.	0	25

Solid-Phase "Sandwich" ELISA

Detection of Rotavirus

Standard Curve for Dose Response. A dose response test was performed in duplicate in serial twofold dilutions on a highly purified NCDV suspension. In this test, the virus was treated by ELISA against its homotypic antibody. A sigmoid shaped curve was obtained (Fig. 2); the

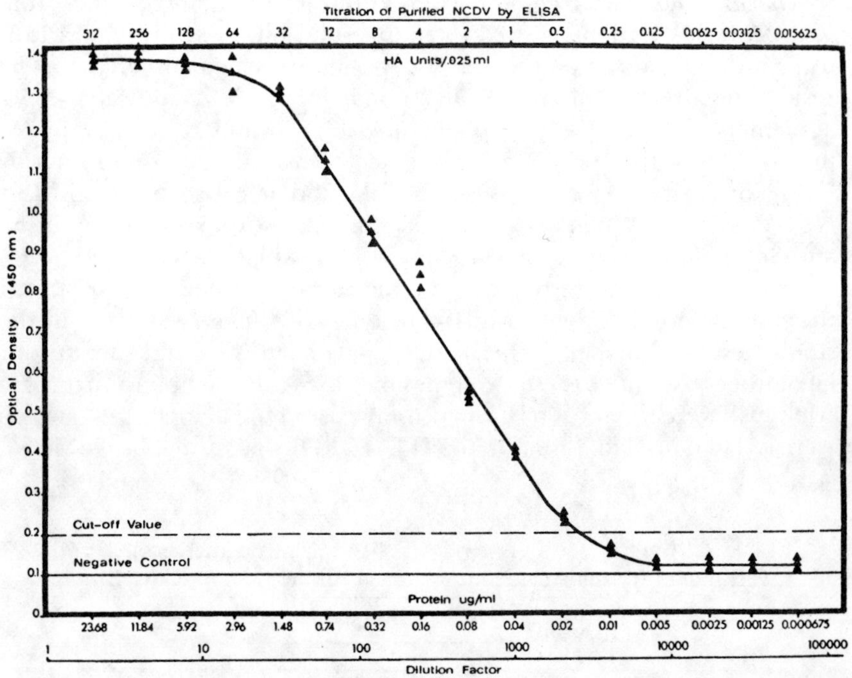

Fig. 2. Titration of highly purified bovine (NCDV) by ELISA. Tubes were coated with IgG fraction of anti-NCDV antiserum prepared in rabbits. The enzyme conjugated was horseradish peroxidase-conjugated anti-NCDV IgG prepared in guinea pigs.

Table 6. Comparison Between EM, CIEP, and ELISA for Detection of Human Rotavirus in Stool Specimens

Stool specimen no.	Endpoint titer[a]		
	EM	CIEP	ELISA
I	16	8	128
II	2	2	128

[a]Reciprocal titer of rotavirus particles (EM) or antigen (CIEP and ELISA).

ELISA test could detect 0.5 HA units per 0.25 μl of NCDV or 20 ng of total protein per ml of virus suspension.

Comparison Between EM, CIEP, and ELISA for the Detection of Human Rotaviruses in Stool Specimens. Two specimens were titrated by the ELISA system, EM, and CIEP techniques (Table 6). The results indicated that endpoint titers obtained by ELISA were 8–64 times higher than those obtained by either EM or CIEP.

Use of the ELISA System for the Detection of Human Rotavirus in Stool Specimens. One hundred and twenty-four specimens collected from gastroenteritis patients were tested by solid-phase sandwich ELISA, using anti-NCDV coated tubes and peroxidase-labeled anti-NCDV. The results obtained, which are illustrated in Table 7, indicated 85% agreement between the results obtained by EM and ELISA. Approximately 10% of the specimens were detected only by ELISA and not by EM. However, 4% were positive by EM and negative by the ELISA NCDV system. When we repeated the 4% (five specimens) using anti-SA11 polystyrene coated tubes and peroxidase-labeled anti-SA11, all five specimens were detected by the second system. This indicated that there were at least two different types of human rotavirus in the stools tested. Further experiments had been carried out in our laboratory to identify these two types by ELISA. It was found that these two types were identical to human rotaviruses type 2 and type 3, which were isolated in a laboratory in the U.K. (F.R. Bishai, unpublished work).

Table 7. Comparison Between ELISA and Electron Microscopy (EM) Techniques for the Detection of Human Rotavirus in Patients' Stools

ELISA	EM	
	Pos.	Neg.
Pos.	32	13
Neg.	5	74

Use of the Solid-Phase Sandwich Procedure to Study the Crossreactivity Between Related Viruses or Related Strains of the Same Virus. Study on crossreactivity between bovine (NCDV) and simian (SA11) rotaviruses: Each of the bovine (NCDV) and simian (SA11) rotaviruses was tested by solid-phase sandwich ELISA using homologous or heterologous antibodies. When 16 HA units of either bovine (NCDV) or simian (SA11) viruses were tested by the sandwich ELISA technique using anti-NCDV coated tubes and peroxidase conjugated anti-NCDV, both viruses were equally well detected. However, when anti-SA11 coated tubes and peroxidase conjugated anti-SA11 system were used, the simian (SA11) virus was readily detected but not bovine (NCDV) virus (Fig. 3). The results indicated that anti-NCDV system could detect both NCDV and SA11 rotaviruses; however, the anti-SA11 system could detect only SA11 rotavirus.

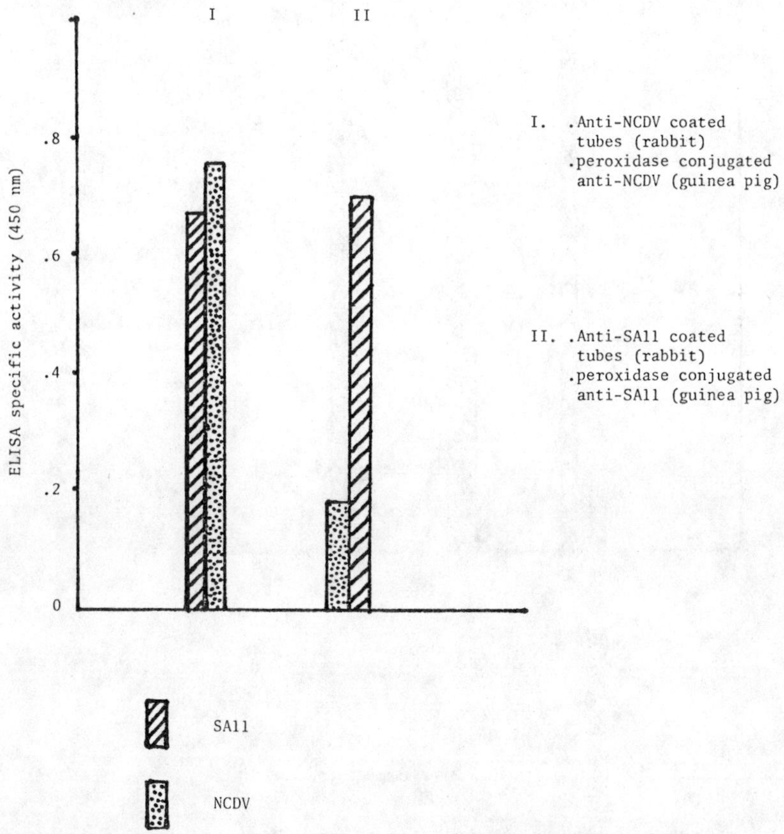

Fig. 3. Crossreactivity between bovine (NCDV) and simian (SA11) rotavirus.

In our study of crossreactivity between different strains of influenza A viruses (A/USSR/90/77 (H_1N_1), A/Singapore/1/57 (H_2N_2), and A/Texas/1/77 (H_3N_2)), each virus was tested by the solid-phase sandwich ELISA system, using homologous and heterologous antibodies. Results showed (Fig. 4) that there was no crossreaction between A/USSR/90/77 (H_1N_1) and either A/Singapore/1/57 (H_2N_2) or A/Texas/1/77 (H_3N_2). However, partial crossreaction was demonstrated between A/Singapore/1/57 (H_2N_2) and A/Texas (H_3N_2).

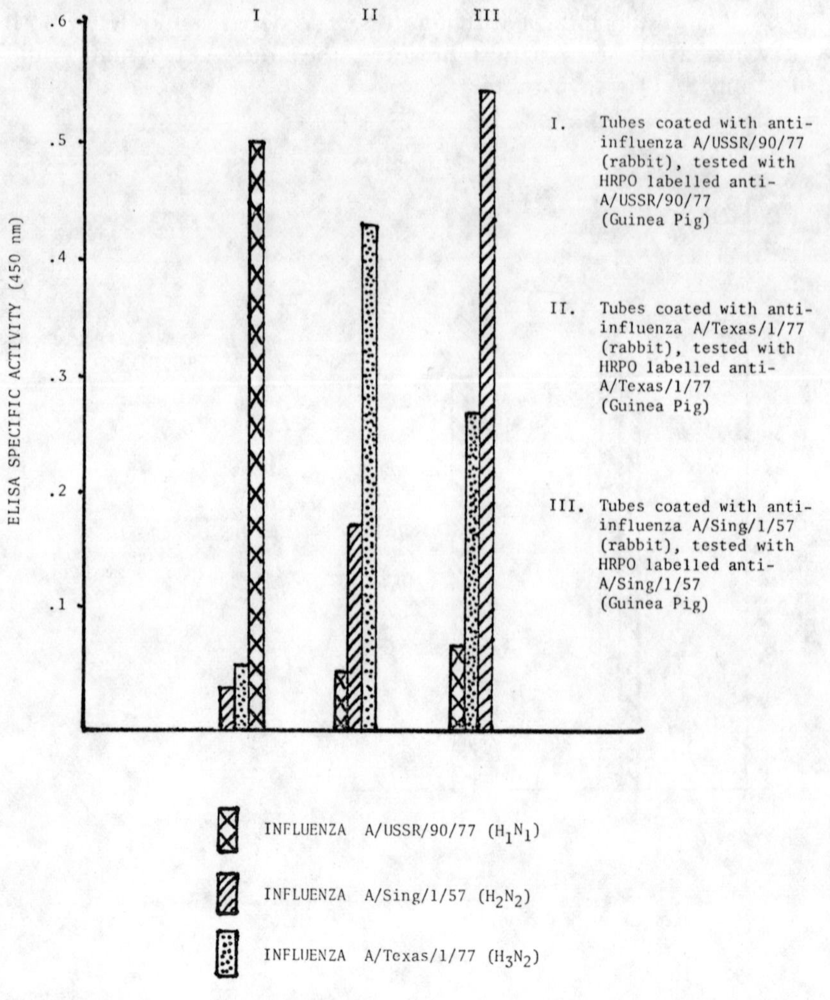

Fig. 4. Crossreactivity between different strains of influenza A viruses [A/USSR/90/77 (H_1N_1); A/Sing./1/57 (H_2N_2); A/Texas/1/77 (H_3N_2)].

From these results, it appears that this ELISA system detected hemagglutinin (H) and neuraminidase (N) located on the surface of the virus but not the nucleoprotein, the common antigen for influenza A viruses.

DISCUSSION

Frequently, patients with viral infections are treated with antibiotics because it is difficult to distinguish viral from bacterial infections, particularly in the early stages of the disease. Prompt differential diagnosis at this stage would assist in avoiding unnecessary antibiotics treatment and thus reduce undesirable consequences such as development of drug resistant bacteria and the sensitization of the patient to the antibiotics involved. Again the recent development of the production of antiviral drugs urges the need for a rapid diagnostic technique for viral infections. Therefore, two ELISA systems, solid-phase amplified ELISA and solid-phase sandwich ELISA, have been developed for use in rapid diagnosis involving the detection of influenza viruses and their antibodies as well as human rotavirus in patients' specimens.

A major factor that has played an important role in any successful solid-phase immunoassay has been the preparation of a uniform solid-phase coupled antigen or antibody. Most previous investigators prepared their solid-phase coupled antigen by physical adsorption of the antigen to the plastic support. It was found that the antigen attached unevenly to the solid support. This could create serious problems in using the method for laboratory diagnosis, especially when acute and convalescent-phase specimens were tested. Differences in titers could be due to an unevenly coated surface rather than to an actual difference in the amount of the specific antibodies in the sera. To circumvent this problem, the solid-phase coupled antigen in the amplified ELISA was prepared by fixing an infected monolayer cell culture to the support surface. This method appeared to be successful, since the results obtained for the detection of influenza viruses and their antibodies were consistent and reproducible. The shelf life of the solid-phase coupled antigen was several months at −70°C. Also, the present technique was found to be highly versatile and was adapted to detect the presence of other viruses in patients' specimens, such as adenoviruses (F.R. Bishai, unpublished work). The solid-phase coupled antibody in the sandwich ELISA was prepared by adsorbing the antibodies to the plastic support after it had been treated with 1% glutaraldehyde solution. This treatment tremendously increased the affinity of the plastic surface for the antibodies. Therefore, the established solid-phase sandwich ELISA is a sensitive and reliable technique for the detection of rotaviruses and for studying the crossreactivity between related viruses such as bovine (NCDV) and simian (SA11) rotaviruses, on the one hand, and studying the crossreactivity between different strains of a virus such as influenza A/USSR/90/77, A/Singapore/1/57, and A/Texas/1/77, on the other.

Another major obstacle in ELISA was the preparation of peroxidase labeled antibody molecules. Although the methods available are limited, we found that Nakane and Kawaoi's method[26] with the minor modifications mentioned above is highly suitable for establishing successfully the ELISA technique. Both ELISA procedures were approximately 8–64 times more sensitive than either CF or HAI tests.

The high sensitivity of ELISA offers a definite advantage in shortening the time span between the acute and convalescent sera to demonstrate specific seroconversion. Again, the test permits the analysis of very small amounts of serum specimens, such as blood specimens collected from infants by heel prick. The droplet of blood obtained from heel prick was collected on filter paper; it was then eluted in 1% BSA solution and tested by the ELISA method described above. The present ELISA method offered, therefore, a new simple way for the detection of maternal viral antibodies in newborn children.

No special treatment of sera is required for the ELISA test. However, sera tested by the HAI procedure should be treated by receptor destroying enzyme (RDE) to remove nonspecific inhibitors of hemagglutinations. The complement fixation test requires daily standardization of the antigen, hemolysis, erythrocytes, and complement, and the test requires overnight incubation. ELISA for the detection of viral antibodies is completed within three hours.

Combination of the tissue culture technique with ELISA in the solid-phase amplified ELISA allowed the detection of minute quantities of the virus (one $TCID_{50}$) in patients' specimens within a short time. One $TCID_{50}$ of influenza A/Victoria/3/75 could be detected within only 48 h. The method proved to be reliable, with 100% agreement between the results obtained by the amplified ELISA and by the isolation method for the detection of influenza A/Texas/1/77 in unknown patients' specimens. The final results were obtained after 48 h when the amplified ELISA method was used; however, it took 15 days when virus isolation methods were used.

ELISA systems were found to be highly specific; the solid-phase sandwich procedure was used to study the crossreaction between related viruses such as bovine (NCDV) and simian (SA11) rotaviruses. When anti-NCDV coated tubes and peroxidase anti-NCDV were used in the ELISA system, both NCDV and SA11 viruses were detected. However, when the anti-SA11 system was used, only SA11 virus was detected. It appeared, therefore, that crossreactivity between NCDV and SA11 was in one direction. Testing routine specimens by both systems (NCDV and

SA11) enabled us to detect and identify both types of human rotaviruses in patients' specimens.

The sandwich technique was also used to study the crossreactivity between infuenza viruses A/USSR/90/77 (H_1N_1), A/Singapore/1/57 (H_2N_2), and A/Texas/1/77 (H_3N_2). The results showed no crossreaction between A/USSR and either A/Singapore or A/Texas. However, there was partial crossreaction between A/Singapore and A/Texas, which shared (N_2). It appeared, therefore, that this ELISA system detected both hemagglutinin and neuraminidase molecules located on the surface of the virus but not the nucleoprotein, the common antigen in the three strains.

This study illustrated that both solid-phase amplified and sandwich ELISA techniques are useful not only for the detection, but also for the identification, of influenza and human rotaviruses in clinical specimens, and the results are obtained within a short period.

ELISA will be readily accepted as a rapid technique for the laboratory diagnosis of viral infections once the type of antibodies and antigens detected by ELISA is clearly identified. This identification should be related to other conventional laboratory tests currently used in diagnostic virology. Laboratories using ELISA as a diagnostic tool should participate in and implement a rigid quality control program. This will ensure a general standardization of the technique, reliability of the results, and their proper interpretation.

REFERENCES

1. G.L. Ada and B.T. Perry, *Austral J Exp Biol Med Sci* **32**:453, 1954.
2. W.H.W. Albert, F. Stachler, and W. Gruber, *Lab Med* **2**:31, 1978.
3. D.J.S. Arora, V. Pavilanis, and P. Robert, *Canad J Microbiol* **19**:633, 1973.
4. F.R. Bishai, *In Proceedings of International Symposium on Enzyme-Labeled Immunoassay of Hormones and Drugs, Ulm, West Germany,* Walter de Gruyter, Berlin, 1978.

4a. F.R. Bishai, 1980 (in preparation).

5. F.R. Bishai and R. Galli, *J Clin Microbiol* **8**:648, 1978.
6. F.R. Bishai and D. Goodwin, Use of ELISA to study the cross-reactivity between bovine (NCDV) and simian (SA11) rotavirus. Canad. Public Health Assoc. Meeting, Nov., 1979.
7. F.R. Bishai, L. Spence, D. Goodwin, and R. Petro, *Canad J Microbiol* **28**:1118, 1979.
8. D. Bout, J.C. Dugimont, H. Farag, and A. Capron, *Lille Med* **20**:561, 1975.
9. H.E. Carlsson, A.A. Lindberg, S.G. Hammarstrom, and A. Lyunggren, *Int Arch Allergy* **48**:485, 1975.
10. S. Comoglio and F. Celada, *J Immunol Methods* **10**:161, 1976.
11. F. Dray, J. Andrieu, and F. Renaud, *Biochim Biophys Acta* **403**:131, 1975.
12. E. Engvall and P. Perlmann, *Immunochemistry* **8**:871, 1971.
13. M. Fauvel, L. Spence, L.A. Babiuk, R. Petro, and S. Bloch, *Intervirology* **9**:95, 1978.
14. B. Forghani and N. Schmidt, *J Clin Microbiol* **9**:657, 1979.

15. S.C. Gilman and J.J. Docherty, *J Infect Dis* **136**(Suppl.):S286, 1977.

16. J.C. Hierholzer, M.T. Suggs, and E.C. Hall, *Appl Microbiol* **18**:824, 1969.

17. D. Hoffman, *J Allerg Clin Immunol* **51**:303, 1973.

18. J. Holmgren and A.M. Svennerholm, *Immunity* **7**:759, 1973.

19. E. Ishikawa, *J Biochem* **73**:1319, 1973.

20. V. Jodal, S. Ahlsledt, B. Carlsson, L. Hanson, U. Lindberg, and A. Sohl, *Int Arch Allergy* **47**:537, 1974.

21. G. Kleinhammer, H. Lenz, R. Linke, and W. Gruber, *Z Anal Chem* **279**:145, 1976.

22. E.H. Lennette and N.J. Schmidt, *Diagnostic Procedures for Viral and Rickettsial Infections*, 4th edn., American Public Health Assoc., New York, 1969.

23. S. Matern, K. Tietjen, H. Matern, and W. Gerok, *In Proceedings of International Symposium on Enzyme-Labeled Immunoassay of Hormones and Drugs, Ulm, West Germany*, Walter de Gruyter, Berlin, 1978.

24. Q.R. Miranda, G.D. Bailey, A.S. Fraser, and H.J. Tenoso, *J Infect Dis* **136**(Suppl.):S304, 1977.

25. K. Miyai, K. Ishibashi, and Y. Kumahara, *Clin Chem Acta* **67**:263, 1976.

26. P.K. Nakane and J.A. Kawaoi, *Cytochemistry* **22**:1084, 1974.

27. E. Ruitenberg, P. Sturenberg, B. Brosi, and J. Buys, *J Immunol Methods* **10**:67, 1976.

28. J.L. Sever, *J Immunol* **88**:320, 1962.

29. A. Shelokov, E.J. Vogel, and I. Chi, *Proc Soc Exp Biol Med* **97**:802, 1958.

30. L. Spence, M. Fauvel, R. Petro, and S. Bloch, *J Clin Microbiol* **5**:248, 1977.

31. E.F. Ullman, J. Blakemore, R.K. Leute, W. Eimstad, and A. Jaklitsch, *Clin Chem* **21**:1011, 1975 (Abstract).

32. B.K. Van Weemen and A.H. Schuurs, *FEBS Lett* **15**:232, 1971.

33. B.K. Van Weemen and A.H. Schuurs, *Immunochemistry* **12**:667, 1975.

34. J. Veldkamp and A.M. Visser, *Br J Vener Dis* **51**:227, 1975.

35. A. Voller, A. Bartlett, and D.E. Bidwell, *Trans Roy Soc Trop Med Hyg* **70**:98, 1976.

36. A. Voller and D.E. Bidwell, *Br Trans Exp Pathol* **57**:243, 1975.

37. C.B. Walberg, *In Proceedings of International Symposium on Enzyme-Labeled Immunoassay of Hormones and Drugs, Ulm, West Germany*, Walter de Gruyter, Berlin, 1978.

38. R.H. Yolken, R.G. Wyatt, G. Zissis, C.D. Brandt, W.J. Rodriguez, H.W. Kim, R.H. Parrott, J.J. Urritia, L. Mata, H.B. Greenberg, A.Z. Kapikian, and R.M. Chanock, *N Engl J Med* **299**:1156, 1978.

Chapter 9

Bacteriophage Immunoassay of Hormones Using β-Galactosidase as a Measure of Phage Infectivity

MICHAEL YOUNG, M.D., and ALBERT L. NICHOLS, M.D.

INTRODUCTION

It has long been known that treatment of bacteriophages with antiphage antiserum renders these viruses noninfective for their host bacterium. This finding led to the idea that if antigens were covalently coupled to bacteriophages, then antibodies to the coupled antigen might block infectivity. This has proved to be the case, and several antigens have been chemically linked to phage. The principal of the assay method is that phage-antigen conjugates are rendered noninfective for bacteria by antisera to the coupled antigen, and free antigen competes for antibody in this reaction. The higher the concentration of free antigen, the fewer phage-antigen particles will be inactivated by antibody. Thus by quantitating the number of viable phages, it is possible to measure the concentration of free uncoupled antigen. For an account of phage biology and immunology the reader is referred to the book by Adams,[1] and for a comprehensive review of phage immunoassays in general, the work of Haimovich and Sela is excellent.[2]

Department of Biochemistry and Molecular Biology, University of Florida, College of Medicine, Gainesville, Fla. 32610, and Nichols Institute, San Pedro, Calif. 90731.

One of the problems with bacteriophage immunoassays in the past is that phage infectivity has been measured by the conventional method of treating host bacteria (*E. coli*) with bacteriophage and then plating these mixtures upon nutrient agar. After about 24 h in culture, lysis plaques are counted as a measure of the number of phages that have remained infective. This procedure is both time consuming and laborious, particularly if one is interested in doing many assays at the same time. Consequently, we have developed a new method for measuring lysis of the host bacteria, utilizing the liberation of the enzyme β-galactosidase into solution when the host bacteria rupture following phage infection and replication.

PRINCIPLE OF THE METHOD

The basic features of the phage assay procedure are as follows. Phage-antigen conjugates are prepared and purified. These conjugates are then treated with antibody to the antigen in the presence of various concentrations of the antigen. After a suitable time period, a second antibody directed against the first is added, and an aliquot of the mixture is plated with the host bacterium onto agar in a petri dish. The basic feature of the β-galactosidase modification is as follows. Mutants of *E. coli* are selected which are constitutive for the enzyme. What this means is that some 10% of the total bacterial protein consists of this single enzyme. Phage infectivity is reflected by the amount of β-galactosidase that is liberated into the medium, this value is then related to the concentration of free antigen, and a standard curve is constructed. The amount of liberated β-galactosidase is proportional to the concentration of infective bacteriophage, and a colorimetric assay (to be described below) is used to relate concentration of free antigen (hormone) to the amount of enzyme activity that is measured.

MATERIALS AND METHODS

For the host bacteria, we utilize the constitutive strain *E. coli* K12 and the wild type strain of bacteriophage T4 (T4Dr$^+$). These organisms can be obtained from the American Type Culture Collection. The preparation of high titer phage stocks and the methods used for growing both bacteriophage and bacteria have been previously described.[3] Thyroid stimulating hormone (TSH) and its antibody-containing serum were obtained from the Nichols Institute for Endocrinology, and it was covalently linked to bacteriophage T4 utilizing gluteraldehyde as the crosslinking reagent, as previously described.[3] For measurement of the enzyme β-galactosidase, the substrate orthonitrophenyl-β-D-galactoside is employed, and hydrolysis of this substrate is measured spectrophotometrically at 420 nm.

RESULTS

Figure 1 illustrates what happens when a rapidly growing midlog culture of *E. coli* K12 is infected at 0 time with T4 phage. For this purpose, 10^7 bacteria/ml were infected with 10^5 phage/ml. Over time, samples were withdrawn and analyzed for liberated enzyme. In this figure, the successive lysis steps are numbered 1, 2, and 3. Step 1 is not seen, because not enough bacteria have been lysed. Lysis steps 2 and 3 reflect the magnification of infectivity that results from successive bacteriophage replication steps. We have chosen to employ the second-state plateau shown in Figure 1 for two reasons. First, utilization of this stage shortens the time required for the assay, and second, sufficient color (due to liberated *o*-nitrophenol) is developed secondary to release of β-galactosidase to permit accurate optical density readings.

Utilizing the second stage of infection shown in Figure 1, we now show that the amount of galactosidase liberated is strictly proportional to the

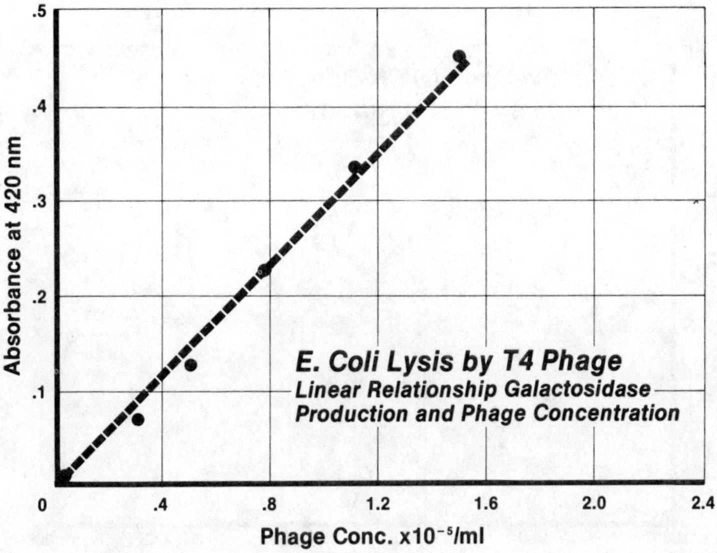

Fig. 1. Lysis of constitutive strain of *E. coli* by T4 phage. A midlog culture of bacteria (5×10^7/ml) was infected with phage to a final concentration of 1×10^5 viruses/ml at zero time. At the indicated times, samples were withdrawn and bacteria were removed by centrifugation. Aliquots of the supernatant solutions were treated with *o*-nitrophenyl β-D-galactoside (1 n*M*) and then incubated for 20 min at 37°C. Liberated *o*-nitrophenol was measured by absorbance at 420 nm.

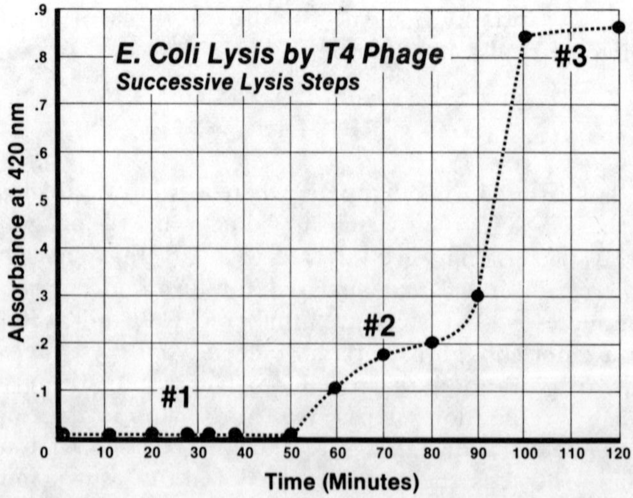

Fig. 2. Liberation of bacterial β-galactosidase as a function of infecting phage concentration. Midlog cultures of *E. coli* were infected with increasing concentrations of T4. After 60 min at 37°C, bacteria were removed by centrifugation, and concentrations of enzyme were measured as described in the legend to Figure 1.

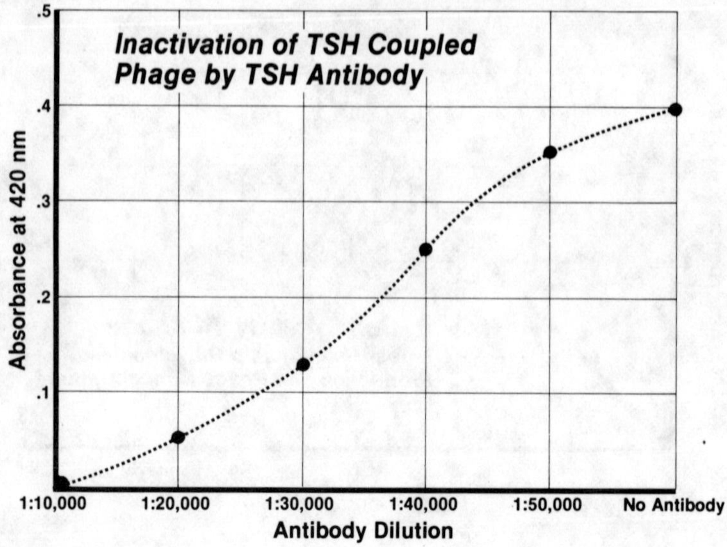

Fig. 3. Inactivation of TSH-T4 conjugates by TSH antibody. Reaction mixtures contained 100 μl each of antiserum and TSH-T4 (1×10^7 phage/ml). These solutions were incubated for 2 h at 37°C, following which 100 μl of a goat anti-IgG antiserum was added for 2 h at 37°C. Aliquots of these solutions were then removed, added to a midlog culture of *E. coli* and liberated enzyme was measured as previously described.

concentration of infecting phage. Figure 2 shows that when a midlog culture of *E. coli* containing approximately 10^7 bacteria/ml is infected with increasing quantities of phage, the absorbance at 420 nm is linear with phage concentration. For purposes of this experiment, the midlog culture was infected with the concentration of phage shown, and after 60–70 min (see Fig. 1), bacteria were removed by centrifugation, orthonitrophenyl-β-D-galactoside was added, and the color developed was measured after 20 min at 37°C.

Figure 3 illustrates what happens when TSH phage conjugates are rendered noninfective by TSH antibody. For this study, T4-TSH conjugates were treated with the dilution of antiserum shown on the *x* axis and incubated for 4 h at 37°C. Aliquots of these solutions were then added to a midlog culture of *E. coli* K12, and the liberation of β-galactosidase was measured as previously described. It will be seen that as the antibody is progressively diluted, the liberated color due to orthonitrophenol increases. This feature reflects decreasing inactivation of the TSH-T4 as the antiserum is diluted.

A standard curve for TSH is shown in Figure 4. For this study, antibody dilutions of 1:40,000 were incubated with TSH phage conjugates in the presence of increasing concentrations of free unconjugated TSH. It will be seen that the color liberated increases as the concentration of TSH increases, and this result stems from the fact

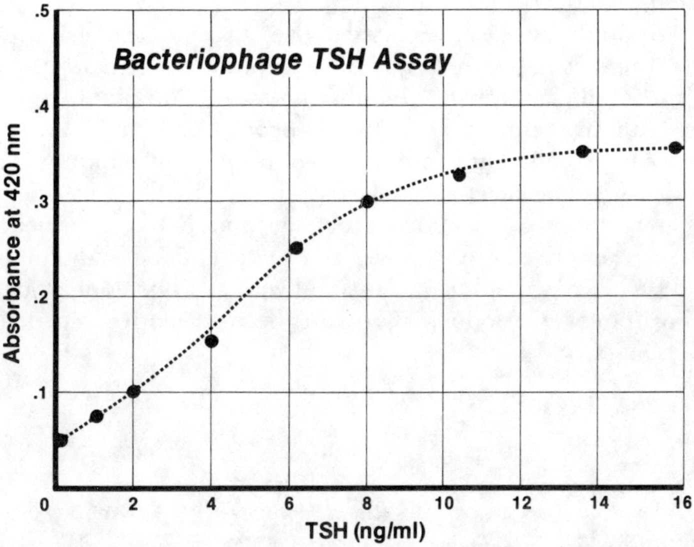

Fig. 4. Standard immunoassay curve for TSH. Solutions of antiserum (1:40,000 dilution), TSH-T4, and several different concentrations of free, unconjugated TSH were reacted as described in the legend to Figure 3. Aliquots were withdrawn and measured for liberated β-galactosidase.

that TSH is competing with the TSH-phage conjugates for the antibody. Standard curves such as this are highly reproducible, and the sensitivity that is achieved here is strictly comparable to that which can be achieved by conventional radioimmunoassay.

DISCUSSION AND CONCLUSIONS

Although the use of bacteriophage as a tracer in immunoassays has been utilized to measure the concentration of a variety of hormones and other substances, it has suffered from the fact that tedious plating assays for phage quantitation have previously been employed. The results presented here demonstrate that the use of a constitutive strain of *E. coli* can be utilized to advantage, since the measurement of liberated β-galactosidase is quantitative, simple, and rapidly performed. For example, following reaction of TSH phage, antibody, and free competing hormone, the time required to complete the galactosidase assay is somewhere between 60 and 90 min. This time could be shortened even further if one were to use a fluorescent substrate for β-galactosidase such as β-umbelliferyl-β-D-galactoside. We have utilized this substrate effectively to measure concentrations of enzyme two orders of magnitude lower than those described in the present study. What this means is that the galactosidase assay time could easily be shortened to about 10 min.

Based upon the studies presented above, it seems clear that the use of mutant strains of *E. coli* in conjunction with the phage assay provides a highly useful alternative to radioimmunoassay. For example, unstable isotopes, gamma counters, and other expensive equipment and reagent expense are virtually eliminated. The only piece of equipment that is required for the galactosidase assay is an inexpensive bench-top colorimeter, and reagents such as phage and *E. coli* are cheap. The assays are as sensitive as those obtained by conventional radioimmunoassay, and the assay should be most useful with any hormone or naturally occurring biologic product that can be covalently joined to the bacteriophage.

REFERENCES

1. M.H. Adams, Bacteriophages. Wiley (Interscience), New York, 1959.

2. J. Haimovich and M. Sela, Antibody reactions with chemically modified bacteriophages. *Methods Immunol Immunochem* **4**:386–398, 1977.

3. M. Young, M.H. Blanchard, and J.D. Saide, Nerve growth factor: radioimmunoassay and bacteriophage immunoassay. *In Methods of Hormone Radioimmunoassay,* B.M. Jaffe and H.R. Behrman (eds.), Academic, New York, 1979, pp. 941–958.

Chapter 10

Polypeptide Hormone Receptors as Binding Agents

BRIJ B. SAXENA Ph.D., D.Sc. AND PREMILA RATHNAM Ph.D.

INTRODUCTION

The single primary event that has led to the actual concept of a "receptor" is the binding of a hormone to a specific recognition site at the target organ to initiate a sequence of steps resulting in the target cell response.[1] A "receptor" is therefore defined as an entity that specifically binds a hormone to mediate target cell response. Receptors to hormones are present in the target organ of the respective hormone. A considerable amount of research has been done on steroid hormone receptors; however, in this paper, we will focus on the receptors of polypeptide hormones. Specific receptors have been recognized for the glycoprotein hormones (FSH, LH, TSH, and hCG) in the mouse, rat, pig, cow, and human ovary, and in rat and human testes.[2]

So far, there appears to be one receptor for LH and hCG. The observation that polypeptide hormones fixed to the tissue are still able to bind to a specific antibody indicated a surface location, such as the plasma membrane, for the site of the initial interaction with the receptor. Purification of tissue homogenates has confirmed the concentration of LH-hCG receptors in the plasma membranes. There is, however, evidence that polypeptide hormones can also enter the cells or that the membrane-bound hormone-receptor complex can be "internalized" by the process of endocytosis.[3] Partial purification of the receptor molecules has been achieved.[2,4,5] Altered secretion, circulation and/or abnormal

Cornell University Medical College, Division of Endocrinology, New York, NY

circulating forms of the hormone, defects in the receptor and its binding to the hormone, as well as additional abnormalities in the intracellular components of the receptor mechanism beyond the target-site uptake lead to eventual end organ failure.[6] Current research on the receptor has been directed to the binding of the hormone by the receptor in order to understand the regulation and the perturbation in the endocrine function. The identification and isolation of hormone receptors has also been undertaken in order to elucidate the intimate biochemical details in the modulation of the hormone-receptor interaction. The immediate

Table 1. Tissue Receptors for Polypeptide Hormones

Hormone	Tissue	Reference
1. hCG/LH	Testis	Dufau et al.[51]
	Ovary	Lee and Ryan[52]; Kammerman et al.[53]
		Rao and Saxena[54]; Haour and Saxena[29]; Saxena[2]
2. FSH	Testis	Bhalla and Reichert[55]
	Ovary	Haour and Saxena[29]
3. TSH	Thyroid	Moore and Wolff[25]
4. Prolactin	Breast	Shiu and Friesen[56]
	Liver	Posner et al.[57]
	Ovary (corpus luteum)	Saito and Saxena[58]
5. Growth hormone	Cultured human lymphocytes	Lesniak et al.[59]
	Liver	Tsushima and Friesen[60]
6. ACTH	Adrenal	Lefkowitz et al.[61]
7. Insulin	Liver	Freychet et al.[62]
	Fat	Cuatrecasas[63]
	Lymphocytes	Gavin et al.[64]
	Placenta	Posner[65]
8. LH-RH	Pituitary	Spona[66]; Park et al.[67]
9. TRH	Pituitary	Barden and Labrie[68]
10. Oxytocin	Uterus	Soloff and Swartz[69]
	Breast	Soloff and Swartz[70]
11. Vasopressin	Kidney	Rajerison et al.[71]
12. Angiotensin	Kidney, adrenal	Glossmann et al.[72]
13. Calcitonin	Kidney	Marx et al.[73]
	Bone	Marx et al.[74]
14. Parathormone	Kidney	Dibella et al.[75]
15. Glucagon	Liver	Tomasi et al.[76]
	β-Cells	Goldfine et al.[77]

and most useful application of receptor research is in the use of receptors as binding agents in receptorassays, in the preparation of hormone-free sera, and in the purification of hormones.

RECEPTORS

Source

The sources of the receptors of the various polypeptide hormones are given in Table 1. The preparation of plasma membranes from bovine corpora lutea, containing receptors, is shown in Diagram 1.

PREPARATION OF PLASMA MEMBRANES

ONE HUNDRED FRESH BOVINE CORPORA LUTEA, 500 g FRESH TISSUE, (PULVERIZED IN LIQUID NITROGEN)

↓

HOMOGENATE (2.5 l OF 10 mM TRIS-HCl, pH 7.4, CONTAINING 0.25 M SUCROSE, 1 mM $CaCl_2$, $MgCl_2$ AND DTT, AND 10,000 IU TRASYLOL AT 4°C).

↓

FILTER THROUGH TWO LAYERS OF CHEESECLOTH TO REMOVE CONNECTIVE TISSUE AND INTACT CELL AGGREGATES (THE LARGER PARTICLES MAY BE PROCESSED AS ABOVE).

↓

THE HOMOGENATE IS FURTHER GROUND IN A TYPE-C TEFLON-GLASS HOMOGENIZER WITH A CLEARANCE SIZE OF 0.12 - 0.17 mm BY 10 TO 15 STROKES.

↓

FIRST CENTRIFUGATION (650xg FOR 20 MIN. AT 4°C)

↓

$PELLET_1$ (INTACT CELLS, NUCLEI, CELL DEBRIS, MAY BE RE-GROUND AS ABOVE: CENTRIFUGED AS IN STEP 2, AND THE SUPERNATE POOLED WITH $SUPERNATE_1$).

$SUPERNATE_1$ (PLASMA MEMBRANES, MITOCHONDRIA AND MICROSOMES).

↓

SECOND CENTRIFUGATION (13,000xg FOR 60 MIN.,4°C)

↓

$PELLET_2$ (HOMOGENIZED AND SUSPENDED IN 500 ml OF TRIS-HCL BUFFER AND INJECTED IN 100 ml ALIQUOTS INTO A ZONAL ROTOR CONTAINING 500 ml OF LINEAR SUCROSE GRADIENT OF 30-50% (W/V) AND SPINNING AT 3000 rpm. THEN CENTRIFUGED FOR 90 min AT 4°C AT 25,000 rpm.

$SUPERNATE_2$

↓

ELUTION (20 ml FRACTIONS)

↓

PLASMA MEMBRANES (ALIQUOTED AND LYOPHILIZED)

Properties of the Gonadotropin Receptors

1. Receptors are molecules that bind the hormone to mediate cell response.

2. Receptors are macromolecules, predominantly protein in nature. Proteolytic enzymes destroy their activity. Carbohydrate moieties of the receptor are involved in the "recognition" process during hormone-receptor interaction. Lipid components at the receptor site stabilize the "steric conformation" necessary for hormone binding.

3. Typical physical features of the receptor are structural specificity, high affinity, usually limited capacity, ready saturability, relatively rapid kinetics, and an appropriate degree of reversibility.

4. The binding of the hormone to the receptor is rapid, saturable, and reversible, and follows a second-order reaction kinetics:

$$H + R \underset{K_d}{\overset{K_a}{\rightleftharpoons}} H \cdot R; \qquad \frac{(H \cdot R)}{(H) \cdot (R)} = K_a$$

From the above equations, one can calculate the affinity constant and the number of binding sites using a Scatchard plot.

5. Molecular weights of the receptor have been found to be in the range of 50,000–300,000 daltons. Intact disulfide (but not free SH groups) and divalent cations, such as Mg^{2+}, Mn^{2+}, and Ca^{2+}, are essential for the activity.

6. Receptorassays provide a measure of biological activity as well as sensitivity and precision higher than the conventional bioassays.

7. Receptors are, in general, "species nonspecific."

8. The hormone-receptor binding has a higher initial association rate at 37°C than at 4°C. At 37°C, steady states of hormone-receptor binding are approached within 30 min. There is a rapid degradation of receptors during incubation at 34° or 37°C. The optimum pH for hormone-receptor binding is in the range of 6–7.

9. The receptor exists in low concentrations in target cells (0.01% of the total cytoplasmic proteins). Receptors occur in two entities: (1) high affinity, low capacity receptors, and (2) low affinity, high capacity receptors. The former entity has a vital physiological role.

10. The specificity and high affinity ($>10^9\ M^{-1}$) of the receptor compensates for the low concentration of hormones in the peripheral circulation, which is sufficient to initiate optimum cell response.

HORMONES: FSH, LH, TSH, AND hCG

Source and Properties

FSH, LH, and TSH are hormones secreted by the anterior pituitary gland. hCG is normally secreted by the placenta during pregnancy. The above hormones are glycoproteins containing 70–80% of protein and 20–30% of carbohydrates. The carbohydrates consist of galactose, mannose, sialic acid, *N*-acetyl galactosamine, *N*-acetyl glucosamine, and fucose. FSH, LH, TSH, and hCG have been isolated in highly purified states, which are suitable for hormone-receptor binding studies.[7-11]

The glycoprotein hormones are composed of a hormone-nonspecific α and a hormone-specific β subunit, which are noncovalently linked. The subunits can be dissociated by reagents like urea, guanidine hydrochloride, or propionic acid, which cause the perturbation of hydrogen bonding. The subunits have little biological activity. The α subunits among the glycoprotein hormones are nearly identical and can be reassociated with the β subunits to regenerate the biological activity of the respective hormone. The β subunits are different from each other and confer hormone specificity. The lack of binding activity of the subunits to the receptor suggests that the specific intrinsic biological activity and recognition properties conferred are manifested during the association of the hormone-specific β subunit to the α subunit. These observations also give credence to the current concepts based on chemical modification studies that the interaction of the hormone to the receptor is via the overlying α subunit, whereas the β subunit is located under the α subunit to provide the hormone-specific conformation.[12,13]

All preparations of α subunits are heterogeneous at the amino terminal region. The entire intact structure at the amino terminal, therefore, may not be necessary in the recombination with the β subunit and thus in the regeneration of the biological activity. There is also heterogeneity in the carbohydrate moieties, where the most notable differences occur in sialic acid at the terminal position of the carbohydrate chains. Loss of sialic acid expedites the hepatic clearance of the glycoprotein hormones; hence the variation in the sialic acid content can be correlated with the variation in the biological activity in *in vivo* bioassays. However, differences in the sialic acid content do not affect the *in vitro* receptor binding of the hormone. These observations suggest that the role of sialic acid lies in the maintenance of the metabolic halflife of the hormone. Desialylated LH and hCG bind to the receptor with equal or enhanced activity compared to that of the respective fully sialylated molecules. Similarly, the removal of galactose does not affect the binding of the hormone to the receptor; however, further sequential removal or modification of carbohydrate moieties may impair the ability of the hormone to elicit cAMP stimulation without impairment of binding ability.[14] A receptor thus provides an essential tool in the evaluation of agonistic and antagonistic analogs of the hormones.

The protein structures of LH and hCG are very similar, and the current evidence suggests that both hormones act at the same receptor but with different affinities. hCG exhibits affinity of binding to the receptor two- to threefold higher than hLH. It may be of interest to note that when hCG and LH are compared in terms of metabolic halflife and relative potency per unit mass, hCG seems to be a more stable molecule in the circulation, which may be due to the higher carbohydrate content of "epitopes." Elucidation of the detailed amino acid sequences of hLH and hCG has led to an appreciation that certain structural differences can potentially be exploited to improve methods for the detection of hCG in the presence of hLH in early pregnancy and in various clinical conditions.

HORMONE-RECEPTOR INTERACTION

Basic Mechanism

The proposed details of the mechanism of hormone action are exemplified in Diagram 2. It has not been established whether the binding component and adenylate cyclase are the same or two different components. There is evidence in the favor of the latter (regulatory vs. catalytic unit). The binding of the cholera toxin to a glycolipid component of the cell membrane, the monosialylganglioside G_{MI}, activates the adenylate cyclase in almost all tissues that possess this enzyme. The activation of adenyl cyclase and the involvement of gangliosides appear to be common components of all the polypeptide hormone-receptor interactions. Binding of cAMP to the regulatory unit of the protein kinase causes the dissociation of the regulatory-catalytic (RC) unit and release of the catalytic subunit, which initiates the phosphorylation of protein substrates like phosphorylase kinase, glycogen synthetase, and adipose tissue glyceride lipase. This event is followed by translocation of cyclic AMP dependent protein kinase from the cytoplasm to the nucleus. The effects of cyclic AMP upon protein synthesis have been found to be more frequently expressed at the translational level, although stimulation of biosynthetic processes by cyclic AMP has been suggested to occur by an effect upon messenger RNA transcription. Protein kinase operates functionally as a single enzyme in mediating numerous roles of cyclic AMP upon cellular function. The diversity in cellular response to cAMP and to peptide hormones is determined by the nature of the protein kinase substrates or by processes that regulate genetic expression and cellular differentiation within the target cell.[15]

Kinetics

In an ideal state, using an isolated hormone and an isolated receptor moiety, the hormone-receptor interaction can be defined as a bimolecular, reversible, reaction:

$$(H) + (R) \underset{K_d}{\overset{K_a}{\rightleftharpoons}} (HR)$$

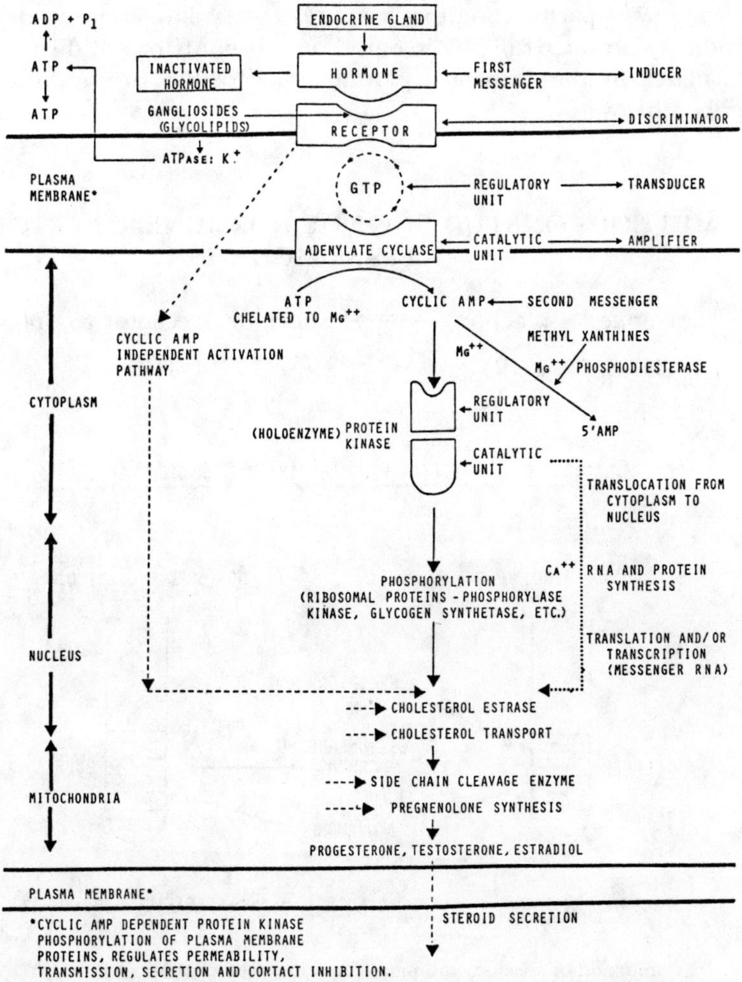

where H is the hormone, R is the receptor, HR is the hormone-receptor complex, K_a is the association rate constant, and K_d is the dissociation rate constant. Affinity is measured as K_D (the equilibrium dissociation constant) of the receptor-hormone interaction.[16] It is numerically equal to the rate of association of the hormone from its receptor divided by its rate of dissociation.

$$K_D = K_a/K_d$$

Therefore, a slow rate of dissociation of hormone from its receptor coupled with a fast rate of association yields high affinity binding. Hence the lower the K_d, the higher the affinity. In addition, the K_D is also the concentration of hormone required to half-saturate the receptor. High affinity, low capacity receptors require a very low concentration of hormone to produce full physiological response. Affinity of the receptor is calculated by the Scatchard plot analysis[17] of the saturation data as described below.

METHODS OF STUDYING THE HORMONE-RECEPTOR INTERACTION

$$\underset{(H)}{\text{hormone}} + \underset{(R)}{\text{receptor}} \rightleftharpoons \underset{(HR)}{\text{hormone-receptor complex}}$$

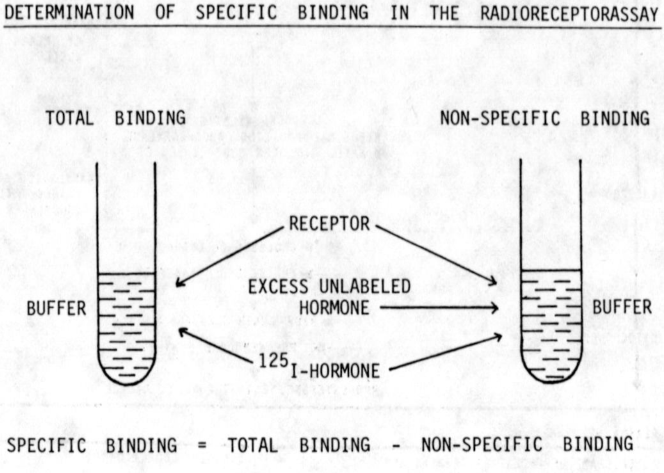

Fig. 1. Determination of specific binding in the radioreceptorassay.

The association constant of this system, K, is given by Eq. (1):

$$K = \frac{(\mathrm{HR})}{(\mathrm{H})\,(\mathrm{R})} \tag{1}$$

Rearranging, we have $K \times (\mathrm{R}) = (\mathrm{HR})/(\mathrm{H})$, and substituting $(\mathrm{R}) = (\mathrm{R})_0 - (\mathrm{HR})$, where $(\mathrm{R})_0$ is the concentration of receptor sites before addition of any hormone, the equation gives:

$$K\,(\mathrm{R})_0 - K(\mathrm{HR}) = (\mathrm{HR/H})$$

A plot of (HR) vs. (HR)/(H) should be linear with a slope of $-K$. When $(\mathrm{HR}) = (\mathrm{R})_0$, all the receptor sites are coupled, and $(\mathrm{HR})/(\mathrm{H}) = 0$. Consequently, the intercept on the (HR) axis gives the total binding capacity of the receptor preparation $(\mathrm{R})_0$. This is the classical Scatchard plot.

A fixed amount of a receptor preparation is incubated with increasing concentrations of radioligand until equilibrium is established. The free hormone is then separated from receptor-bound hormone. Specific binding of the hormone is determined as the difference between total binding and nonspecific binding in the presence of excess unlabeled hormone (Fig. 1). The ratio of bound to free hormone is plotted as the ordinate against the concentration of the bound as the abscissa. A straight line is indicative of a single class of binding sites. The reciprocal of the negative slope is K_D, and the intercept on the abscissa is the number of high affinity binding sites (Fig. 2).

However, in the absence of ideal ingredients of hormone-receptor binding, such as an isolated receptor moiety, it becomes difficult to interpret the data in terms of the kinetics of a simple bimolecular reaction. Damaged tracer leads to the high nonspecific binding and erroneous specific activity in terms of the biologically active molecules. The lack of information on the ratio of labeled to unlabeled molecules, and of active to inactive molecules, does not permit an accurate calculation of their molar concentration. Other factors, such as the separation of bound hormone, cooperative binding, and alterations taking place in receptors during transfer from *in vivo* to *in vitro* systems, may affect the ideal kinetics of hormone-receptor binding.

Regulation of the Receptor

The appearance of receptors is related to cell differentiation during development and maturation. Response or resistance of a given cell to hormonal stimulation has been related to the presence of the hormone receptor, and the responsiveness of the receptor is modulated by the

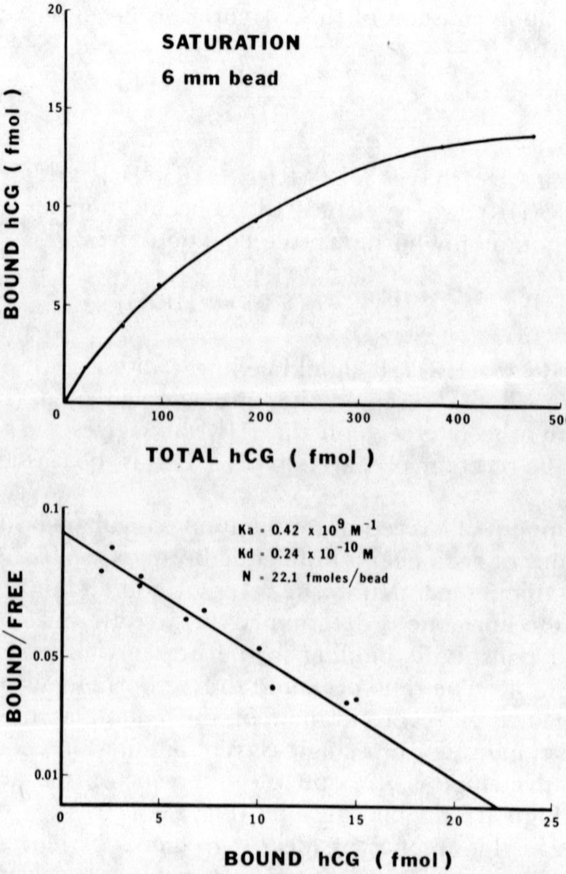

Fig. 2. Saturation of anti-hCG-β-globulin coupled glass bead with ^{125}I-hCG. Scatchard plot of saturation data.

exposure to the hormone.[6,18] For example, refractiveness can be induced in the ovarian receptors for hLH and hCG, which is associated with a decrease in the number of receptors in the target cell. The phenomenon of a "down-regulation" or "desensitization" of the receptor by the hormone has also been shown for insulin, calcitonin, hGH, TRH, vasopressin, and catecholamines, but not for ACTH and TSH.[19] Prolactin, on the other hand, does not induce desensitization of its own receptors, but may affect the receptor of other hormones, e.g., LH and hCG in the Leydig cells.[20]

The desensitization phenomenon cannot be explained by receptor occupancy, since a normal concentration of the receptor exists in the presence of high levels of hCG. Further, a lower number of rat Leydig cell receptors are also encountered in the presence of low concentration of hCG. There is a paradoxical recovery of receptor loss following down-regulation. At present, there are indications that the mechanism of down-regulation is controlled by the suppression of the synthesis of the receptor, or under acute stimulation the receptor is either actively destroyed or removed from the plasma membrane and may be internalized into the cell.

Negative Cooperativity

The affinity of receptors is high when they are unoccupied but decreases sharply when the occupancy by the hormone increases. Site-site interactions (bioactive site and cooperative site) accelerate the rate of dissociation and result in a decrease in the affinity, which is designated as negative cooperativity. This phenomenon is exhibited when the binding of the hormone to the receptor does not behave as expected from a single class of receptors obeying the law of mass action.[21] The reverse phenomenon is called positive cooperativity.

APPLICATION OF RECEPTORS AS BINDING AGENTS

Radioreceptorassays

The introduction of RIA techniques by Yalow and Berson,[22] the availability of highly purified hCG for labeling with radioisotopes with the retention of native conformation and biological activity, and the property of the receptor to specifically bind to a hormone resulted in the development of specific radioreceptorassays of LH-hCG,[23] FSH,[24] and TSH,[25] as well as of other hormones.[26] The radioreceptorassay for LH-hCG has been applied in the development of a rapid, sensitive, and biospecific pregnancy test, as well as a test for the diagnosis and management of trophoblastic disease and ectopic tumors.[27]

Satisfactory tracer, e.g., hCG, has a specific activity of one atom of ^{125}I per molecule. The labeling of tyrosines with ^{125}I is confined to the α subunit. Purification of the tracer is performed by gel filtration on Sephadex G-100, cellulose adsorption chromatography, and by chromatography on Sepharose-Concanavalin A columns. The most appropriate determination of the specific activity of the ligand is obtained by self-displacement in the radioligand receptorassay for hCG, or by *in vitro* bioassay.[28]

The principle of RRA is shown in Fig. 3. The plasma membranes from bovine corpora lutea, containing the receptor to LH-hCG, are isolated in large quantities by the use of zonal ultracentrifugation in sucrose density gradient,[23,29] aliquoted and lyophilized. The reference or the unknown serum and labeled ^{125}I-hCG are added to the tubes with the lyophilized

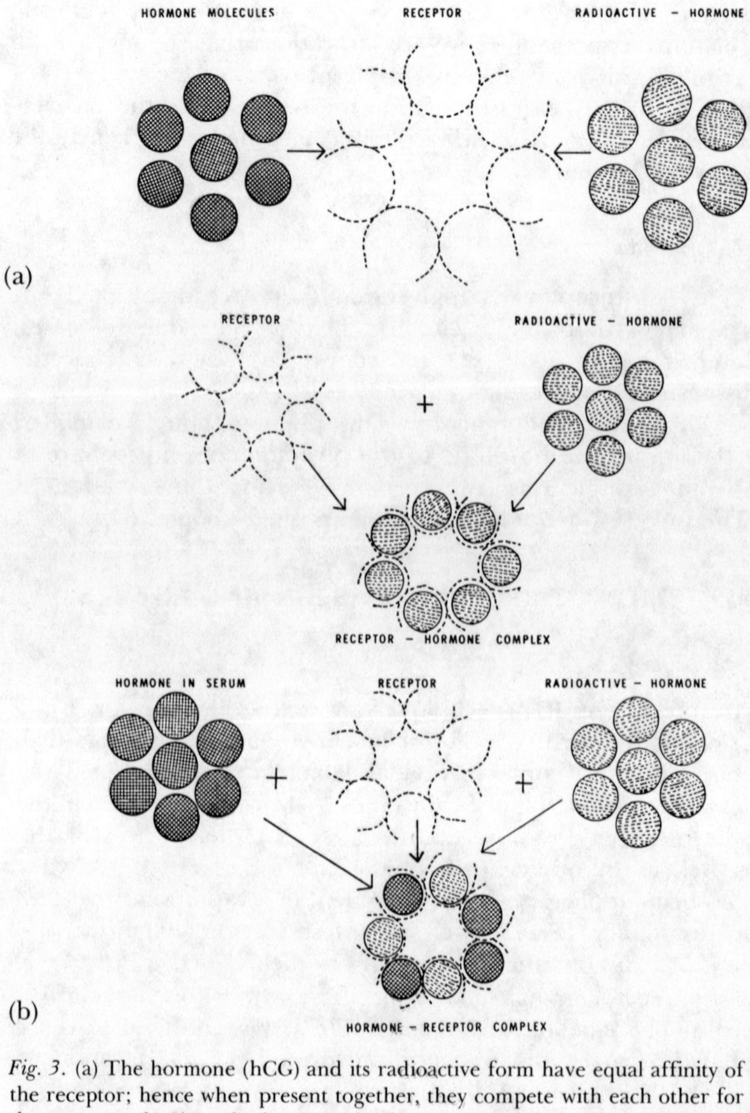

Fig. 3. (a) The hormone (hCG) and its radioactive form have equal affinity of binding to the receptor; hence when present together, they compete with each other for binding to the receptor. (b) Since the hormone in the serum and the radioactive hormone have the same affinity of binding to the receptor, fewer radioactive hormone molecules are bound to the receptor; hence the hormone-receptor complex has less radioactivity. This change in radioactivity indicates the presence of hCG in the serum and, thus, pregnancy.

receptor. After 30 min of incubation at 37°C, 1.0 ml of chilled distilled water is added and the tubes are centrifuged at 3,000 rpm for 15 min. The plasma membranes containing the receptor, being a solid phase, can be separated by a simple centrifugation step to yield the quantity of the bound labeled hormone. Following the decantation of the supernates, the precipitates are counted for one minute in an autogamma counter with approximately 51% of efficiency for ^{125}I. The entire assay could thus be completed within one hour. For quantitation, several concentrations of hCG standards are included in the assay. The unknowns are compared to the standard. The logit-log transformation of the dose-response curve of the RRA of hCG is given in Fig. 4. In the presence of normal serum, the sensitivity or the lower limit of detection of hCG in the RRA is 0.5 ng or 6 mIU per ml, with a precision of ±15%. Various dilutions of serum of a pregnant woman yielded a slope parallel to that of hCG, confirming the validity of the assay.

The receptor discriminates the active hormone from all other molecules and thereby determines the specificity of the hormone–target cell system. A receptorassay, therefore, combines the high sensitivity, precision, and reproducibility of saturation analysis procedures of radioimmunoassays and the specificity of biological assays. Due to the variations in the affinity, titer, and specificity of the antisera used in the radioimmunoassay, the immunoreactive estimates of the hormone may or may not show a correlation coefficient with the levels obtained by the receptorassay. Values obtained by the receptorassay are generally two- to threefold higher than those obtained by radioimmunoassay. The sensitivity of the receptorassay for LH and hCG is 0.5 ng per ml, which is

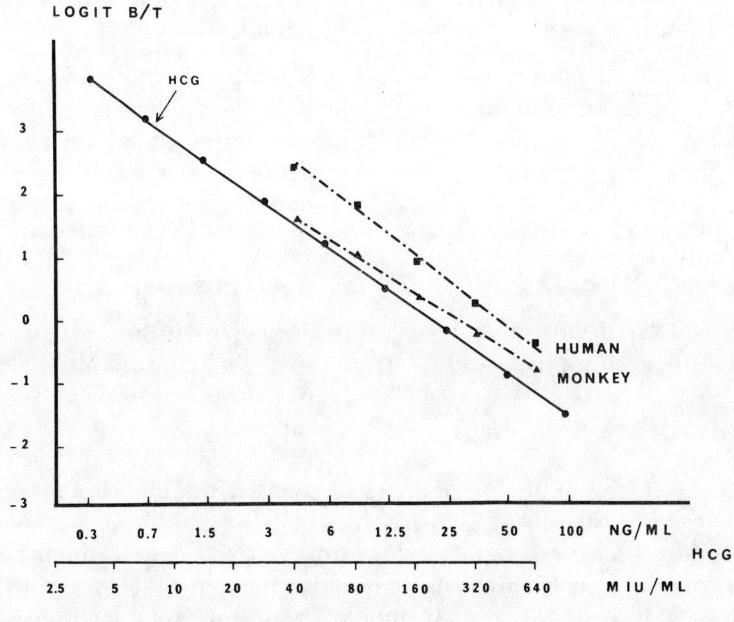

Fig. 4. Computer output of the logit-log plot of the dose-response curve of the RRA of hCG.

consistent with the equilibrium constant of $2.4 \times 10^{10}\ M^{-1}$, which is equal to or one order of magnitude above the sensitivity attainable by the radioimmunoassay, provided high affinity antisera are used. A comparison of the radioreceptorassay with the radioimmunoassay is presented hereunder.

Radioreceptorassay	*Radioimmunoassay*
1. Biological activity of the ^{125}I-hormone is essential (biologic sites are extremely susceptible to denaturation during labeling).	1. Biological activity not essential (antigenic sites are less susceptible during labeling).
2. Receptors are homogeneous and stable in the lyophilized state for extended periods.	2. Antibodies are heterogeneous and are stable for extended periods.
3. Binding affinity of the receptor is high and consistent.	3. Binding affinity of the antibody is variable (requires pure antigen and immunization of a large number of animals to select appropriate antibody).
4. Equilibrium is approached with 1-h incubation.	4. Requires 24–48 h to approach equilibrium.
5. Separation of bound and free is rapid (centrifugation).	5. Separation of bound and free is by precipitation and is time consuming; however, antibody coupled to a solid phase renders the separation simple and rapid.
6. Good precision.	6. Good precision.
7. Measures biological activity (physiological significance).	7. Measures immunological activity (may be of physiological or nonphysiological significance).

The development of quantitative RIA and RRA of hCG has permitted the detection of hCG as early as one week after documented conception,[27] and has significantly improved the management of the first trimester of pregnancy. A quantitative Biocept-G kit for the RRA is commercially available from Wampole Laboratories. Other uses of the receptorassay include detection of antibodies to the receptor and evaluation of the antifertility vaccine as described later.

Clinical Application of the Radioreceptorassay of hCG

PREGNANCY AND/OR AMENORRHEA

The RRA of hCG is virtually 100% reliable on the day of the first missed period or at four weeks from the last menstrual period in a 28–30 day cycle.[27] False negative results can occur if the day of ovulation is delayed. If the quantitative RRA is performed during the LH peak or delayed LH peak, a level of 15–20 ng or 180–240 mIU per ml may be obtained. A repeat assay after 24–48 h will be necessary to confirm or rule out pregnancy. During ovulation as well as during the pre- and postmenopausal periods, the RRA may yield LH levels in the range of 10–30 ng/ml. In these cases, a repeat assay is necessary to rule out pregnancy. The declining and the plateauing of the hormone levels will indicate ovulation and menopause, respectively, whereas rising levels of hCG will indicate pregnancy (Fig. 5). However, the sensitivity of the Biocept-G, the commercialized pregnancy test, is set at 200 mIU, which permits the detection of pregnancy on day 10 after ovulation with virtually no interference with LH (Table 2).

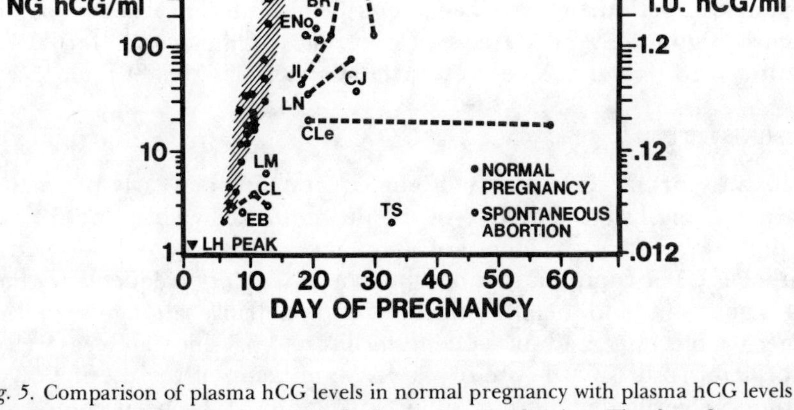

Fig. 5. Comparison of plasma hCG levels in normal pregnancy with plasma hCG levels in 15 patients who subsequently experienced spontaneous abortion. The day of pregnancy was based on the last menstrual period and the usual length of cycle reported by the patient.

Table 2. Sensitivities of Various Pregnancy Tests

Test	Sensitivity (IU/liter)
Tube tests:	
Biocept-G (RRA) (quantitative)	6
Biocept-G (RRA) (Wampole Labs.)[a]	200
Accusphere (Organon, Inc.)	750
Pregnostic (Organon, Inc.)	750
Pregnosis Placentex (Roche Labs.)	1,000
UCG-Lyphotest (Wampole Labs.)	1,250
E.P.T. (Warner-Chilcott Labs.)	1,250[b]
Slide tests:	
Dri-Dot (Organon, Inc.)	1,500
Pregnosis (Roche Labs.)	1,500
Pregnosticon (Organon, Inc.)	1,500
UCG (Wampole Labs.)	2,000
Gravidex (Ortho Pharm. Corp.)	3,500

[a]Sensitivity of quantitative RRA and RIA: 0.6 IU per liter.
[b]Estimated.

Spontaneous Abortion

The high sensitivity of the RRA (0.5 ng or 6 mIU of hCG/ml) has revealed many abnormal pregnancies, which are indicated by levels of hCG that are significantly lower than the normal values for the duration of gestation (Fig. 5).[30] These pregnancies result in inevitable abortions. The RRA has also detected very early pregnancies that abort before the first missed period and have been described as subclinical abortions[31] or occult pregnancies.[32] The frequencies of such pregnancies in fertile and unprotected women has been estimated to be much greater than 15%.[33]

Miniabortion

Because of the unreliability of current tests in very early pregnancy with no clinical signs, 30–40% of the procedures have been performed in the absence of any evidence of pregnancy, as verified by endometrial pathology. The complications of miniabortion are not frequent, but they are significant, and include infection, endometritis, salpingitis, uterine synechia, bleeding, and subsequent sterility and psychic trauma as well as exorbitant cost.[34] By the use of the RRA, invasion of the uterine cavity without a verified indication of pregnancy has thus been completely eliminated. In addition, the early confirmation of pregnancy has permitted selective and optimum scheduling for miniabortion.

Ectopic Pregnancy

The clinical value of the RRA of hCG has been demonstrated in the diagnosis of ectopic pregnancy, which continues to be one of the most frequent cases of maternal morbidity and death in the United States. The hCG levels are lower in ectopic pregnancy (Fig. 6) than in normal gestation of the same duration with no clinical signs of pregnancy from either palpation or curettage of the uterus. In a total of 50 suspected ectopic pregnancies, two negative RRAs performed on subsequent days virtually exclude the diagnosis of ectopic pregnancy. It has lessened hospital admissions by eliminating indications for diagnostic procedures including curettage, colpotomy, and laparoscopy. Earlier antenatal care in the first trimester with the use of the quantitative RRA for hCG has been invaluable in reducing the morbidity and deaths associated with ectopic pregnancy.

Hydatidiform Mole and Choriocarcinoma

Human chorionic gonadotropin (hCG) is synthesized by trophoblastic tumors and has been established as a reliable index of tumor activity. Serum hCG was measured by RRA as well as hCG, and its free α and β subunits were measured by RIA, in 14 patients with hydatidiform mole and in three patients with choriocarcinoma.[35] From our study of these four indicators of hCG activity in trophoblastic disease, the following conclusions were drawn. The RRA, because of its biospecificity,

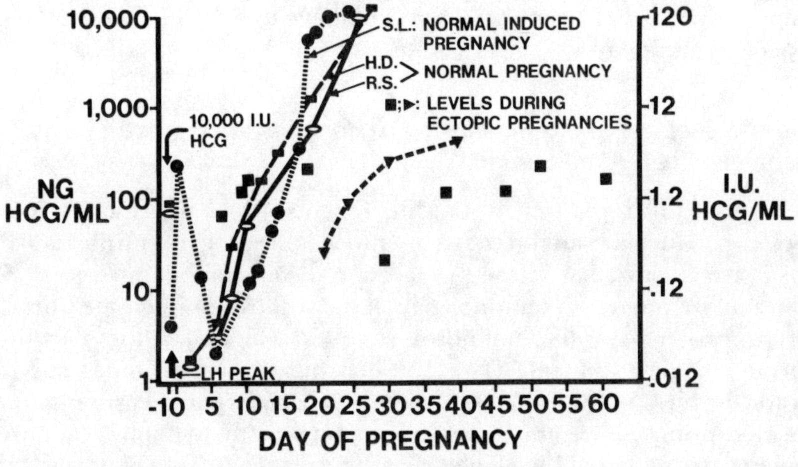

Fig. 6. Comparison of the plasma levels of hCG during two normal pregnancies (H.D. and R.S.) and one induced ovulation resulting in intrauterine pregnancy (S.L.) with the hCG levels of 10 patients with ectopic pregnancies. The day of pregnancy was based on the last menstrual period reported by the patient.

simplicity, and rapidity, is the most useful diagnostic tool and should be performed frequently during the initial stages of treatment in trophoblastic neoplasia, until the levels fall within the sensitivity range of the assay. At this stage, assays of hCG by both RRA and RIA, and assays of hCG-β and hCG-α by RIA are performed and treatment is continued until hCG and hCG-β are negative and hCG-α has declined to within normal limits.

Detection of Ovulation

The RRA has the double advantage of detecting the midcycle LH peak and hCG rise six to eight days later in serum (Fig. 5) and eight to ten days later in an unextracted morning sample of urine.[36] The RRA may be used to supplement the basal body temperature curve to further pinpoint ovulation. The RRA also recognizes LH. However, the receptor has one-third or lesser affinity for the LH as compared to hCG. The rapidity and sensitivity of the RRA for determining the ovulatory LH surge have proved valuable tools in artificial insemination and in determining the efficacy of ovulatory drugs.

Animal Husbandry

The RRA for hCG is species nonspecific and is a potential tool in livestock breeding and animal experimentation. The detection of equine, murine, canine, and human pregnancy LH-hCG-like material by the same receptor (Fig. 7), suggests that the receptor and the biological "active core" of LH from various species have undergone little mutation during evolution.

Use of Receptors in the Purification of Hormones and in the Preparation of LH-free Serum

The use of receptors as binding agents for a specific hormone provides a novel and effective method in the final purification of hormones,[37] as well as in the preparation of hormone-free serum[38] for addition to the radioimmunoassay standards to compensate for the serum proteins in the unknown samples. Generally, the need for hormone-free serum in RIA is fulfilled by the sera of other species. However, the species nonspecificity of RRA limits the measurement of hormone only above the basal levels. Sera from hypophysectomized subjects are not readily available and are rarely totally free of hormones.

Plasma membranes containing the "receptors" are isolated from bovine corpora lutea by zonal ultracentrifugation in sucrose density gradient.[29] hCG containing 12,000 IU/mg was used as standard and for iodination with ^{125}I-Na to a S.A. of 30–50 μCi/μg.[39] Serum pools from

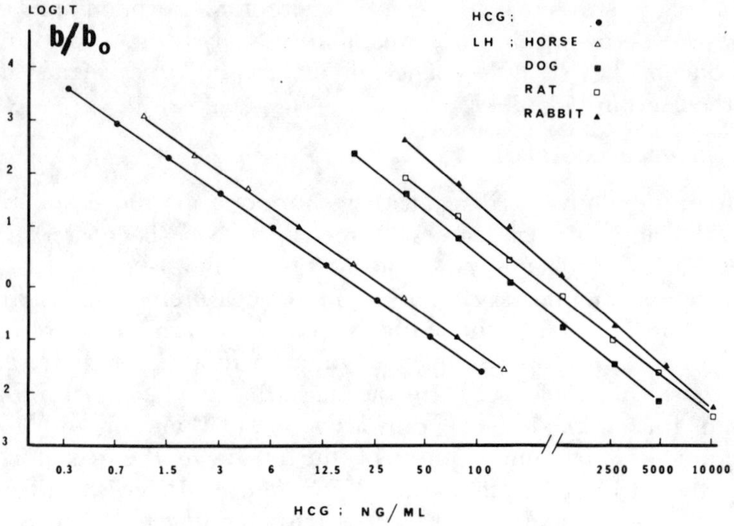

Fig. 7. Competitive inhibition of the binding of ^{125}I-hCG by hCG and LH from various species in the radioreceptorassay. The biological potencies of human, horse, dog, and rabbit LH were 8.9, 5.5, 0.023, and 0.9 units, respectively, in terms of NIH-LH-S1.

luteal phase were used for the preparation of LH-free serum. Five ml of receptors, usually stored in sucrose solution, are diluted five times with 10 m*M* Tris-HCl buffer of pH 7.2, containing 1 m*M* $MgCl_2$ and 1 m*M* $CaCl_2$, and centrifuged at 5,000 rpm for 15 min. The pellet is washed thrice as above to remove soluble material. Aliquots of 0.625, 1.25, 2.5, and 5.0 mg protein of washed receptor are incubated in 1 ml serum for 30 min at 37°C and centrifuged. The serum is decanted and analyzed for LH by RRA and RIA.[40] Total protein and its components in sera before and after receptor adsorption were analyzed by Refractometer[41] and Micro Zone electrophoresis.

In the presence of unadsorbed serum, the lowest quantity of ^{125}I-hCG is bound to the receptor, indicating competition by endogeneous LH with ^{125}I-hCG (Fig. 8). However, bound ^{125}I-hCG is increased in direct proportion to the amount of receptor used for adsorption, indicating removal of LH from the serum. At 2.5 mg receptor, the quantity of bound ^{125}I-hCG reached a plateau, with no further increase up to 5 mg receptor. The LH dissociation from pellets obtained after incubation with 1.25, 2.5, and 5 mg receptor was 4.75 ± 0.25 and 8.0 ± 0.5 ng/ml, respectively. The maximal LH is recovered from the pellet of 2.5 mg receptor. By RIA, the LH was undetectable in receptor-adsorbed serum, whereas PRL, GH, and FSH were not removed by the receptor. The content of total protein before and after receptor adsorption was 7.0 and 6.5 g%, respectively. Similarly, quantitative analysis of various protein components showed little change in the protein components of the adsorbed serum (Fig. 9).

Receptorimmunoassay

The antisera produced against the hormone-specific β subunit of hCG, showing varying degrees of specificity, have been used in the measurement of hCG in the blood by RIA in the presence of LH.[43,33] The receptorimmunoassay[42] is based on the measurement of binding of ^{125}I-hCG or ^{125}I-hLH to the antibody to hCG-β in the presence of the receptor, and provides a simple and rapid method to select antisera to hCG-β, which are biospecific in the sense that they compete with the receptor for binding to biologically active ^{125}I-hCG and not to ^{125}I-hLH (Diagram 3). Maximum binding of the tracer to the receptor and antibody is achieved in 20 min at 37°C. Figure 10 shows competition between receptor and anti-hCG-β sera for binding to ^{125}I-hCG. The ^{125}I-hCG showed a total specific binding of 22% to the receptor. At increasing concentrations of the anti-hCG-β sera, a concomitant increase in the binding of ^{125}I-hCG to the antiserum and a corresponding decrease in the binding of ^{125}I-hCG to the receptor were observed. These observations indicated that anti-hCG-β sera competed with the receptor for binding to ^{125}I-hCG.

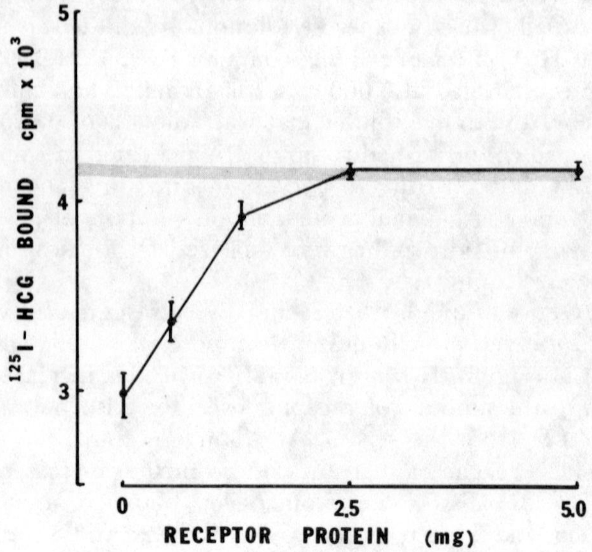

Fig. 8. Binding of ^{125}I-hCG to receptor vs. the quantity of receptor used to adsorb LH per ml serum. The hatched line represents the cpm ^{125}I-hCG bound to receptor in the presence of LH-free serum prepared by immunoadsorption.[38]

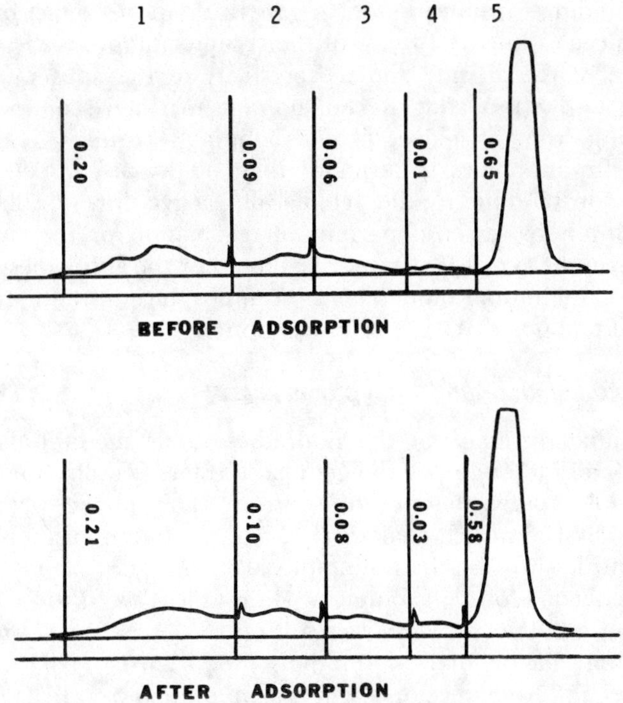

Fig. 9. Micro Zone electrophoresis of serum: 1, γG; 2, β-G; 3, α_2-G; 4, α_1G; 5, albumin.

RECEPTOR-IMMUNOASSAY PROTOCOL

RECEPTOR (100 µl) (160 µg Protein) + ANTI-hCG-β-SERA (100 µl) (Various Dilutions) + ^{125}I-hCG OR ^{125}I-hLH (100 µl) (50,000 cpm)

↓

INCUBATION (20 MIN, 37°C)

↓

ADD 1 ml OF CHILLED 10 mM TRIS-HCl BUFFER (pH 7.2)

↓

CENTRIFUGE 5,000 rpm, 15 MIN.

↓ PELLET ('Receptor' Bound Labelled Hormone)

↓ SUPERNATANT (400 µl Aliquot)

↓

Add 20 µl Horse Serum And 2 ml 6.6% Ammonium Acetate in 66% Ethanol*, Centrifuge 5000 rpm, 15 min.

↓

PELLET (Antibody-Bound Lablled Hormone)

*Römmler and Saxena: Acta Endocrinol. 72:643, 1973.

Since binding to the receptor, in general, requires intact biologically active molecules, the usefulness of the receptorimmunoassay lies in the estimation of the affinity and biospecificity of the antisera produced against hCG-β or its analog. Recent attempts to achieve contraception by immunizing women against hCG-β subunit[45] requires a method to evaluate the antibodies in terms of their ability to compete with the receptor for binding to the biologically active form of hCG. The receptorimmunoassay also permits an estimation of the quantity of endogeneous hCG or LH that may be bound by the antibodies produced during active immunization. This is of importance in the regulation of antibody titers necessary for contraception.

Nonisotopic Immuno- and Receptorassays

The main advantage of the nonradioisotopic methods lies in the elimination of radioisotopes and gamma counters as well as difficulties in the use of rapidly deteriorating tracer. The phage plaque assay developed by Haimovich et al. in 1970[46] as the first nonisotopic assay is tedious and less precise than the radioassays. Also, an automatic colony counter is needed for high volume work, as well as access to an autoclave. Use of an enzyme as a marker can provide an equal or greater amplification factor than the radioisotope. Yorde et al.[47] and Van Weemen et al.[48] have developed enzyme immunoassays (EIA) for hCG.

We have utilized purified receptor from bovine corpus luteum (BCL) or from rat testes (RLC), immobilized on Sepharose-4B or glass beads,

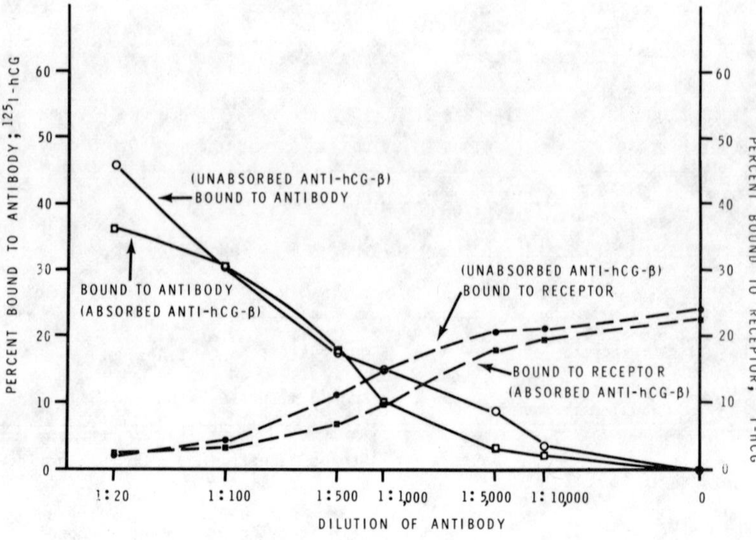

Fig. 10. Percent ^{125}I-hLH bound to unabsorbed and absorbed antisera to hCG-β.

and horseradish peroxidase (HRP)-conjugated or hCG, in the development of a rapid and nonradioactive enzyme receptorassay (ERA), which has been used for the detection of ovulation and pregnancy.[69]

PREPARATION OF "IMMOBILIZED RECEPTOR

The soluble receptor was coupled to CNBr activated Sepharose-4B (2 g) (Pharmacia Fine Chemicals, N.J.) in 0.1 *M* $NaHCO_3$, pH 8.3.[50] The Triton X-100 solubilized gonadotropin receptor exhibited rapid degradation when stored in the presence of the detergent at 4°C. In contrast, if the soluble receptor was immediately coupled to Sepharose 4-B in the presence of Triton X-100, the "activity" of the immobilized receptor remained unchanged up to a period of 6–8 weeks when stored at 4°C. Immobilization of the "purified" receptor on Sepharose 4-B after removal of Triton X-100 using biobeads (a procedure that removed 98% of the initial concentration of Triton) gave similar results. Thus immobilization of the receptor molecule on a solid support such as Sepharose 4-B or glass beads appears to stabilize the activity.

HRP-LH CONJUGATE

The HRP-LH conjugate was prepared[48,51] and purified by gel filtration on Sephadex G-100 (Fig. 11).[30] Each fraction was analyzed for

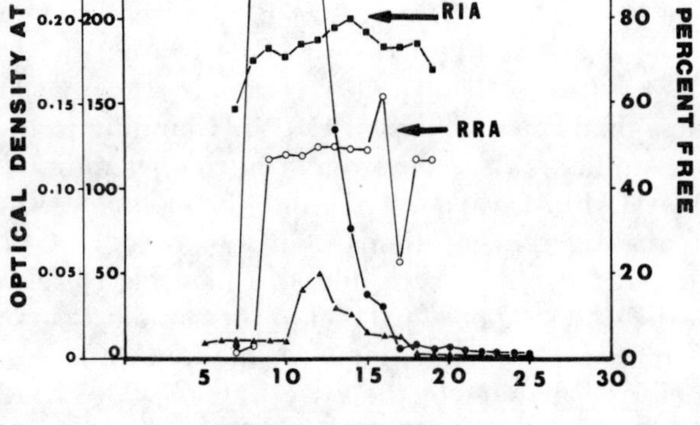

Fig. 11. Fractionation of HRP-LH conjugate on Sephadex G-100. Fractions 11–14 showed activity in ERA. EIA: Enzyme immunoassay.

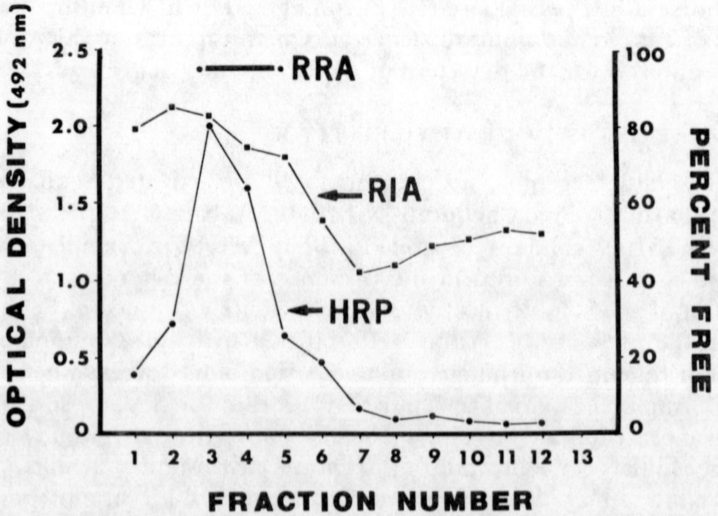

Fig. 12. Purification of fractions 11–14 from Sephadex G-100 column on sucrose density gradient. Fractions 3–5 were used in the ERA.

HRP activity[51] and for the immunological and biological activities of LH by RIA and RRA. Fractions 11–14 were pooled and further purified by centrifugation in a 20–60% sucrose density gradient (Fig. 12). Fractions 3–5 gave 25–30% specific binding with the receptor, and were used in the ERA (Diagram 4).

The dose-response curves obtained by using HRP-LH and affinity purified receptor preparations from bovine corpora lutea and rat Leydig cells immobilized on Sepharose 4-B are given in Figure 13. The sensitivity of the assay was 1 ng LH with BCL. Nonspecific serum effects were not observed, since blank tubes containing up to 100 μl serum resulted in less than 2% of the total HRP-LH binding to the receptor. Crossreaction studies with other protein hormones indicate that both receptors, hFSH, hPRL, and hTSH did not compete with ^{125}I-LH. However, increasing concentrations of hCG showed a dose response parallel to the LH curve. Serum dilutions of a high hCG containing sample gave the dose-response parallel to the standard curve.

Three serum samples containing low, medium, and high concentrations of LH were analyzed by the ERA (Table 3). The values obtained by ERA using BCL or RLC were in reasonable agreement. The interassay variation was less than ±10%. Using the same assay procedure with HRP-hCG as the labeled ligand, the ERA could also be used for detection of hCG in early pregnancy.

ENZYMERECEPTORASSAY

100 μl OF IMMOBILIZED "PURIFIED" RECEPTOR
100 μl OF LH-HRP LABEL
100 μl OF BUFFER OR STANDARD LH OR SERUM SAMPLE
IN 12x75 mm PYREX TUBES COATED WITH 5% BSA

↓

INCUBATE FOR 1 hr AT 37°C

↓

PLACE IN ICE-BATH AT 4° TO TERMINATE THE REACTION

↓

ADD 1 ml OF A 2 mg/ml CELLULOSE SUSPENSION
OR GRABIT (UPDATING, INC., TEXAS)

↓

CENTRIFUGE FOR 30 MIN AT 4,000xg

↓

ASPIRATE SUPERNATANT AND RESUSPEND PELLET IN 0.5ml PBS pH 7.0

↓

CENTRIFUGE FOR 15 MIN AT 4,000xg

↓

SUSPEND PELLET IN 2ml OF 0.1M SODIUM PHOSPHATE BUFFER
CONTAINING 2.5mM O'PHENYLINEDIAMINE 0.06% H_2O_2·SUBSTRATE

↓

INCUBATE FOR 1HR IN THE DARK

↓

CENTRIFUGE FOR 10 MIN AT 2,000xg

↓

MEASURE OPTICAL DENSITY AT 492 nm

Table 3. Comparison of Serum LH Levels Obtained by Enzyme Receptorassay (ERA)

	Enzyme receptorassay (ERA)	
Serum sample	BCL	RLC LH (ng/ml)
No. 1a[a]	31	20
1b	29	15
No. 2a	45	40
2b	40	35
No. 3a	80	70
3b	75	60

[a]Nos. 1, 2, and 3 represent low, medium, and high LH containing sera (a and b), respectively.

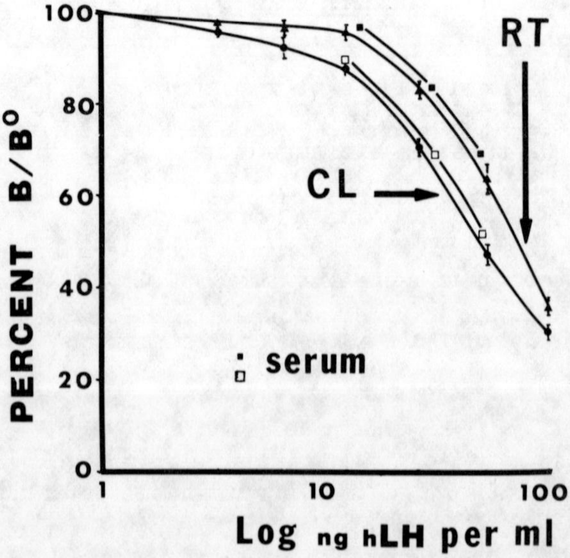

Fig. 13. Standard dose-response curves for LH in ERA using bovine corpus luteum receptor (CL) and rat testes Leydig cell receptor (RT). ■, □, dilutions of serum with high LH activity.

ACKNOWLEDGMENTS

The participation of Dr. Firyal Khan, Ph.D., Dr. Robert Landesman, M.D., Dr. Klaus Post, M.D., and Miss Kazuko Jibiki, M.Sc., in the investigations is greatly appreciated.

REFERENCES

1. O. Hechter, Concerning the mechanisms of hormone action. *In Vitamins and Hormones.* Academic, New York, 1955, p. 293.

2. B.B. Saxena, Gonadotropin receptors. *In Methods in Receptor Research,* M. Blecher (ed.), Marcel Dekker, New York, 1976, p. 252.

3. C.M. Szego, Parallels in the modes of action of peptide and steroid hormones: membrane effects and cellular entry. *In Structure and Function of the Gonadotropins,* K.W. McKerns (ed.) Plenum, New York, 1978, p. 431.

4. K.J. Catt, Receptors for gonadotropic hormones. *In Methods in Receptor Research,* M. Blecher (ed.), Marcel Dekker, New York, 1976, p. 176.

5. K. Khan and B.B. Saxena, in preparation.

6. P. DeMeyts, et al., *Metabolism* **25**(S1):1365, 1976.

7. P. Rathnam and B.B. Saxena, *J Biol Chem* **242**:3769, 1967.

8. P. Rathnam and B.B. Saxena, *J Biol Chem* **245**:3725, 1970.

9. J.S. Cornell and J.G. Pierce, *J Biol Chem* **248**:4327, 1973.

10. O.P. Bahl, *In Hormone Proteins and Peptides,* C.H. Li (ed.), 1973, p. 171.

11. R.E. Canfield and F.J. Morgan, *In Investigative and Diagnostic Endocrinology,* S.A. Berson and R.E. Yalow (eds.), North-Holland, Amsterdam, 1974, p. 727.

12. P. Rathnam and B.B. Saxena, *Biochim Biophys Acta* **576**:81, 1979.

13. D.N. Ward, Chemical approaches to the structure-function relationships of luteinizing hormone (lutropin). *In Structure and Function of the Gonadotropins,* K.W. McKerns (ed.), Plenum, New York, 1978, p. 31.

14. M.R. Pandian and O.P. Bahl, *Arch Biochem Biophys* **182**:420, 1977.

15. T.A. Langan, Protein kinases and protein kinase substrates. *In Advances in Cyclic Nucleotide Research*, Vol. 3, P. Greengard and G.A. Robison (eds.), Raven Press, New York.

16. R.G. Smith, *Int J Fertil* **21**:159, 1976.

17. G. Scatchard, *Ann NY Acad Sci* **51**:660, 1949.

18. J. Roth et al., *Recent Progr Horm Res,* 31, 1975.

19. M.A. Lesniak and J.J. Roth, *J Biol Chem* **251**:3720, 1976.

20. P. Morris and B.B. Saxena, submitted for publication.

21. P. DeMeyts, Insulin and growth hormone receptors in human cultured lymphocytes and peripheral blood monocytes. *In Methods in Receptor Research*, M. Blecher (ed.), Marcel Dekker, New York, 1976, p. 301.

22. R.S. Yalow and S.A. Berson, *J Clin Invest* **39**:1157, 1960.

23. B.B. Saxena et al., *Science* **184**:793, 1974.

24. L.E. Reichert and H. Abou-Issa, The interaction of follitropin (FSH) with membrane-bound and solubilized gonadal receptors and adenylate cyclase. *In Structure and Function of the Gonadotropins,* K.W. McKerns (ed.), Plenum, New York, 1978, p. 259.

25. W.V. Moore and J. Wolff, *J. Biol Chem* **249**:6255, 1974.

26. M. Blecher, (ed.), *Methods in Receptor Research,* Parts I and II, Marcel Dekker, New York, 1976.

27. B.B. Saxena and R. Landesman, *Am J Obstet Gynecol* **131**:97, 1978.

28. K.J. Catt and M.L. Dufau, *Biol Reprod* **14**:1, 1976.

29. F. Haour and B.B. Saxena, *J Biol Chem* **249**:2195, 1974.

30. T.P. Rosal, *Fertil Steril* **26**:1105, 1975.

31. C.G. Beling, et al., *Am J Obstet Gynecol* **125**:855, 1976.

32. S.K. Block, *Obstet Gynecol* **48**:365, 1976.

33. G.D. Braunstein et al., *Obstet Gynecol* **50**(Suppl):41, 1977.

34. R. Landesman et al., *Contraception* **8**:527, 1973.

35. M.Y. Dawood et al., *Obstet Gynecol* **50**:172, 1977.

36. B.B. Saxena et al., *Fertil Steril* **28**:163, 1977.

37. P. Rathnam and B.B. Saxena, The structure and function of follicle-stimulating hormone. *In Structure and Function of the Gonadotropins.* K.W. McKerns (ed.), Plenum, New York, 1978, p. 183.

38. T. Saito and B.B. Saxena, *J Clin Endocrinol Metab* **43**:1186, 1976.

39. J.I. Thorell and B.G. Johansson, *Excerpta Medica International Congress Series 241*, Part 2, Amsterdam, 1972, p. 531.

40. Römmler A. and B.B. Saxena, *Acta Endocrinol (kbh)* **72**:642, 1973.

41. A.V. Wolf, *Aqueous Solutions and Body Fluids*, Harper & Row, New York, 1966.

42. K. Jibiki and B.B. Saxena, *Acta Endocrinol* **87**:838, 1978.

43. O.P. Bahl et al., *Biochem Biophys Res Commun* **70**:525, 1976.
44. J.L. Vaitukaitis et al., *Am J Obstet Gynecol* **113**:751, 1972.
45. S.J. Segal, *Contraception* **13**:125, 1976.
46. Haimovich et al., *Biochim Biophys Acta* **207**:115, 1970.
47. D.E. Yorde et al., *Clin Chem* **22**:1372, 1976.
48. B.K. Van Weemen and A.H.W.M. Schuurs, *FEBS Lett* **24**:77, 1972.
49. S.K. Khan and B.B. Saxena, Use of purified gonadotropin receptor in the development of an enzyme receptorassay (ERA) for luteinizing hormone (LH) and human chorionic gonadotropin (hCG). *In Enzyme Labelled Immunoassay of Hormones and Drugs*, S.B. Pal (ed.), Walter de Gruyter, Berlin, 1978, p. 257.
50. R. Axen et al., *Nature* **214**:1302, 1967.
51. M.L. Dufau et al., *Biochem Biophys Res Commun* **44**:1022, 1971.
52. C.Y. Lee and R.J. Ryan, *Endocrinology* **89**:1515, 1971.
53. S. Kammerman et al., *Endocrinology* **91**:65, 1972.
54. Ch.V. Rao and B.B. Saxena, *Biochim Biophys Acta* **313**:372, 1973.
55. V.K. Bhalla and L.E. Reichert, *J Biol Chem* **249**:43, 1974.
56. R.P.C. Shiu and H.G. Freisen, *Biochem J* **140**:301, 1974.
57. B.I. Posner et al., *Proc Natl Acad Sci* **71**:2407, 1974.
58. T. Saito and B.B. Saxena, *J Lab Clin Med* **85**:487, 1975.
59. M.A. Lesniak et al., *Nature New Biol* **241**:20, 1973.
60. T. Tsushima and H.G. Friesen, *J Clin Endocrinol Metab* **37**:334, 1973.
61. R.J. Lefkowitz, *Proc Natl Acad Sci* **65**:745, 1970.
62. P. Freychet et al., *Proc Natl Acad Sci* **68**:1833, 1971.
63. P. Cuatrecasas, *Proc Natl Acad Sci* **68**:1264, 1971.
64. J.R. Gavin et al., *J Biol Chem* **248**:1973.
65. B.I. Posner, *Clin Res* **20**:922, 1972.
66. J. Spona, *FEBS Lett* **39**:221, 1974.
67. K.R. Park et al., *Acta Endocrinol* **82**:62, 1976.
68. N. Barden and F. Labrie, *J Biol Chem* **248**:7601, 1973.
69. S. Soloff and T.L. Swartz, *J Biol Chem* **249**:1376, 1974.
70. S. Soloff and T.L. Swartz, *J Biol Chem* **248**:6471, 1973.
71. R. Rajerison et al., *J Biol Chem* **249**:6390, 1974.
72. H. Glossman et al., *J Biol Chem* **249**:428, 1974.
73. S.J. Marx et al., *J Biol Chem* **248**:4794, 1973.
74. S.J. Marx et al., *Science* **178**:999, 1972.
75. F.P. Dibella et al., *Proc Natl Acad Sci* **71**:723, 1974.
76. V. Tomasi et al., *Biochim Biophys Acta* **211**:31, 1970.
77. I.D. Goldfine et al., *J Biol Chem* **247**:1211, 1972.

Chapter 11

Competitive Protein Binding Assays Monitored with Bioluminescence and Chemiluminescence

HARTMUT R. SCHROEDER, M.D., ROBERT C. BOGUSLASKI, M.D., ROBERT J. CARRICO, M.D., KWOK-KAM YEUNG, M.D., AND RICHARD D. FALB, M.D.

INTRODUCTION

Many substances are measured at very low levels with competitive protein binding (CPB) assays, which are monitored with radiolabeled ligands.[1,2] Alternatively, the radiolabels have been replaced by enzymes,[3-5] substrates,[6] and fluorescent dyes.[7] In addition, cofactors[8,9] and chemilumigenic compounds[10-12] have been used as labels, which are detected in light generating reactions. Since very low levels of light can be readily measured, these methods offer the possibility of providing very sensitive CPB assays.

Two bioluminescent methods were investigated and both used cofactors for labeling the ligands. One method used an NADH derivative coupled covalently to the ligand, and this NADH-ligand conjugate could be determined quantitatively with the bacterial luciferase system. The second method used an ATP-ligand conjugate,

Ames Research Laboratory, Ames Division, Miles Laboratories, Inc., P.O. Box 70, Elkhart, Ind. 46515.

which could be measured at nanomolar levels with firefly luciferase.

A simplified CPB reaction can be illustrated by

$$\underset{\text{(Free)}}{\text{L—C} + \text{L} + \text{P}} \rightleftharpoons \underset{\text{(Protein Bound)}}{\text{P}\cdots\text{L—C} + \text{P}\cdots\text{L}}$$

where L is the ligand being assayed, P is the binding protein such as the antibody, and L—C is the ligand coupled covalently to the cofactor. While the L—C conjugate is active in the appropriate bioluminescence system, the protein bound form, P · · · L—C, is much less active. If P is present in limited quantity, L—C and L will compete for binding sites on P, and the light produced with L—C is a measure of the concentration of L in the reaction mixture. Thus both bioluminescent systems provide homogeneous methods for monitoring CPB assays, i.e., without separation of protein bound and free labeled ligand.

The chemiluminescence method uses labels that participate in efficient light-emitting reactions. Measurement of the light allows the labels to be determined at remarkably low levels. In some situations the binding protein influences the light production from the labeled conjugate, and this effect has been used to develop homogeneous CPB assays. However, it is usually more practical to use heterogeneous CPB methods with chemiluminescence. These novel immunoassay methods are discussed individually in more detail below.

CPB REACTIONS MONITORED WITH BACTERIAL LUCIFERASE

Luciferase from *Photobacterium fischeri* has been used for quantitative measurement of NADH at nanomolar levels.[13,14] Bacterial extracts contain both enzymes necessary for light production from NADH according to the reactions

$$NADH + FMN + H^+ \xrightarrow{\text{FMN reductase}} NAD^+ + FMNH_2$$
$$FMNH_2 + O_2 \xrightarrow[\text{(long-chain aldehyde)}]{\text{luciferase}} \text{light} + FMN$$

These reactions were first used to monitor CPB assays using the ligand biotin, coupled covalently through a bridging arm to NAD (Fig. 1). Biotinyl-AENAD[8] was active with several dehydrogenases and was reduced to biotinyl-AENADH with alcohol dehydrogenase and ethanol. The reduced cofactor produced light with the bacterial luciferase system. The light reached peak intensity within 2 s after addition of the cofactor to the enzymes, and the peak light intensity (PLI) varied linearly with the reduced cofactor concentration. The sensitivity was about

10 n*M* biotinyl-AENADH (10^{-13} mol) in the solution before mixing with the luciferase.

An avidin solution was titered by incubating various amounts with a fixed level of the biotinyl-AENAD. After reduction of the cofactor with alcohol dehydrogenase, aliquots of the binding reactions were added

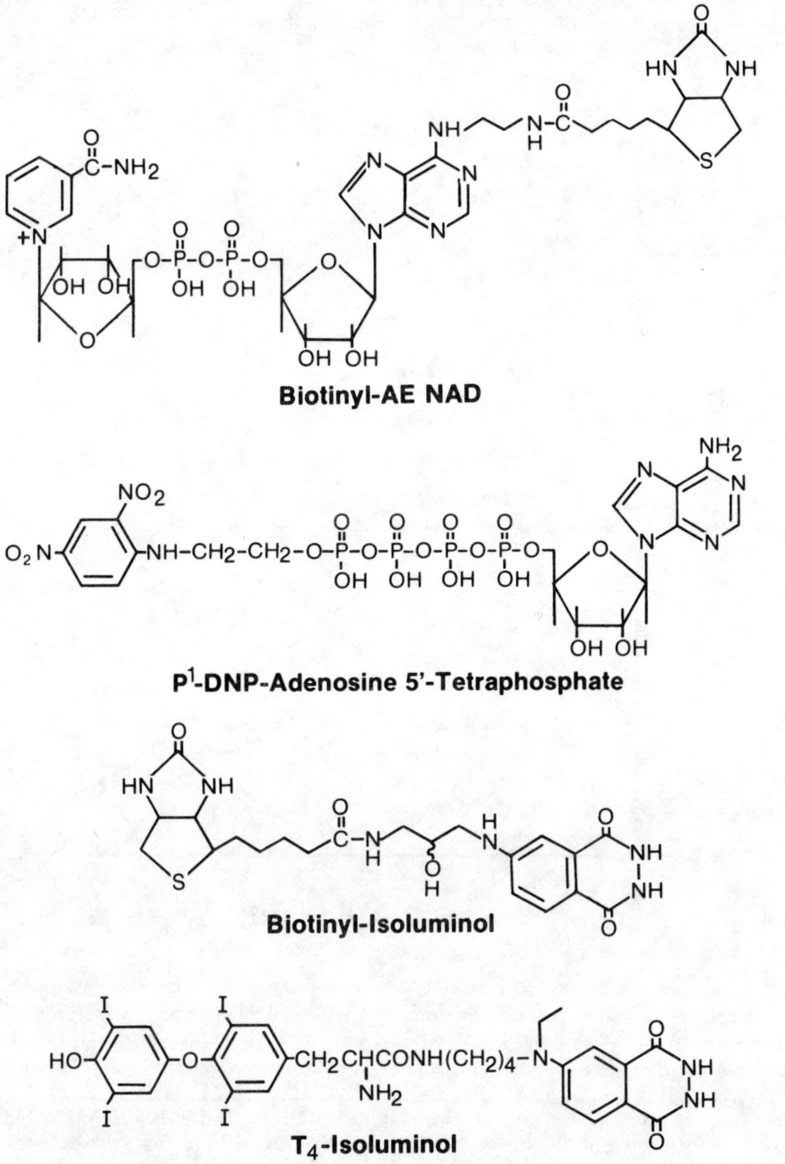

Fig. 1. Structures of labeled ligands used in CPB assays.

rapidly to the luciferase, and the PLI was recorded. The PLI decreased as the avidin level increased, indicating that the avidin prevented the biotinyl-AENAD(H) from reacting with the enzyme(s) (Fig. 2). Results of control experiments showed that avidin inhibits the reaction of biotinyl-AENADH with FMN reductase. Since only the free biotinyl-AENAD(H) is active with the enzymes, the bacterial luciferase could be used to monitor homogeneous CPB reactions.

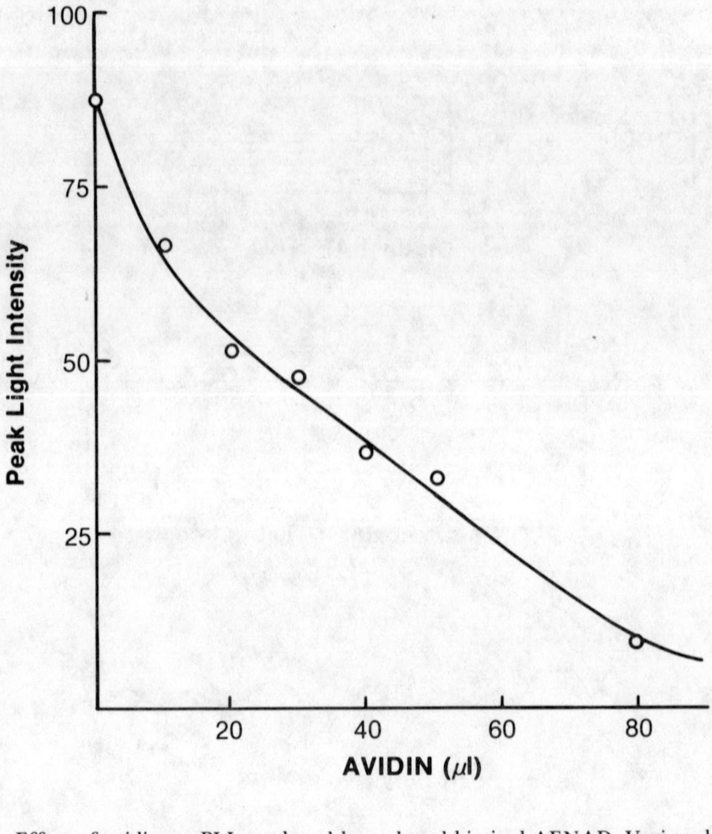

Fig. 2. Effect of avidin on PLI produced by reduced biotinyl-AENAD. Various levels of avidin were incubated for 10 min with 383 n*M* biotinyl-AENAD in 180 μl of 0.1 *M* Tris-HCl, pH 8, containing 0.6 *M* ethanol and 0.01 *M* semicarbazide·HCl. Then the cofactor was reduced on addition of 20 μl (0.02 U) of alcohol dehydrogenase. After 20 min incubation, 10-μl aliquots were injected into 100 μl of light generating solution in 6 × 50-mm glass tubes mounted in a custom-built photometer, and PLIs were measured. The assay solution contained luciferase extract from *P. fischeri* at 15 mg/ml, 0.5% bovine serum albumin, 12 m*M* FMN, 5 μl of dodecanal emulsion, and 10 m*M* sodium acetate in 0.1 *M* potassium phosphate, pH 7. Values represent the average of duplicates.

CPB reactions were conducted with a fixed level of biotinyl-AENAD, a limiting level of avidin, and various levels of biotin. The PLI produced by the biotinyl-AENADH from these reaction mixtures increased as the biotin level increased (Fig. 3). The sensitivity was about 30 n*M* biotin. These studies were carried out with a crude enzyme extract and a relatively insensitive photometer. Improvements in the instrumentation and the luciferase preparation[15] would probably improve the sensitivity.

Endogeneous NAD and degradative enzymes in the sample being assayed would interfere with this assay system. For example, some fresh serums contain nanomolar levels of NAD, which is completely inactivated as a cofactor in 24 h at 25°C. The enzymes that inactivate the endogeneous NAD might also inactivate the cofactor in ligand-NAD conjugates. These problems are serious impediments to the practical use of bacterial luciferase for monitoring CPB assays.

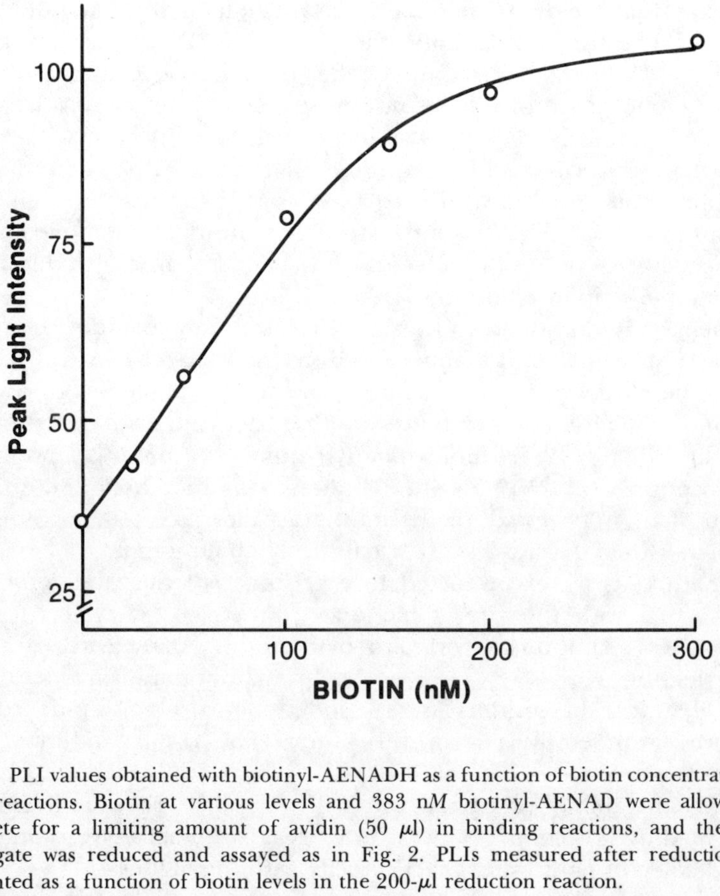

Fig. 3. PLI values obtained with biotinyl-AENADH as a function of biotin concentration in CPB reactions. Biotin at various levels and 383 n*M* biotinyl-AENAD were allowed to compete for a limiting amount of avidin (50 μl) in binding reactions, and then the conjugate was reduced and assayed as in Fig. 2. PLIs measured after reduction are presented as a function of biotin levels in the 200-μl reduction reaction.

CPB REACTIONS MONITORED WITH FIREFLY LUCIFERASE

Since ATP can be measured quantitatively at subnanomolar levels with firefly luciferase,[9] we investigated the possibility of labeling ligands with ATP for use in CPB assays. The basic reactions for light production with firefly luciferase are as follows:[15]

$$LH_2 + ATP + E \xrightarrow{Mg^{++}} E\text{—}LH_2\text{—}AMP + PP_i$$
$$E\text{—}LH_2AMP + O_2 \rightarrow E\text{—}L\text{—}O^- + AMP + CO_2 + \text{light}$$

where E and LH_2 are the luciferase and reduced luciferin, respectively. Light production was initiated by injecting ATP, ligand-ATP conjugate, or aliquots of CPB reaction mixtures into a bioluminescence assay system consisting of luciferase, luciferin, and necessary cofactors.

Several ligand-ATP conjugates were synthesized to determine the structure that yields greatest light production in the bioluminescent reaction. The ligand 2,4-dinitrophenyl residue (DNP) was coupled to either the C8 or the N6 position of the adenine moiety, and also at the terminal phosphate of adenosine tetraphosphate.[9] ATP was detected with the bioluminescence assay at lower levels (1×10^{-10} *M* or 1×10^{-15} mol) than the DNP-ATP conjugates (Fig. 4). P^1-DNP-adenosine-5′-tetraphosphate was measurable at 0.5 n*M*, whereas the limit for measurement of N^6[2(2,4-dinitrophenyl) aminoethyl]adenosine-5′-triphosphate and C^8[2(2,4-dinitrophenyl) aminoethylamino]-adenosine-5′-triphosphate was 5 n*M*.

When ATP was added to firefly luciferase, the maximum light yield occurred in less than 1 s and then decreased sharply. With P^1-DNP-adenosine-5′-tetraphosphate as the cofactor, light emission reached maximum intensity in 0.5 min and then decayed with a halflife of 1.2 min. When C^8[2(2,4-dinitrophenyl) aminoethylamino]adenosine-5′-triphosphate and N^6[2(2,4-dinitrophenyl) aminoethyl]adenosine-5′-] triphosphate were tested, the light intensity increased to a maximum in 2 min and then decreased with a halflife of about 4 min.

Experiments were conducted to determine whether the conjugates were active with the firefly luciferase directly or enzyme(s) in the luciferase preparation converted them to products that participate in the light-yielding reaction.[9] Thin-layer chromatography for identifying ATP degradation products and also inhibitors for ATP-dependent enzymes were employed for this study. The results indicated that P^1-DNP-adenosine-5′-tetraphosphate was degraded to N-DNP-ethanolamine phosphate and ATP, which then initiated the light-yielding reaction. It was not clear whether the other two ligand-cofactor conjugates react directly with the luciferase.

The conjugate P[1]-DNP-adenosine-5′-tetraphosphate was employed for titration of antiserum to DNP. Figure 5 shows that increasing levels of antibody decreased the light production by this conjugate in the bioluminescent reaction. Control experiments indicated that the light production by ATP was not affected by antibody and that immunoglobulin from a nonimmunized rabbit had no effect on light production by P[1]-DNP-adenosine-5′-tetraphosphate. Thus the inhibition of the bioluminescent reaction by the antibody was specific for the ligand-ATP conjugate.

The specificity of the inhibition of the DNP-ATP conjugate by antibody to DNP provides a means for monitoring homogeneous CPB assays. Addition of increasing levels of N(DNP)-β-alanine to the binding reaction relieved the inactivation of the ligand-ATP conjugate, and this inhibition was fully reversed by excess N(DNP)-β-alanine (Fig. 6). This CPB assay measured N(DNP)-β-alanine at levels as low as 10 n*M*.

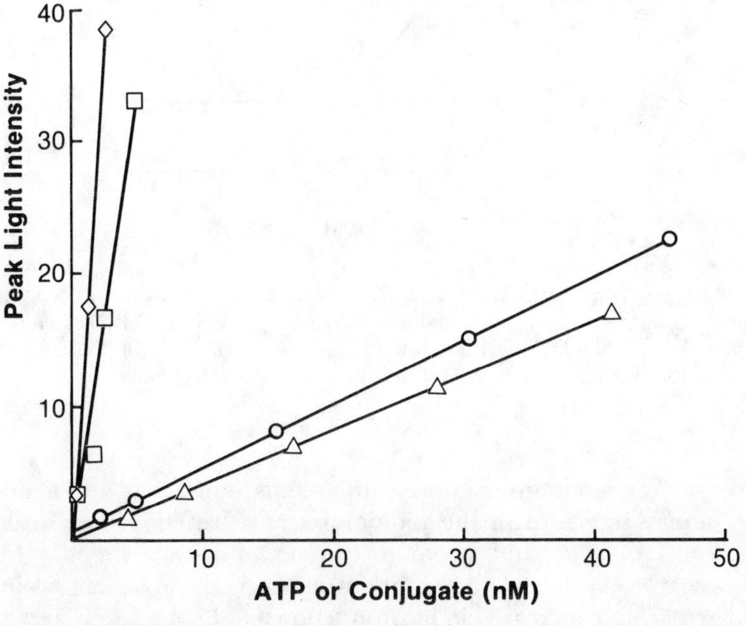

Fig. 4. PLIs obtained with various levels of ATP and ligand-ATP conjugates. A light generating solution was prepared containing partially purified firefly luciferase, 0.7 m*M* luciferin, 10m*M* $MgSO_4$, and 0.15% bovine serum albumin in 10 m*M* morpholinopropane sulfonate buffer, pH 7.4. Aliquots (100 μl) of this solution were dispensed into 6 × 50-mm test tubes, which were then mounted in the Model 760 DuPont Luminescence Biometer. Light production started on addition of 10 μl of ATP or ligand-ATP conjugate solution. The average PLI of duplicates are presented as a function of the levels of ATP (◇), P′-DNP-adenosine-5′-tetraphosphate (□), [8][2,(2,4-dinitrophenyl)aminoethyl amino] adenosine-5′-triphosphate (○), and N[6][2(2,4-dinitrophenyl)aminoethyl]adenosine-5′-triphosphate (△).

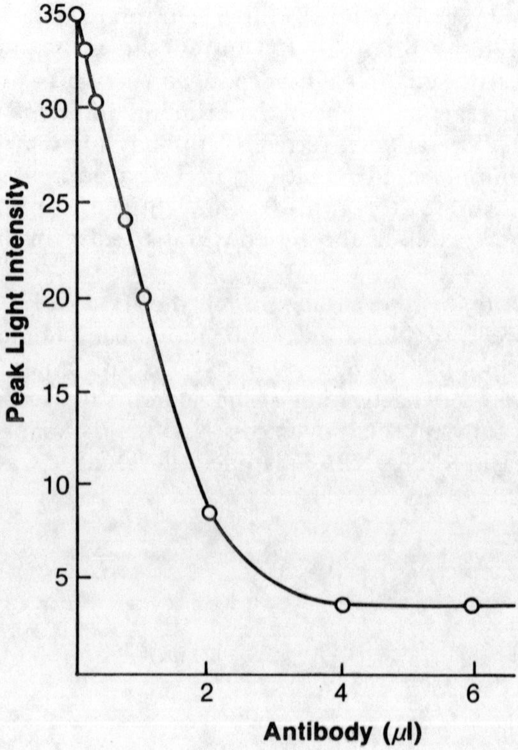

Fig. 5. Titration of P′-DNP-adenosine-5′-tetraphosphate with antibody to DNP. Various amounts of antibody were incubated for 1.5 h at 25°C with P′-DNP-adenosine-5′-tetraphosphate in 20-mM Tris-HCl buffer, pH 7.4, containing 10 m*M* EDTA. Then 10 μl aliquots of the binding mixture (100 μl) were assayed with the bioluminescence reaction as in Fig. 4.

In practical situations, sample components other than the ligand of interest may interfere in the bioluminescence reaction. For instance, high levels of salts and proteins can be inhibitory for the firefly luciferase.[16,17] We found that proteins at levels up to 15 mg/ml in the simulated sample increased light production and higher levels decreased it. Addition of 1.5 mg bovine serum albumin/ml to the firefly luciferase eliminated the effects of protein in the sample on light production.

Furthermore, endogenous ATP in biological samples could lead to interference with measurement of ligand-ATP conjugates. However, serum and plasma contain ATP-degrading enzymes that rapidly destroy the ATP. EDTA at 10 m*M* in the binding reaction prevented these endogenous enzymes from degrading the ligand-ATP conjugates without interfering with subsequent bioluminescence reactions.

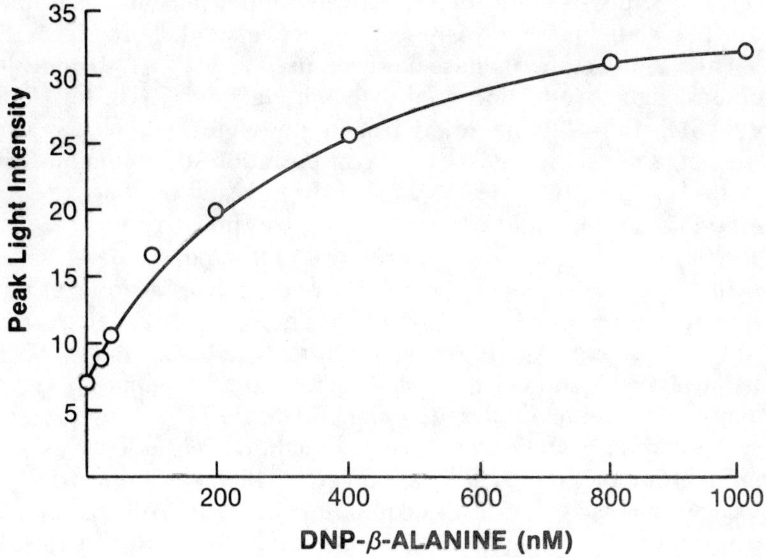

Fig. 6. CPB reactions monitored with P′-DNP-adenosine-5′-tetraphosphate and firefly luciferase. N(DNP)-β-alanine at indicated concentrations and 45 n*M* P′-DNP-adenosine-5′-tetraphosphate were incubated at 25°C for 2 h with 2 μl of antibody to DNP. Then 10-μl aliquots of the reaction were assayed as in Fig. 4. The levels of N(DNP)-β-alanine shown are those in the binding reaction.

CPB REACTIONS MONITORED WITH CHEMILUMINESCENCE

Among the many chemiluminescent reactions, the oxidation of certain aminophthalhydrazides and aminonaphthalhydrazides yields light with relatively high efficiency.[18-20] Since light measurements are very sensitive and require only rather simple equipment, chemilumigenic compounds are attractive labels for monitoring immunoassays.

Hydrogen peroxide is an effective and convenient oxidant for chemiluminescent reactions, and a catalyst such as metal ion, hematin, or a peroxidase is usually employed:

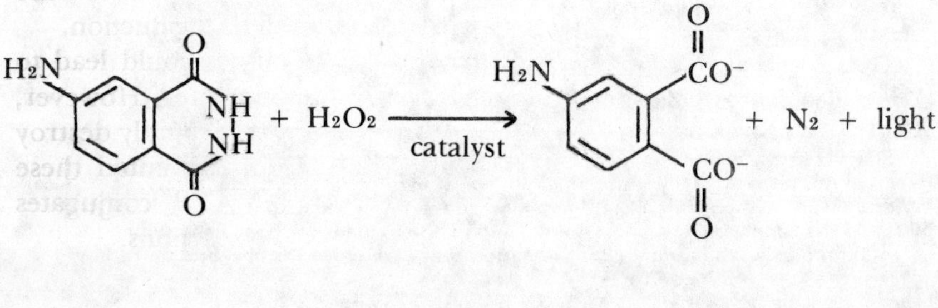

All of the catalysts function effectively under alkaline conditions, pH 10–13, while microperoxidase is effective in the broader range, pH 7.4–13, and lactoperoxidase has been used at pH 7.4.[11] Under these conditions, light production attains maximum intensity in less than a second after the addition of hydrogen peroxide and decays with a halflife of several seconds. The concentration of chemilumigenic compounds is linearly related to the PLI over greater than two orders of magnitude, and total light measurements give similar results.

Detection limits for chemilumigenic compounds depend on the efficiency of light production, which is based on the reaction conditions and the structures of the compounds.[11] The heme catalyzed reactions give the lowest limit of detection for luminol (1 p*M*) among several oxidation systems shown in Table 1. The detection limits of several compounds in heme catalyzed reactions at pH 13 are presented in Table 2. Isoluminol (I) can be measured quantitatively at levels as low as 30 p*M*. Akylation of the primary amino group increases the sensitivity of the measurements as shown with compounds III and V (Table 2). Thus it is convenient to couple a ligand to isoluminol using one of the alkyl chains as a bridging arm. Attachment of biotin to isoluminol provided a conjugate (VI), which could be measured at levels similar to the original label, II (Table 2). The thyroxine conjugate (VII) had a light yield which was only about 2% of that obtained with compound V. This ligand is unusual because it bears iodine atoms that quench light.

An aminonaphthalhydrazide can be measured quantitatively at lower levels than the aminophthalhydrazide (e.g., isoluminol) derivatives. The lower limit for measurement of this compound was 0.1 p*M* (1.5×10^{-17} mol) using the H_2O_2-microperoxidase oxidation system at pH 12.6 (Fig. 7). Thus immunoassays monitored with chemiluminescence are potentially capable of sensitivities similar to radioimmunoas-

Table 1. Detection Limit of Luminol in Various Oxidation Systems[a]

Oxidation system	pH	Detection limit (pM)
H_2O_2-hematin	13.0	1
H_2O_2-microperoxidase	12.6	1
H_2O_2-microperoxidase	8.6	1
Hypochlorite-$CoCl_2$	13.0	10
$NaIO_4$	13.0	20
KO_2	10.5	10
H_2O_2-lactoperoxidase	8.8	50
H_2O_2-lactoperoxidase	7.4	300

[a]Reaction mixtures (150 μl) containing luminol at varying levels and the catalyst at the pH indicated were assembled in 6 x 50-mm glass tubes. After a short incubation they were placed in the Biometer, and addition of 10 μl of the oxidant initiated light production. The detection limit was the luminol concentration that gave twice the background PLI.

says. The sensitivities were not changed significantly by measurement of total light production.

The reproducibility of measurements of chemilumigenic compounds was determined with the H_2O_2-microperoxidase system, since this was the most versatile system investigated. Reaction mixtures consisting of chemilumigenic compound and catalyst were assembled in 150 μl of aqueous solution at pH 12.6 in 6 × 50-mm test tubes. Each tube was then mounted in the Biometer, and hydrogen peroxide was injected from a 25-μl Hamilton syringe. When the peak light intensities produced by N,N-diethylisoluminol in 15 individual reactions were measured, the mean PLI for the five triplicate averages had a coefficient of variation of 12.7%. The variability was only 5% for the thyroxine-isoluminol conjugate, perhaps because the PLI occurs later.[11] After a syringe was used for an unpredictable period, PLI values became irreproducible, evidently because metal(s) from the syringe plunger interfered with the chemiluminescent reaction. When a syringe with a Teflon-tipped plunger was employed to add 20 μl of hydrogen peroxide, the coefficient of variation improved to ±2%. Measurements conducted with a custom-built automatic injection device which allowed hydrogen peroxide to contact only Teflon and glass, gave coefficients of variation of 2–5%. The reproducibility of total light measurements was not significantly different from that for peak light measurements.

Table 2. Relative Light Yields of Isoluminol Derivatives in the H_2O_2-Hematin System[a]

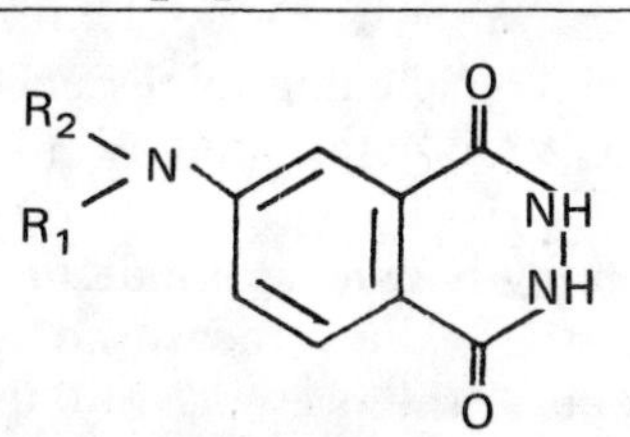

Compound	R_1	R_2	Detection limit (p*M*)
I	-H	-H	30
II	-H	$-CH_2CH(OH)CH_2NH_2$	20
III	-H	$-(CH_2)_4-NH_2$	20
IV	$-CH_2CH_3$	$-CH_2CH(OH)CH_2NH_2$	5
V	$-CH_2CH_3$	$-(CH_2)_4NH_2$	82
VI	-H	$-CH_2CH(OH)CH_2NHCO$-biotin	10
VII	$-CH_2CH_3$	$-(CH_2)_4NHCO-T_4$	100

[a]Reaction mixtures (150 μl) containing the indicated compound at several levels in 50 m*M* NaOH with 0.07 μ*M* hematin were incubated for 10 min and then injected with 10 μl of 90 m*M* H_2O_2 to produce light. Measurements with biotinylisoluminol employed 0.27 μ*M* microperoxidase instead of hematin in mixtures that also contained 55 m*M* barbital, giving a final pH of 12.6.

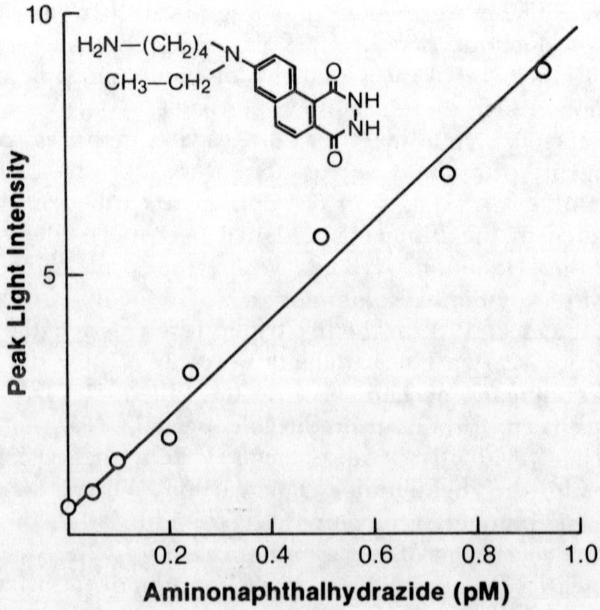

Fig. 7. PLI values obtained on oxidation of an aminonaphthalhydrazide. Reaction mixtures (150 μl) contained the aminophthalhydrazide at indicated concentrations, 0.27 μ*M* microperoxidase, 57 m*M* barbital, and 50 m*M* NaOH (final pH 12.6). Manual addition of 10 μl of 90 m*M* H_2O_2 initiated light production, which was measured in the Biometer. PLI values are averages from reactions performed in triplicate.

The effects of protein on chemiluminescence were evaluated with bovine serum albumin and compound V (Table 2) in the H_2O_2-microperoxidase system, pH 12.6. Peak light intensities measured in the presence of 0.8 and 8.3 mg bovine serum albumin per ml were 86 and 43%, respectively, of the values measured without the protein.[21] Additional measurements in the presence of 0.01 and 0.1% serum (v/v) gave peak light intensities that were 80 and 50%, respectively, of the control value. Apparently, serum contains materials besides proteins that interfere with chemiluminescence. These problems with practical samples can be circumvented in heterogeneous immunoassays.

HETEROGENEOUS IMMUNOASSAY FOR SERUM THYROXINE MONITORED BY CHEMILUMINESCENCE

We evaluated a chemiluminescent immunoassay for serum thyroxine that was monitored with the T_4-isoluminol conjugate (Fig. 1).[12] Competitive binding reactions were carried out on 1-ml columns of Sephadex G-25, which binds both thyroxine and T_4-isoluminol. Serum samples were diluted in 0.1 N NaOH and applied to individual columns that contained adsorbed T_4-isoluminol. The serum components other than thyroxine were washed from the column with 75 mM sodium barbital buffer, pH 8.6. Then aliquots of antibody were allowed to flow into the columns. After 1 h incubation, the antibody-bound T_4-isoluminol was eluted with an aliquot of buffer, and PLIs produced with aliquots of the effluent in the H_2O_2-microperoxidase system at pH 12.6 were measured.

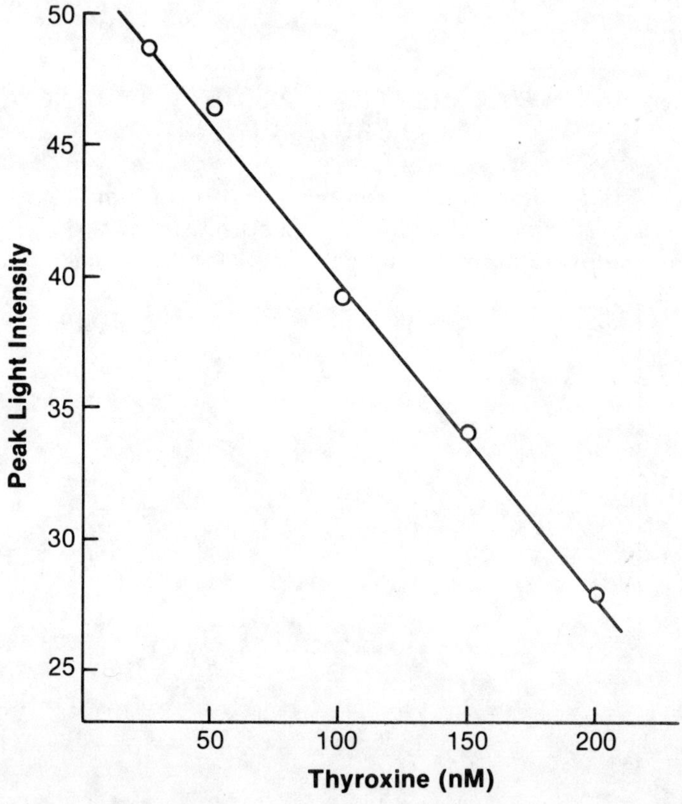

Fig. 8. Heterogeneous chemiluminescence immunoassays for serum thyroxine. Five pmol of T_4-isoluminol in 200 μl of 0.1 M NaOH were applied to columns packed with 1 ml of Sephadex G-25 and washed into the bed with 1 ml of 0.1 N NaOH. Serum standards were diluted 1:10 in 0.1 N NaOH and 200-μl aliquots were added. The columns were washed with 4 ml of 75 mM barbital, pH 8.6, to remove interfering serum components. The CPB reaction was initiated with the addition of 0.3 ml of an antibody to T_4 (sufficient to bind 60% of the label in the absence of competing T_4). After 1 h incubation, the antibody was eluted with 0.8 ml barbital buffer. Antibody-bound T_4-isoluminol was determined from the PLI produced by 95-μl aliquots of the eluate as in Fig. 7. CPB reactions were performed in triplicate, and each chemiluminescence measurement was also in triplicate to give the indicated mean PLI.

A standard curve was generated for conversion of PLI to thyroxine concentration. As the thyroxine level increased, the amount of T_4-isoluminol bound to antibody decreased, and consequently the PLI decreased (Fig. 8). The chemiluminescence method was useful for determining 25–200 n*M* thyroxine, which is the range typically found in clinical samples. Results obtained with 28 serums correlated reasonably well with the results of a reference method (Fig. 9). Although this example demonstrates the feasibility of monitoring immunoassays with chemiluminescence, it is not as convenient for routine use as radioimmunoassays.

A HOMOGENEOUS COMPETITIVE PROTEIN BINDING ASSAY FOR BIOTIN

An interesting homogeneous competitive protein binding assay for biotin was investigated.[10] Chemiluminescence was generated by oxidation of the biotinyl-isoluminol conjugate (Fig. 1) with hydrogen peroxide

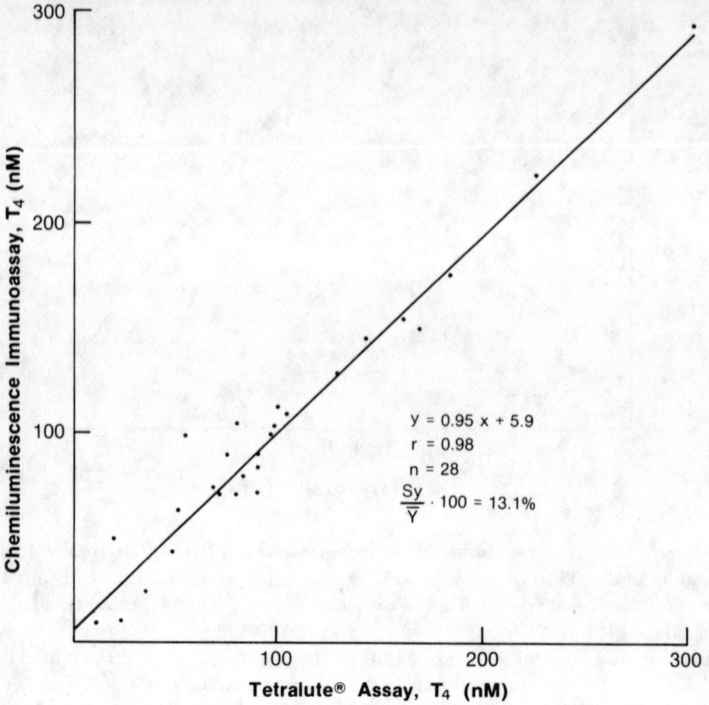

Fig. 9. Evaluation of the chemiluminescence immunoassay for T_4. Thyroxine concentrations of 28 clinical serums were measured in triplicate with the chemiluminescence immunoassay as in Fig. 8 and compared to values obtained in duplicate by the Tetralute® method, which employs a radiolabel.

at pH 7.4 in the presence of lactoperoxidase. A constant amount of biotinyl-isoluminol was incubated with increasing levels of avidin in individual reactions. Then the PLI, as well as the total light production during the oxidation reaction, increased 10-fold as the avidin level increased to 14 μg/ml (Fig. 10). Higher levels of avidin decreased the chemiluminescence, possibly due to interference by the protein. In control reactions avidin did not have an effect on the peak light intensity produced by compound III (Table 2).

The enhancement of light production by avidin provided a means for performing a homogeneous CPB assay for biotin. In this model system, avidin and biotinyl-isoluminol were used at levels that gave the enhanced light production, and various levels of biotin were included in the reactions to compete with biotinyl-isoluminol for avidin binding sites. The chemiluminescence measured with these binding reaction mixtures decreased as the biotin level increased (Fig. 11). This assay determined 50 to 400 n*M* biotin. Further optimization of the reaction conditions might increase the sensitivity.

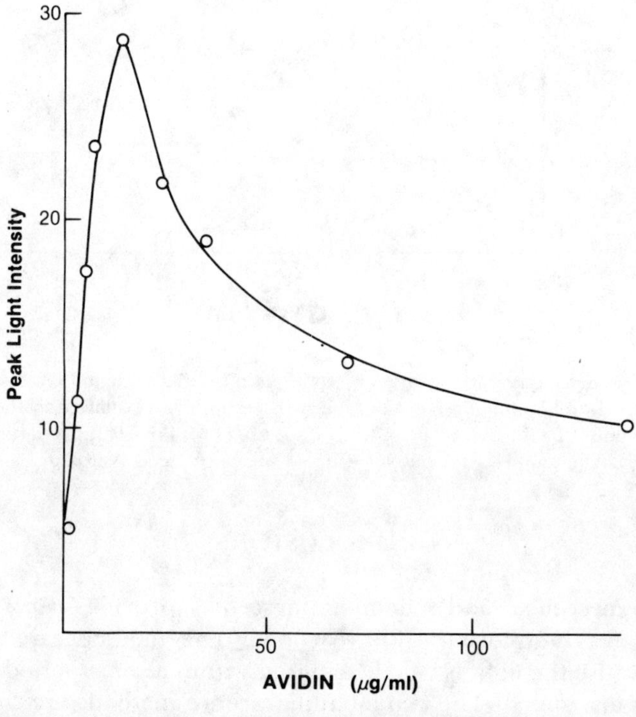

Fig. 10. Effect of avidin on PLI produced with biotinyl-isoluminol. Binding reactions (140 μl) containing 84 n*M* biotinyl-isoluminol and various levels of avidin in 0.1 *M* Tris-HCl, pH 7.4, were incubated for 15 min. Then 10 μl of lactoperoxidase (2 U) was added and after 2 min, 10 μl of 0.95% H_2O_2 was injected to initiate light production. PLI values measured with the Biometer are averages of triplicate assays.

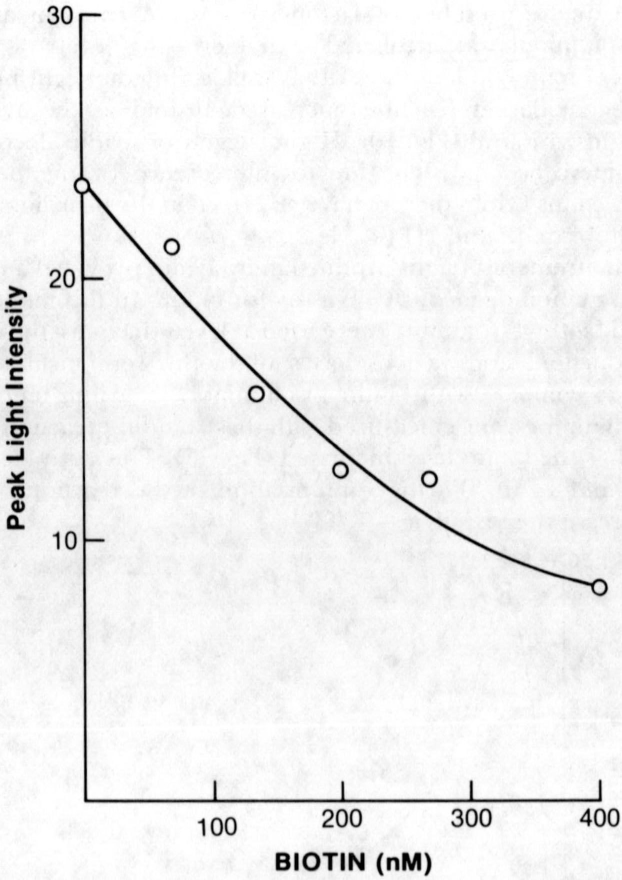

Fig. 11. Homogeneous CPB assay for biotin monitored by chemiluminescence. The indicated levels of biotin and 90 n*M* of biotinyl-isoluminol were allowed to compete for a limiting amount of avidin (3.65 μg/ml) in 140 μl of 0.1 *M* Tris-HCl, pH 7.4. After 5 min incubation, chemiluminescence measurements were performed as in Fig. 10.

CONCLUSIONS

Bioluminescence and chemiluminescence provide very sensitive methods for monitoring CPB reactions. The methods are relatively rapid because the light is usually emitted within a short period after the reactants are mixed. The two bioluminescence methods are convenient because separation of protein bound and free labeled ligands is not necessary. The most prominent shortcoming is interference by endogenous cofactors and degradative enzymes in the sample being assayed. This problem is very significant with serum.

The chemiluminescence method is particularly notable for its sensitivity and the stability of the chemilumigenic labels. The sensitivity is similar to that achieved with radiolabels. Although a homogeneous chemiluminescence CPB method has been demonstrated, interference by materials in the sample being assayed could be a serious problem. However, heterogeneous chemiluminescence CPB assays offer considerable promise because of their sensitivity and the stability of the labels.

REFERENCES

1. R.S. Yalow, *Pharmacol Rev* **25**:161, 1973.
2. J.P. Ransom, *Practical Competitive Binding Assay Methods,* C.V. Mosby, St. Louis, 1976.
3. K.E. Rubenstein, R.S. Schneider, and E.F. Ullman, *Biochem Biophys Res Commun* **47**: 846, 1972.
4. G.B. Wisdom, *Clin Chem* **22**, 1243, 1976.
5. A. Schuurs and B.K. Van Veemen, *Clin Chim Acta* **81**:1, 1977.
6. J.F. Burd, R.J. Carrico, M.C. Fetter, R.T. Buckler, R.D. Johnson, R.C. Boguslaski, and J.E. Christner, *Anal Biochem* **77**:56, 1977.
7. R.A.A. Watson, J. Landon, E.J. Shaw, and D.S. Smith, *Clin Chim Acta* **73**:51 (1976.
8. H.R. Schroeder, R.J. Carrico, R.C. Boguslaski, and J.E. Christner, *Anal Biochem* **72**:283, 1976.
9. R.J. Carrico, K-K Yeung, H.R. Schroeder, R.C. Boguslaski, R.T. Buckler, and J.E. Christner, *Anal Biochem* **76**:95, 1976.
10. H.R. Schroeder, P.O. Vogelhut, R.J. Carrico, R.C. Boguslaski, and R.T. Buckler, *Anal Chem* **48**:1933, 1976.
11. H.R. Schroeder and F.M. Yeager, *Anal Chem* **50**:1114, 1978.
12. H.R. Schroeder, F.M. Yeager, R.C. Boguslaski, and P.O. Vogelhut, *J Immunol Methods* **25**:275, 1979.
13. S.E. Brolin, E. Borglund, L. Teguer, and G. Wettermark, *Anal Biochem* **42**:124, 1971.
14. P.E. Stanley, *Anal Biochem* **39**:441, 1971.
15. J.W. Hastings, *Ann Rev Biochem* **37**:597, 1968.
16. L.M. Aledort, R.I. Weed, and S.B. Troup, *Anal Biochem* **17**:268, 1966.
17. H. Holmsen, I. Holmsen, and A. Bernhardsen, *Anal Biochem* **17**:456, 1966.
18. U. Isacsson and G. Wettermark, *Anal Chim Acta* **68**:339, 1974.
19. R.B. Brundrett, D.F. Roswell, and E.H. White, *J Am Chem Soc* **94**:7536, 1972.
20. K.-D. Gundermann and M. Drawert, *Chem Berichte* **95**:218, 1962.
21. H.R. Schroeder, R.C. Boguslaski, R.J. Carrico, and R.T. Buckler, *In Methods Enzymol, Vol. 57,* M. DeLuca (ed.), Academic, New York 1978, p. 424.

Chapter 12

Nephelometric Immunoassay Techniques*

JOHN SAVORY, Ph.D.

INTRODUCTION

Quantitative immunochemical methods involving the direct reaction of antigen and antibody are the most direct, technically simple, and rugged of all immunochemical techniques. Although these methods have not made much impact on hormone analysis due to sensitivity problems, they have contributed considerably to the measurement of specific proteins in biological fluids. Quantitative immunochemistry was introduced by Heidelberger and Kendall in their classic work on the precipitin reaction between Type III pneumococcus polysaccharide and its homologous antibody.[1-3] These investigations provided the theoretical basis for the development of a series of analytical methods for the determination of specific proteins. The technique was first applied in a clinical situation by Goettsch and Kendall[4] for the estimation of albumin and globulin in human serum. Subsequent studies involved estimation of protein in other body fluids of interest in a variety of diseases,[5-7] and the diagnostic value of protein measurements became well established.

Beginning in 1946, several procedures were developed that were based on the migration of the antigen and an antibody molecule through an agar gel matrix. The simple diffusion system of Oudin[8] was the first to employ this principle; this method can be both precise and sensitive, and is still a useful tool for measurement of proteins in dilute solutions. The Oudin system was followed by the technique of immunoelec-

*This chapter is based in part on a paper presented by the author at a College of American Pathologists' meeting on Diagnostic Immunology: Current and Future Trends, Aspen, Colorado, September, 1978.

trophoresis,[9,10] used extensively in the classification of monoclonal gammopathies of various types, and deficiencies of certain serum proteins.[11,12] Radial immunodiffusion, introduced by Mancini et al.[13] and other workers,[14,15] brought about a new era in the immunochemical measurement of proteins in biological fluids. This method gained wide popularity not attained by those described previously, and has retained that popularity to the present time. Radial immunodiffusion is deficient, however, in that it is imprecise, time consuming, and lacks the sensitivity required to detect most proteins in unconcentrated cerebrospinal fluid and urine.

Determination of the concentration of proteins by electrophoresis into antibody-containing agarose gel was introduced by Laurell[16,17] at about the same time that Mancini et al.[13] published their work on radial immunodiffusion. The technique, known as electroimmunodiffusion, differs from radial immunodiffusion in that an electrical field is employed to force migration of the antigen into the gel. In some cases, as little as 0.1 μg of antigen can be detected. Many human proteins have been measured by electroimmunodiffusion in a few specialized laboratories, but it has not attained widespread use since numerous technical details must be mastered in order to obtain acceptable results. However, electroimmunodiffusion has many advantages over radial immunodiffusion.

As an alternative to the analysis of proteins through their migration in a gel, the precipitin reaction may be quantitated by optical measurements of aqueous solutions. In 1947, Boyden and coworkers[18] introduced the concept that precipitin curves could be characterized through the measurement of the turbidity that developed in mixtures of antigen and antibody. Their studies showed that turbidity values correlated closely with the actual amounts of precipitate formed in the immunochemical reaction.

This approach was not applied to clinical measurements until Schultze and Schwick[19] published their turbidimetric methods for determining several plasma proteins. Ritchie[20] later improved this technique so that very small amounts of sample and antiserum could be utilized, and measurements could be made on a standard spectrophotometer. Alper et al.[21] also utilized turbidimetric analysis in studies on the inherited deficiency of the third component of complement (C3), but did not discuss details of the procedure. The use of turbidimetric analysis in immunochemistry has been discussed by Leone[22] and Li and Williams.[23]

Interest in quantitation of immunochemical reactions by optical measurements of aqueous solutions has increased in the past few years. The need to automate diagnostic immunochemical tests has resulted in several procedures based on nephelometric measurements of immune complexes. Nephelometric, or light-scattering, procedures usually detect light at a 90° angle to the incident light, and can be performed on slightly modified filter fluorometers; however, recently other angles of detection have been employed. These nephelometric techniques are capable of greater sensitivity than those employing turbidimetry, and are easily automated in either discrete sample or continuous-flow systems.

Eckman et al.[24] reported the first automated immunoprecipitin technique for use with continuous-flow modules. Existing components of the Autoanalyzer system were used to dilute serum samples, provide mixing with antiserum, and make light-scattering measurements for the determination of human transferrin. Analyses were performed at a rate of 60 per hour with good precision and accuracy. This initial study provided the impetus for several other groups of investigators to develop additional manual and automated procedures for analysis of proteins in human serum,[25-31] cerebrospinal fluid,[32-34] and urine.

PRINCIPLE

The specific protein (antigen) in the body fluid reacts with antibody in a specific antiserum to form antigen-antibody (Ag/Ab) complexes, which can be detected by light-scattering techniques. The Ag/Ab reaction can be characterized by a precipitinlike curve such as that shown in Figure 1, which reflects the change in particle size and number caused by increasing Ag/Ab ratios. In this specific example, a series of serum samples containing IgG at concentrations ranging from 500 to 3,000 mg/dl was diluted 1:700 with dust-free physiologic saline. One part of diluted sample was mixed with one part of diluted goat antihuman IgG and, after 40 min at room temperature, Ag/Ab complex formation achieved an equilibrium state and light-scattering measurements were made in a fluorometer with identical excitation and emission wavelengths (360 nm). The first section of the precipitin curve (Fig. 1), where light-scattering intensity increases with concentration of IgG, is termed the antibody excess zone. There is an equivalence zone at the apex of the curve and an antigen excess zone where intensity decreases with increasing IgG concentration. Qualitative data dealing with all zones of the precipitin curve have revealed that Ag/Ab complex size and/or concentration increases through antibody excess, reaching a limiting value at equivalence and then dropping in antigen excess. The pattern is thought to be a function of the antigen-to-antibody site ratio. As the number of antigen sites increases, a greater number of complexes are formed in antibody excess, until site equivalence is reached and a limiting particle size and concentration result. The further addition of antigen results in smaller complexes due to the excess of antigenic sites, and reduced cross-linking between aggregates occurs.

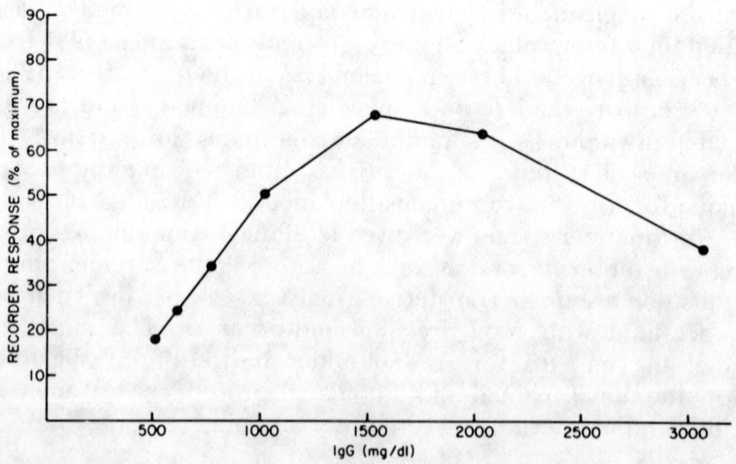

Fig. 1. Precipitin curve for the IgG anti-IgC complex. (Reproduced by permission, *Clin Chem* **18**:337, 1972).

FACTORS AFFECTING LIGHT-SCATTERING PROCEDURES

Reagent Preparation

Exogenous particulate matter such as dust causes serious interferences in light-scattering measurements. All diluent buffer solutions and diluted antisera must be filtered prior to use. Filters with an average pore size of 0.22 μm provide satisfactory results.

Antiserum

Most laboratories rely on antiserum from commercial sources. In all cases the monospecificity of the antiserum should be confirmed by observation of a single precipitin arc on immunoelectrophoresis against whole human serum. The degree of dilution of the antiserum prior to the immunochemical reaction depends on the avidity of the antiserum. Thus a precipitin curve should be constructed with each new batch of antiserum and the dilution adjusted to give adequate sensitivity and a broad range of antigen concentrations in the antibody excess zone.

Wavelength

For nonpolarized incident light, Rayleigh's law states that the intensity of scattered light is inversely proportional to the fourth power of the wavelength, and for this reason a wavelength of 360 nm is used on most commercially available instruments. Higher wavelengths may be used if the source possesses greater intensity. Usually, adequate sensitivity can be achieved up to 650 nm, provided a high intensity source is used. The limiting feature is not the actual total intensity of light scattered but the difference in intensity of the sample in relation to the sample blank. Most biological fluids possess relatively high background light scattering, and reaction conditions must be adjusted so that the immunochemical reaction gives considerably more scatter than the background.

Angular Variation

Traditionally, light-scattering photometers used for measurements of proteins using immunochemical methods measured light scattering at 90°; however, it has been known for many years that increases in scattering intensity can be obtained at angles <90° when large particles are involved. According to Rayleigh, the intensity of scatter from a particle, which is small relative to the wavelength, should be distributed symmetrically about an axis that is at right angles to the incident beam. However, for particles whose dimension is comparable to the wavelength of light used for analysis, destructive interference of the light scattered from individual elements can occur, resulting in a decrease in total scattering measured. Phase difference between scattered radiation, which causes the destructive interference, is reduced as the angle of observation approaches zero, resulting in an asymmetrical scattering envelope and significant angular dependence. Shown in Figure 2 are

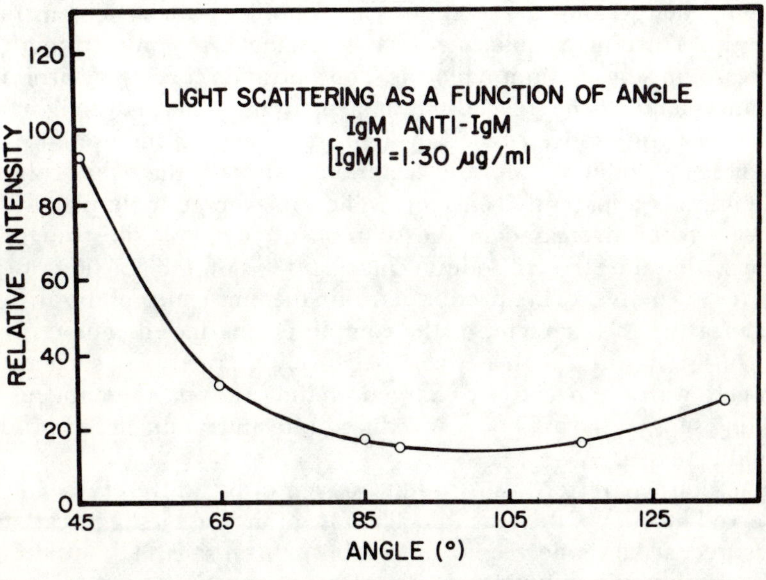

Fig. 2. Change in light scattering intensity as a function of angle for IgM anti-IgM reaction products. (Reproduced by permission, *Clin Chem* **21**:1738, 1975)

angular dependent scattering intensity measurements for a particular Ag/Ab ratio, using the IgM anti-IgM reaction as an example. It is obvious that the scattering measured is least intense at 90° and markedly increased in intensity at smaller angles. If the particles were homogeneous with respect to size and shape, a series of light-scattering maxima and minima should have been observed as a function of the angle of observation, according to the Mie theory. However, no intensity maxima or minima are observed as a function of angle, indicating that the complex population is a polydisperse system with respect to size.

Effects of Temperature, pH, and Urea

Using an IgG anti-IgG model system, the effects of temperature, pH, and a variety of urea concentrations have been studied in our laboratory,[35] and we demonstrated that temperature and pH, if controlled within reasonable limits, causes minimal variations in the Ag/Ab reaction. Urea, which is present in body fluids, sometimes at relatively high levels, has an appreciable effect of inhibiting the reaction. Thus for urine analysis, attention must be paid to the urea concentration of the final reaction mixture in order to ensure that pronounced inhibition of the Ag/Ab reaction does not occur.

Effects of Ions in the Reaction Medium

Using the IgG anti-IgG reaction as an example, it can be demonstrated that this reaction is quite sensitive to changes in ionic strength. A decrease in the sodium chloride concentration exerts a profound enhancement of the reaction rate. Apparent molecular weight and radius of gyration determined by light scattering[36] in the presence and absence of sodium chloride has demonstrated that the complex dimension is apparently constant, while the average molecular weight appears to be decreased in the solution of higher ionic strength. It appears that the effect of sodium chloride is to slow the reaction rate, so that fewer complexes are produced within the time frame of the analysis, while leaving the character of the complexes unaffected. These results are consistent with the theory that negatively charged ions, such as Cl^-, compete with the negatively charged binding sites on the antigens for binding sites on the antibody. A reduced rate and an unaltered product would be expected.

The ion character also produces significant differences in the observed kinetics of the reaction. The rate of increase in light scattering measured at 90° is decreased by certain neutral salts. The efficacy of reduction is in the order $NO_3^- > Br^- > F^-$ (with the same cation) using the IgG anti-IgG systems.[35]

Effect of Polymers and Proteins

Water soluble straight chain polymers have been used to enhance the signal for the Ag/Ab reaction, thereby increasing sensitivity and reducing analysis time.[37] Studying the IgG and anti-IgG system with polyethylene glycol (PEG, molecular weight 6,000) in the reaction medium, there is a lag period in the rate of change in light scattering during the first 5 s of the reaction. After the initial 5 s, however, the rate increases markedly, and the reaction proceeds much more rapidly in PEG (40 g/liter) plus phosphate buffered physiological saline than in phosphate buffered physiological saline alone.

MATERIALS AND METHODS

Instrumentation

The original manual procedures[30,31] involved dilutions made with an automated pipetting device and with light-scattering measurements being carried out on either a filter or grating spectrophotofluorometer. Because of the relative lack of dependence of the measurement on the wavelength of the incident light, filter instruments were found to be quite satisfactory. Most of the early instruments used 90° light scattering on a conventional spectrophotofluorometer. Recently, an instrument dedicated to nephelometry has been introduced, where 90° light scattering is measured, but the incident light appears through the bottom of the cuvette (Kallestad Laboratories, Inc., Chaska, Minn. 55318).

The introduction of near forward light scattering with laser light sources[38,39] has led to the development of two commercial laser nephelometers. The lasers employed are inexpensive helium-neon lasers, which emit light at a wavelength of 632.8 nm. The advantages of using lasers are the intensity of the light, a simplified optical system, and adaptability to forward light-scattering measurements. The Hyland Laser Nephelometer (Hyland, Division of Travenol Laboratories, Inc., Costa Mesa, Calif. 92626) uses an optical configuration with an angle of measurement of 31°. The Behring Laser Nephelometer (Behring Diagnostics, American Hoechst Corp., Somerville, NJ 08876) uses a dark field similar to the first near forward light-scattering system developed in the author's laboratory and which is described later. The angle of measurement with the Behring instrument is from 5 to 12°.

Many tedious dilutions are required for manual systems, and computation of results also is time consuming. For these reasons, the tendency in present-day instrumentation is to use some type of semiautomatic dilutor and to integrate the nephelometer with a microprocessor for calculation of results.

A manual nephelometer that performs analyses using kinetic measurements recently has become available from Beckman Instrument Company (Fullerton, Calif. 92634). This rate nephelometer uses a tungsten/iodine light source, and scattered light is detected at a 70° angle. The instrument measures the rate of increase in intensity of scattered light, and a microprocessor converts the peak rate into concentration. The microprocessor is programmed by a card, which for a specific test carries information for curve fitting, analysis time, antigen excess detection criteria, analyte identification, and instrument gain.

The most widely used automated approaches to nephelometry have been with the centrifugal analyzer and with continuous-flow systems. The first description of the use of a centrifugal analyzer for the measurement of specific proteins was by Tiffany et al.[40] These workers used a miniature centrifugal analyzer modified for fluorescence and light-scattering measurements, the latter being carried out at 410 nm. The cuvettes held 120–150 μl of reaction mixture, with mixing of reactants being accomplished at a Y-junction following acceleration of the rotor with rapid acceleration and deceleration used to ensure complete mixing. Light-scattering measurements could be made approximately 6 s after constant speed was attained. Computer control of the instrument enabled readings of light scatter to be made at any predetermined time.

The major problems with the instrument used by Tiffany et al.[40] are its lack of availability on the commercial market and, even assuming access to the miniature centrifugal analyzer, the extensive modifications necessary for 90° light scattering. In order to adapt kinetic methods to an available commercial centrifugal analyzer, investigations in the author's laboratory led to the modification of existing equipment to measure near 0° angle light scattering.[38,39–43] This approach involved a simple modification of the optical system of a commercial centrifugal analyzer equipped for conventional visible and ultraviolet spectroscopic analysis, with changes being made to allow only scattered light to reach the detector, while blocking out all light coming directly from the source. An Aminco Rotochem II centrifugal analyzer (American Instrument Company, Silver Spring, Md. 20910) was modified with the following three basic changes: replacement of the tungsten-halogen lamp with a helium-neon gas laser (alignment of the laser is most easily accomplished with the rotor removed from the instrument), removal of both lenses located in the optical path, and placement of a dark field between the cuvettes and the detector.

A schematic diagram of the apparatus and dark field disk is shown in Figures 3A and 3B. The optical system consisted of a helium-neon gas laser (Spectra Physics, Mountain View, Calif. 94049, Model 155,

632.8 nm), which has a peak power output of 0.5 mW and is, therefore, a relatively safe laser to use on a routine basis. Long-term stability is rated at 5% of output power drift. A constant-voltage transformer (Sola Electric, Elk Grove Village, Ill. 60007) was used to reduce variation in line voltage reaching the laser. The laser beam was directed through the cuvettes to the detector by means of a mirror positioned at a 45° angle to the incident beam (see Fig. 3A). The primary reason for use of the laser was to minimize the modification of the optical system. The cuvette assembly, made up of 15 cuvettes, was formed from a stainless steel heat pack, which was sandwiched between two pieces of quartz. A dark field was interposed between the cuvettes and the detector, to block out light coming directly from the source, thereby allowing only scattered light to reach the detector.

The dark field was made up of a circular piece of quartz 1.4 cm in diameter and 1.0 mm thick (Fig. 3B). Optical black paint was used to block out an area 4.5 mm wide and 2.5 cm long across the center of the quartz disk. The detector was a custom photodiode with a radiometrically determined optimum range of 250–620 nm. The signal was passed directly from the photodiode through a bandpass-limited amplifier and processed by an analog-digital converter. Data accumulation and averaging were controlled by a PDP/8M minicomputer (Digital Equipment Corp., Maynard, Mass. 01754). A single absorbance or transmittance reading for a cuvette was obtained by averaging the digital signal over eight consecutive revolutions of the rotor to improve the signal-to-noise characteristics. Data were processed by the computer and then displayed by a high-speed 30-character printer terminal.

The concept of a dark field and focused source beam is currently in use in the field of microscopy. The need to use lenses to focus the output

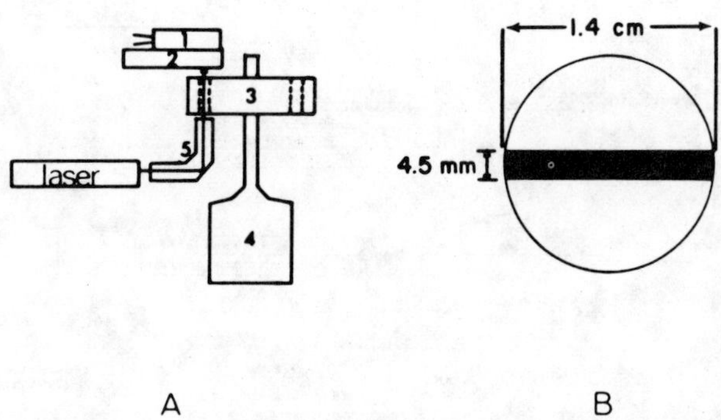

Fig. 3. (A) Schematic diagram of laser-modified parallel fast analyzer: 1, photodiode; 2, interference filter wheel; 3, rotor assembly; 4, centrifuge motor; 5, shielded optical path containing mirror. (B) Dark field design used in present modification of parallel fast analyzer system. (Reproduced by permission, *Anal Chem* **46**:2047, 1974)

from a conventional incandescent source can be eliminated if a laser source is employed. The laser source provides a highly collimated and intense beam, allowing dark field size to remain at a minimum. The combination of a highly collimated source beam and minimum field size allows maximization of the signal-to-noise ratio. Several dark field designs were tested. A relatively high signal-to-noise ratio should be obtainable with a small circular field; however, the use of this type of field resulted in an asymmetrical signal, with large spikes being seen on one edge of the signal from each cuvette. The asymmetrical signals were produced by the intersection of the laser beam with the edge of a cuvette, causing a brilliant flash of light. Other field designs were tested in an attempt to correct this problem. These fields prevented the light flash from reaching the detector but resulted in a decrease in the signal-to-noise ratio. A rectangular dark field, centered on the disk as shown in Figure 3B, provided an acceptable signal-to-noise ratio and eliminated the asymmetrical signal.

The stability of a laser-modified centrifugal analyzer was tested by measuring the light scattered from a stable starch suspension at 30-s intervals over a 5-min time period. The mean relative standard deviation (RSD) for a 5-min interval for 14 cuvettes was 0.68%, which demonstrates exceptional instrument stability.

The earliest approach to automated nephelometric techniques was to use continuous-flow systems (Technicon Instruments, Co., Tarrytown, N.Y. 10591). Continuous-flow techniques provide excellent timing of standards and samples, and it is a simple matter to keep the equipment free of contaminating reagents. Complex multichannel systems have been used in the author's laboratory and are capable of measurement of several antigens simultaneously. A simple system[44] is shown in Figure 4,

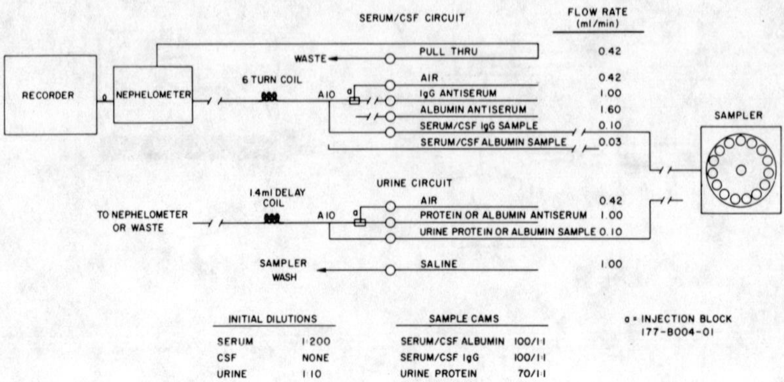

Fig. 4. Multiuse continuous-flow manifold for measurement of specific proteins in serum, CSF, and urine. (Reproduced by permission, *Advances in Automated Analysis,* Mediad Inc., 1977, pp. 274–277)

which is a multiuse manifold for serum, urine, and cerebrospinal fluid analysis. The system consists of a sampler, proportionating pump, time delay coils, fluoronephelometer with 355-nm filters, flow-through cuvette, and recorder. This system is not adaptable to rate measurements but gives excellent results with steady state analysis. Some continuous-flow systems use a predilution circuit; however, in the author's laboratory, it has been found more convenient to make any predilution of the sample with a semiautomated dilutor.

PROCEDURES

The early manual methods using nephelometric techniques involved conventional fluorometers for the final detection of the complexes and used equilibrium measurements without polymer enhancement. Methods were developed for the measurement of specific proteins in serum, urine, and cerebrospinal fluid and involved an initial dilution of the sample, followed by gentle mixing with diluted antiserum and incubation for 15–60 min to allow the Ag/Ab reaction to attain equilibrium. Serum blanks without antiserum were required and light-scattering measurements made in a fluorometer. Light-scattering readings of blanks were subtracted from those of reactions containing Ab/Ab complexes. A multipoint standard curve was constructed and concentrations of unknown samples were obtained by interpolation from this standard curve. The earlier manual methods did not contain PEG in the reaction medium and a relatively long period of time was required for the reaction to achieve equilibrium. Similar approaches have been used recently, using nephelometers with laser excitation sources, with times of one to three hours required for incubation in the absence of PEG. In the presence of PEG, these times are reduced to 30 min.[45]

The first kinetic procedures that were developed employed centrifugal analyzers. As described earlier, Tiffany et al.[40] used a fixed-time kinetic approach with readings at 6 and 60 s on a miniaturized centrifugal analyzer adapted for 90° light-scattering measurements. Methods for serum IgG, IgM, C3, and alpha-1-antitrypsin were described. The rate of the reaction was controlled by varying the amount of PEG in solution. A concentration of PEG of 20 g/liter was used to enable the reaction to proceed to equilibrium fast enough for convenient analysis time, but still allow for an early reading to be used. Fixed-time kinetics can provide for increased throughput and improved precision. In a pseudo-first-order reaction, the change in absorbance between two fixed times is directly proportional to concentration. In monitoring the aggregation phase of an antigen-antibody reaction by light-scattering measurements, the change in intensity (ΔI) is not directly proportional to antigen concentration. However, a plot of ΔI versus antigen concentration produces a plot with characteristics of the precipitin curve, which can be used as an analytical working curve. Advantages of such a kinetic approach are the speed of analysis, which is often less than 2 min, and the elimination of separate sample blank measurements.

Similar procedures have been developed in the author's laboratory for the laser modified centrifugal analyzer,[42,46] with determinations of IgG, IgA, IgM, and C3 and C4 being made using a fixed-time kinetic approach as shown in Table 1. Standardization for all protein assays was accomplished by use of commercial reference sera. Standard curves of change in relative intensity (ΔI) between T_1 and T_2 to concentration of antigen again followed a similar pattern to conventional precipitin curves.

The Beckman rate nephelometer uses a similar approach to that described above and monitors continuously the rate of formation of the complexes. The first derivative of the nephelometric signal is taken as a function of time and is roughly gaussian in shape. This peak signal is used to quantitate the antigen. Under suitable conditions, a maximum reaction rate is obtained within 10–40 s after mixing the antigen with the antibody. There is a subtle change in the rate curve as the concentration changes from antibody excess to antigen excess, making it possible to detect antigen excess samples without reanalyzing a diluted sample.

Continuous-flow systems have been used more extensively than any other light-scattering technique for specific protein measurement. The first procedures developed were carried out in 0.9% saline or phosphate buffered saline, but the use of PEG now has become widespread and offers advantages of speed of analysis and sensitivity over the use of saline alone. In the continuous-flow methods, the Ag/Ab reaction is allowed to achieve equilibrium before the light-scattering measurement is made. Blanks must also be run to correct for intrinsic light scattering of the biological samples. Nonlinear standard curves are constructed in a

Table 1. Fixed-Time Kinetic Determination of IgG, IgA, IgM, C3, and C4 Using a Laser Modified Centrifugal Analyzer

Protein	Sample dilution[a]	Antiserum vol.	T_1	T_2
IgG	1:100	250 μl	15 s	115 s
IgA	1:40	250 μl	15 s	115 s
IgM	1:15	250 μl	15 s	185 s
C3	1:20	250 μl	10 s	150 s
C4	1:9	250 μl	10 s	310 s

[a]All tests used 50 μl of the diluted sample. Reactions were carried out in phosphate buffered saline with a final concentration of 2% PEG.

manner similar to the manual methods. The rate of analysis usually is 60 samples per hour but the necessity of blank measurements halves the throughput.

DETECTION OF ANTIGEN EXCESS SAMPLES

All of the analytical methods have the inherent problem of requiring the detection of antigen excess samples. The precipitin curve shown in Figure 1 demonstrates that two widely varying antigen concentrations will give the same light-scattering response. One concentration is in antibody excess and the other in antigen excess. Since the standard curve is constructed in the zone of antibody excess, it is imperative that antigen excess samples be detected in order that dilution of the sample can be made. The manual discrete sample and centrifugal fast analyzer methods can only detect antigen excess by making a dilution of all samples to see if the response characterizes an antibody or an antigen excess zone. Some mention already has been made of the antigen excess detection on the Beckman instrument. In practice for serum proteins, the method conditions can be adjusted so that zone electrophoresis can be used to screen for those samples that might exhibit antigen excess for any specific protein. In many laboratories, serum samples for protein measurements are subjected to agarose gel electrophoresis, and only in the case of patients with profound hyperimmunoglobulinemia, such as in plasma cell dyscrasias, will antigen excess occur. For urine and CSF proteins, it is advisable to screen for antigen excess using the dilution method.

Continuous-flow analysis possesses a convenient means of detecting antigen excess, since these samples will give a bimodal recorder peak. The reason for this bimodal response is that there is a gradient dilution of sample as it enters the antiserum stream. Thus the reaction starts in antibody excess but soon achieves antigen excess.

STANDARDIZATION

No primary standards exist for nephelometric assays; this is a common difficulty of all methods for measuring specific proteins. Where possible, secondary standards in a serum matrix that have been standardized against the International Reference Standard prepared by the World Health Organization should be used.

SENSITIVITY LIMITS OF NEPHELOMETRY

Many variables enter into estimation of sensitivity limits of nephelometry, such as the nature of the antigen, clarity of the specimen, etc. Using the laser nephelometer, limits of detection of IgE and C-reactive protein in serum appoach 10^{-10} *M*.[47]

APPLICATIONS OF NEPHELOMETRY

A wide variety of analyses have been adapted to the nephelometric technique. A listing of applications from one commercial source (Hyland Diagnostics, Division of Travenol Laboratories, Costa Mesa, Calif. 92626) is shown in Table 2. From this extensive list, the immense potential of this technically simple analytical system is evident.

Serum Proteins

The main contribution of nephelometry to serum protein measurements is in the quantitation of the immunoglobulins, where the accuracy and precision of the analyses probably are superior to those with any other technique. Besides the serum immunoglobulins, some other proteins of importance are alpha-1-antitrypsin for detection of

Table 2. Methods Developed for Laser Nephelometer

Immunoglobulins	Complement	Acute phase protein
IgG	C3	C-Reactive protein
IgA	C4	α_1-Acid glycoprotein
IgM	C3PA	α_1-Antitrypsin
IgD	c1q	Ceruloplasmin
Coagulation	Autoimmune	Carrier proteins
Plasminogen	Rheumatoid factor	Ceruloplasmin
Antithrombin III		Haptoglobin
		Transferrin
		Prealbumin
		Albumin
		TBG
Protease inhibitors	CSF	Miscellaneous
α_1-Antitrypsin	IgG	CSF total protein
α_2-Macroglobulin	Albumin	Urine total protein
CI Esterase inhibitor		Amylase
		Lipase
		Triglycerides
		Antiserum titer
		Human plasma fibrinogen

individuals with a hereditary deficiency of this protein, and haptoglobin, where low values are seen in *in vivo* hemolysis. Some laboratories measure transferrin in place of total iron binding capacity and, obviously, the transferrin results are slightly lower. Albumin may be measured by nephelometric immunochemical techniques, but it is easier to use dye binding methods, provided care is taken to avoid interference from the globulins.[48,49] The acute phase proteins, C-reactive protein, orosomucoid, alpha-1-antitrypsin, haptoglobin, transferrin, and albumin frequently are observed to be altered in hospital patients. The significance of these changes in affecting patient care is still obscure and requires further clinical investigations. Of particular interest is C-reactive protein, which now can be measured using commercially available instrumentation and reagents (Hyland). The third component of complement is of importance in detection of autoimmune disease. A comprehensive summary of changes in serum proteins in disease is shown in Figure 5, which was compiled by L. M. Killingsworth, working in the author's laboratory.

Urine Proteins

The secretion of albuminous urine was recognized by Richard Bright almost 150 years ago as being the hallmark of serious renal disease. Today the examination of the urine for protein is still an important test for renal disease. Measurement of proteins in the urine provides many difficulties for the analyst. In 1914 Folin and Denis reported a procedure utilizing sulfosalicylic acid.[50] Various other techniques have been evaluated since that time to measure albumin and other proteins in urine. The turbidimetric method of Schultze and Schwick[51] was adapted to urinary albumin measurements in 1961, but preconcentration of the sample was required.[52] Concentrated urine also was needed for the semiquantitative detection of albumin, transferrin, and alpha-2-macroglobulin by immunoelectrophoresis[53,54] or radial immunodiffusion.[55-57] Radioimmunoassay procedures possess the sensitivity for quantitation of urinary proteins and have been used to study proteinuria associated with juvenile diabetes.[56-60]

Nephelometric immunochemical methods are extremely useful as routine procedures for measuring proteins in the urine. Work in the author's laboratory led to the development of such procedures for the measurement of urinary albumin, transferrin, and alpha-2-macroglobulin.[61] The methods used the appropriate goat antiserum, and in all cases the precision was better than 5%. Similar automated continuous-flow methods have been developed for urinary total protein and albumin.[62] These methods are sensitive enough to detect protein in normal individuals and have been extremely valuable in providing an accurate assessment of the extent of proteinuria. Also, the differentiation of selective from nonselective proteinuria can be made by measuring these urinary proteins of widely differing molecular weights.

Cerebrospinal Fluid Proteins

The measurement of protein fractions or specific proteins in cerebrospinal fluid (CSF) has been used clinically for many years in the diagnosis of some neurological diseases. Kabat and coworkers[63] first

GUIDE TO PLASMA PROTEIN INTERPRETATIONS

PATHOLOGIC CONDITION	PRE ALB	ALB	OROS	α1 AT	α2 MACRO	HAPTO	TRANS	C3	C4	IgG	IgA	IgM	COMMENTS
INFLAMMATORY RESPONSE													
Acute	↓	↓	↑	↑		↑	↓						The inflammatory response should be considered a fluid process characterized by dynamic changes in the "acute phase reactants". Immunoglobulins increase with infection and/or antigenic stimulation.
Subacute	↓	↓					↓	↑	↑				
Chronic	↓	↓					↓			↑	↑	↑	
LIVER DISEASE													
Chronic Hepatocellular	↓	↓	↑,N	↑,N		↓,N	↓	↓,N		↑	↑	↑,N	β
Biliary Obstruction						↑		↑					β-Lipoprotein is also increased.
PROTEIN-LOSING DISORDERS													
Nephrotic Syndrome	↓	↓	↓	↓	↑	↓↑	↓	↓,N		↓,N	N	↑	β-Lipoprotein is usually increased Haptoglobin loss depends on genetic type.
Diffuse Hypoproteinemia	↓	↓	↓	↓	↓	↓	↓	↓	↓	↓	↓	↓	This pattern can result from nonselective renal or GI protein loss, hemodilution, or malnutrition
PLASMA CELL DYSCRASIAS													
G-Myeloma										↑	↓	↓	
A-Myeloma										↓	↑	↓	These are usually monoclonal increases. Active tumor growth can produce an acute phase reaction.
Waldenstrom's Disease										↓	↓	↑	
ANEMIA													
Iron Defiency						N	↑						
Hemolytic						↓	N						Decreases in C3 and C4 with increases in IgG and IgM can be observed in immune hemolysis.
AUTOIMMUNE DISEASE						↓,N		↓	↓	↑	↑,N	↑,N	SLE can give a cathodal IgG increase.
HYPERESTROGENISM	↓	↓	↓		↑		↑						Ceruloplasmin is also increased.
NEWBORNS			↓		↑	↓		↓		N	↓	↓	IgG is of maternal origin

LEGEND: PRE ALB—Prealbumin; ALB—Albumin; OROS—Orosomucoid; α_1-AT—α_1-Antitrypsin; α_2-Macro—α_2-Macroglobulin; HAPTO—Haptoglobin; TRANS—Transferrin; C3—Complement component 3; C4—Complement component 4; IgG—Immunoglobulin G, IgA—Immunoglobulin A; IgM—Immunoglobulin M; N—Normal; ↑—Increased; ↓—Decreased.

Fig. 5. Summary of plasma protein changes in disease (Reproduced by permission, *Laboratory Management,* March, 1975, pp. 30–34)

noted the importance of elevated CSF gamma-globulin fraction, which was abnormally increased in demyelinating disease.[64] It was further noted that the analytical data most characteristic of multiple sclerosis were those of an increased percentage of IgG relative to the CSF total protein. Other studies have confirmed this observation and have established quantitation of CSF IgG as an aid in the diagnosis of multiple sclerosis, subacute sclerosing panencephalitis, and neurosyphilis.[65-67] Infections of the central nervous system also result in increases of CSF immunoglobin concentration.

Various methods have been used for the determination of CSF protein fractions. In 1948 Kabat et al.[68] utilized immunoprecipitation to quantitate CSF immunoglobulins and achieved excellent results. The complexity of the immunoprecipitation technique makes it unsuitable, however, for routine clinical work. Immunoelectrophoresis has been employed for the estimation of CSF IgG, but these semiquantitative data are of limited value. Electrophoresis of CSF on cellulose acetate or agar gel usually requires concentration of the sample. The sensitivity of electroimmunodiffusion has allowed several investigators to measure specific proteins in small volumes of CSF without prior concentration. Simultaneous measurement of albumin and IgG by electroimmunodiffusion provides an IgG/albumin quotient that is as discriminative for multiple sclerosis as the IgG/total protein ratio.[69] Radial immunodiffusion of CSF has met with some success, but the lack of sensitivity of this technique makes it less than ideal. A simple procedure was introduced in 1970 by Laffin,[70] who measured IgG in unconcentrated CSF by simple immunodiffusion in narrow-bore glass tubes, as originally described by Oudin.[8] This diffusion technique has been refined in our laboratory[71] and used to measure IgG, IgA, and IgM in CSF. Nephelometric methods that measure immunochemical reactions in aqueous solutions are easily adapted for analysis of CSF proteins.[72-74] Even though the quantity of protein in CSF is very small, the samples are usually clear and cause little background light scattering. This property enables the analyst to obtain sensitivity from the nephelometric technique not attained by other methods.

As stated previously, the main contribution of nephelometric specific protein measurements in the CSF involves the measurement of IgG. Elevation of the percentage of IgG (upper limit of normal is 11%) is indicative of demyelinating disease. Unfortunately, the IgG in the CSF is related to the concentration in serum and, therefore, efforts have been made to minimize this effect. Ganrot and Laurell[75] introduced the simultaneous measurement of IgG and albumin in CSF and serum and plotted the results on a graph as shown in Figure 6. Individuals without demyelinating disease fall within the area outlined by the broken line. Patients with local production of IgG within the central nervous system

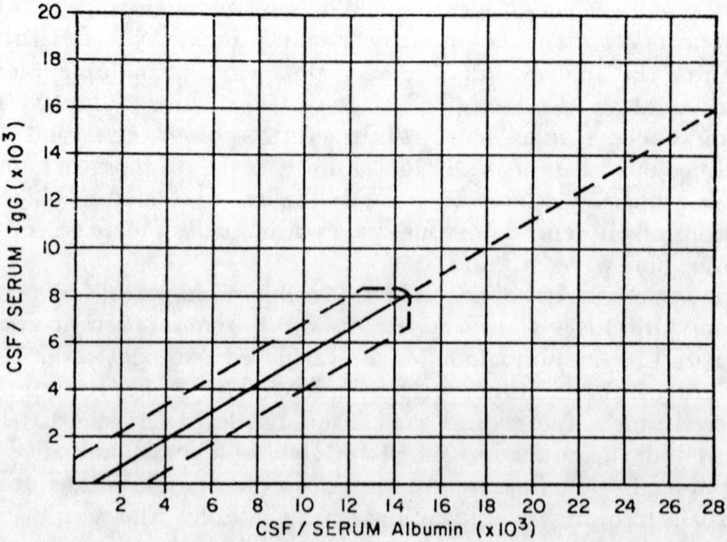

Fig. 6. Plot of CSF/serum IgG against CSF/serum albumin. Hatched line encloses patients with no local production of IgG in the central nervous system.

fall above the broken line area. The reason for this type of analysis is to eliminate the effects of serum proteins crossing the "blood-brain barrier" into the CSF. Albumin is not synthesized locally within the central nervous system and provides an adequate means of assessing serum protein passage into the CSF. Nephelometry provides a convenient means of measuring all of these proteins both in the serum and CSF.

CONCLUSIONS

Many factors must be taken into consideration in choosing a system for the nephelometric measurement of specific proteins. Since the standard curve is nonlinear, several standards are required and the tedium of analyzing all of the standards as well as unknowns makes automated techniques appear extremely attractive. The choice between continuous-flow and kinetic discrete sample analytical techniques will depend on the availability of equipment. Both have advantages and disadvantages. The continuous-flow methods require sample blanks but offset this inconvenience by providing ready detection of antigen excess samples. The kinetic centrifugal fast analyzer procedures do not require blanks but require a separate analysis for detecting antigen excess. Some innovative development obviously is necessary to detect antigen excess for these kinetic techniques, and it is possible that monitoring reaction rates over the first few seconds of the reaction might be used. It has been demonstrated[76] that reactions carried out with antigen in large excess exhibit a very rapid initial rate (0–5 s), which subsequently becomes constant, while a reaction in which the antigen concentration is low (antibody excess) proceeds much slower initially (0–5 s), but continues to show increases in light scattering over a longer time period.

Polymer enhancement of reactions increases both the speed and sensitivity of the Ag/Ab reaction and now is used with all systems. The angle of measurement usually is 90°, although advantages of increased sensitivity come with other angles, and one centrifugal fast analyzer system employs 180° as the angle of measurement.

Because of the sensitivity, simplicity, and low consumption of antiserum, the use of nephelometric methods for measuring specific proteins should continue to increase in popularity. The precision of the technique is excellent and enhances greatly the clinical value of specific protein measurements in biological fluids.

ACKNOWLEDGMENTS

The author wishes to acknowledge the contributions of his colleagues Drs. G. M. Buffone and L. M. Killingsworth, whose work plays a prominent role in the present review.

REFERENCES

1. M. Heidelberger and F.E. Kendall, A quantitative study of the precipitin reaction between type III pneumococcus polysaccharide and purified homologous antibody, *J Exp Med* **50**:809, 1929.

2. M. Heidelberger and F.E. Kendall, Quantitative studies on the precipitin reaction. The determination of small amounts of specific polysaccharide. *J Exp Med* **55**:555, 1932.

3. M. Heidelberger, F.E. Kendall, and T. Teorell, Quantitative studies on the precipitin reaction: effect of salts on the reaction. *J Exp Med* **63**:819, 1936.

4. E. Goettsch and F.E. Kendall, Analysis of albumin and globulin in biological fluids by the quantitative precipitin method. *J Biol Chem* **109**:221, 1935.

5. K. Goettsch and E.B. Reeves, Observations on the nature of serum proteins in nephrosis. *J Clin Invest* **15**:173, 1936.

6. F.E. Kendall, The use of immunochemical methods for the identification and determination of the serum proteins. *Cold Spring Harbor Symp Quant Biol* **6**:376, 1938.

7. E.A. Kabat, M. Glusman, and V. Knaub, Quantitative estimation of the albumin and gamma globulin in normal and pathological cerebrospinal fluid by immunochemical methods. *Am J Med* **4**:653, 1948.

8. J. Oudin, Méthode d'analyse immunochimique par précipitation spécifique en milieu gélifié. *CR Acad Sci* **222**:115, 1946.

9. P. Grabar and C.A. Williams, Méthode permettant l'étude conjugée des propriés électrophorétiques et immunochimique d'un mélange de protéines: application au serum sanguin. *Biochim Biophys Acta* **10**:193, 1953.

10. J.J. Scheidegger, Une micro-méthode de l'immunoélectrophorèse. *Int Arch Allergy Appl Immunol* **7**:103, 1955.

11. P. Grabar and P. Burtin, *Immunoelectrophoretic Analysis; Applications to Human Biological Fluids,* Elsevier, New York, 1964.

12. M.H.G. Clarke and T. Freeman, Quantitative immunoelectrophoresis of human serum proteins. *Clin Sci* **35**:403, 1968.

13. G. Mancini, A.O. Carbonara, and J.F. Heremans, Immunochemical quantitation of antigens by single radial immunodiffusion. *Immunochemistry* **2**:235, 1965.

14. J.L. Fahey and E.M. McKelvey, Quantitative determination of serum immunoglobulins in antibody-agar plates. *J Immunol* **94**, 84, 1965.

15. K. Lou and E. Shanbron, Immunodiffusion techniques in clinical medicine. II. Radial immunodiffusion. *JAMA* **200**:323, 1967.

16. C.B. Laurell, Antigen-antibody crossed electrophoresis. *Anal Biochem* **10**:358, 1965.

17. C.B. Laurell, Quantitative estimation of proteins in agarose gel containing antibodies. *Anal Biochem* **15**:45, 1966.

18. A. Boyden, E. Bolton, and D. Gemeroy, Precipitin testing with special reference to the measurement of turbidity. *J Immunol* **57**:211, 1947.

19. H.E. Schultze and G. Schwick, Quantitative immunologische Bestimmung von Plasmaproteinen. *Clin Chim Acta* **4**:15, 1959.

20. R.F. Ritchie, A simple, direct, and sensitive technique for measurement of specific protein in dilute solution. *J Lab Clin Med* **70**:512, 1967.

21. C.A. Alper, R.P. Propp, M.R. Klemperer, and F.S. Rosen, Inherited deficiency of the third component of human complement (C'3). *J Clin Invest* **48**:553, 1969.

22. C.A. Leone, Turbidimetric analysis of precipitation reactions. *In Methods in Immunology and Immunochemistry*, Vol. III, C.A. Williams and M.W. Chase (eds.), Academic, New York, 1971, pp. 86–94.

23. I.W. Li and C.A. Williams, Estimation of antigen concentration in complex mixtures by optical density of turbid suspensions. *In Methods in Immunology and Immunochemistry,* Vol. III, C.A. Williams and M.W. Chase (eds.), Academic, New York, 1971, pp. 94–102.

24. I. Eckman, J.B. Robbins, C.J.A. Van den Hamer, J. Lentz, and I.H. Scheinberg, Automation of a quantitative immunochemical microanalysis of human serum transferrin: a model system. *Clin Chem* **16**:558, 1970.

25. L.M. Killingsworth, J. Savory, and P.O. Teague, Automated immunoprecipitin technique for analysis of the third component of complement (C'3) in human serum. *Clin Chem* **17**:374, 1971.

26. L.M. Killingsworth and J. Savory, Automated immunochemical procedures for measurement of immunoglobulins IgG, IgA, and IgM in human serum. *Clin Chem* **17**:936, 1971.

27. C. Larson, P. Orenstein, and R.F. Ritchie, An automated method for quantitation of proteins in body fluids. *In Advan. Automat. Anal. Technicon International Congress, 1970,* Vol. 1, E.C. Barton et al. (eds.), Thurman Assoc., Miami, Fla., 1971, p. 9.

28. C.A. Alper, Automated nephelometric determination of serum haptoglobin, C'3 and alpha-1 antitrypsin. *In Advan Automat Anal Technicon International Congress, 1970,* Vol 1, E.C. Barton et al. (eds.), Thurman Assoc., Miami, Fla., 1971, p. 13.

29. P.F. Wegfahrt, M.B. Fish, F.B. Aldana, and S.B. Aronson, Automated immunoprecipitin determination of albumin in serum. *In Advan Automat Anal Technicon International*

Congress, 1970, Vol. 1, E.C. Barton et al. (eds.), Thurman Assoc., Miami, Fla., 1971, p. 21.

30. L.M. Killingsworth and J. Savory, Manual nephelometric methods for immunoglobulins IgG, IgA, and IgM in human serum. *Clin Chem* **18**:335, 1972.

31. J. Savory and L.M. Killingsworth, Determination of alpha-1 antitrypsin by a nephelometric procedure. *Ann Clin Lab Sci* **3**:43, 1973.

32. R.F. Ritchie and J. Graves, Automated analysis of cerebrospinal fluid proteins. *In Advan Automat Anal Technicon International Congress, 1970,* Vol. 1, E.C. Barton et al. (eds.), Thurman Assoc., Miami, Fla., 1971, p. 25.

33. J. Savory, M.G. Heintges, L.M. Killingsworth, and J.M. Potter, Manual and automated determination of immunoglobulins in unconcentrated cerebrospinal fluid. *Clin Chem* **18**:37, 1972.

34. L.M. Killingsworth and J. Savory, Measurement of immunoglobulins in cerebrospinal fluid employing nephelometric immunoprecipitin techniques. *Clin Chem Acta* **43**:279, 1973.

35. L.M. Killingsworth and J. Savory, Nephelometric studies of the precipitin reaction: a model system for specific protein measurements. *Clin Chem* **19**:403, 1973.

36. G.J. Buffone, J. Savory, and J. Hermans, Evaluation of kinetic light scattering as an approach for the measurement of specific proteins using the centrifugal fast analyser II. Theoretical considerations. *Clin Chem* **21**:1735, 1975.

37. K. Hellsing, Influence of polymer on the antigen-antibody reaction in a continuous-flow system. *Colloquium on A.I.P. and Technicon International Congress,* Vol. 17, 1972.

38. G.J. Buffone, R.E. Cross, J. Savory, and C. Soodak, Measurement of laser-induced near front surface light-scattering with a parallel fast analyzer system. *Anal Chem* **46**:2047, 1974.

39. G.J. Buffone, J. Savory, and R.E. Cross, Use of a laser modified centrifugal analyzer for kinetic measurement of serum IgG. *Clin Chem* **20**:1320, 1974.

40. T.O. Tiffany, J.M. Parella, W.F. Johnson, and C.A. Burtis, Specific protein analysis by light-scatter measurement with a miniature centrifugal analyser. *Clin Chem* **20**:1055, 1974.

41. G.J. Buffone, M.G. Heintges, J. Savory, and L.M. Killingsworth, The kinetic nephelometric measurement of IgG and albumin in serum and CSF using a laser modified Aminco Rotochem centrifugal fast analyzer. *Clin Chem* **21**:943, 1975.

42. G.J. Buffone, J. Savory, A.E. Cross, and J.E. Hammond, Evaluation of kinetic light-scattering as an approach to the measurement of specific proteins with the centrifugal analyzer I. Methodology. *Clin Chem* **21**:1731, 1975.

43. G.J. Buffone, J. Savory, and J. Hermans, Evaluation of kinetic light-scattering as an approach to the measurement of specific proteins with the centrifugal fast analyzer. II. Theoretical considerations. *Clin Chem* **21**:1735, 1975.

44. C.E. Britain, J.D. Butts, and L.M. Killingsworth, CSF/serum specific protein ratios in the diagnosis of neurological disease. *In Advances in Automated Analysis,* E.C. Burton et al (eds.), Mediad, Inc., Tarrytown, N.Y., 1977, pp. 274–277.

45. G.J. Buffone, S. Lewis, J. Savory, and J.M. Hicks, Measurement of proteins in serum, urine and cerebrospinal fluid using laser nephelometry, *In Seminar on Proteins and Proteinopathies,* F.W. Sunderman, Sr. (ed.), Institute for Clinical Science, 1977, pp. 73–79.

46. R.E. White, G.J. Buffone, J. Savory, and L.M. Killingsworth, A rapid nephelometric method for the measurement of C_3 and C_4 in serum using a laser-modified Aminco Rotochem centrifugal fast analyzer. *Ann Clin Lab Sci* **6**:525, 1976.

47. R.J. Russeau, personal communication.

48. J. Savory, M.G. Heintges, M. Sonowane, and R.E. Cross, Measurement of total protein and albumin in serum with a centrifugal analyzer. *Clin Chem* **22**:1102–1104, 1976.

49. S.W. King, R.E. Cross, and J. Savory, Improved specificity of the bromcresol green (BCG) dye method for serum albumin using an early (6 seconds) absorbance reading. *Clin Chem* **23**:1136, 1977.

50. O. Folin, and W. Denis, The quantitative determination of albumin in urine. *J Biol Chem* **18**:273, 1914.

51. H.E. Schultze and G. Schwick, Quantitative immunologische Bestimmung Von Plasmaporteinen. *Clin Chim Acta* **4**:15, 1959.

52. I. Berggard and C. Risinger, Quantitative immunochemical determination of albumin in normal human urine. *Acta Soc Med Upsal* **66**:217, 1961.

53. H.E. Schultze and J.F. Heremans, *Moleculary Biology of Human Proteins,* Vol. 1, Elsevier, Amsterdam, 1966, pp. 670–731.

54. I. Berggard, Studies on the plasma proteins in normal human urine. *Clin Chim Acta* **6**:413, 1961.

55. P.A. Petersson, P.E. Evrin, and I. Berggard, Differentiation of glomerular, tubular, and normal proteinuria: determinations of urinary excretion of beta-2 microglobulin, albumin, and total protein. *J Clin Invest* **48**:1189, 1969.

56. C.R. Joachim, J.S. Cameron, M. Schwartz, and E.L. Becker, Selectivity of protein excretion in patients with nephrotic syndrome. *J Clin Invest* **43**:2332, 1964.

57. J. Poortmans, and R.W. Jeanloz, Quantitative immunological determination of 12 plasma proteins excreted in human urine collected before and after exercise. *J Clin Invest* **47**:386, 1968.

58. H. Keen, M.B. Lond, and C. Chlouverakis, An immunoassay method for urinary albumin at low concentrations. Lancet **ii**:913, 1963.

59. C.E. Mogenson and E. Vittinghus, Urinary albumin excretion during exercise in juvenile diabetes, a provocation test for early abnormalities. *Scand J Clin Lab Invest* **35**:295–300, 1975.

60. D.W. Miles, C.E. Mogenson, and H.J.G. Gundersen, Radioimmunoassay for urinary albumin using a single antibody, *Scand J Clin Lab Invest* **26**:5–11, 1970.

61. L.M. Killingsworth and J. Savory, Nephelometric methods for the determination of urinary albumin, transferrin, and alpha-2 macroglobulin. *Ann Clin Lab Sci* **4**:46–52, 1974.

62. L.M. Killingsworth, C.E. Britain, and L.L. Woodard, Automated immunochemical method for determination of urinary protein of plasma origin, *Clin Chem* **21**:1465, 1975.

63. E.A. Kabat, D.H. Moore, and H. Landow, An electrophoretic study of the protein components in cerebrospinal fluid and their relationship to the serum proteins. *J Clin Invest* **21**:571, 1942.

64. T.F. Hartley, D.A. Merrill, and H.N. Claman, Quantitation of immunoglobulins in cerebrospinal fluid. *Arch Neurol* **15**:472, 1966.

65. H. Link, Immunoglobulin G and low molecular weight proteins in human cerebrospinal fluid. *Acta Neurol Scand* **43**(Suppl. 28): 1, 1967.

66. D. Riddoch and R.A. Thompson, Immunoglobulin levels in the cerebrospinal fluid. *Br Med J* **1**:396, 1970.

67. H. Link and R. Muller, Immunoglobulins in multiple sclerosis and infections of the nervous system. *Arch Neurol* **25**:326, 1971.

68. E.A. Kabat, M. Glusman, and V. Knaub, Quantitative estimation of the albumin and gamma globulin in normal and pathological cerebrospinal fluid by immunochemical methods. *Am J Med* **4**:653, 1948.

69. W.W. Tourtellotte, B. Tavolato, J.A. Parker, and P. Comiso, Cerebrospinal fluid electroimmunodiffusion. *Arch Neurol* **25**:345, 1971.

70. R.J. Laffin, A simple immunologic method for the quantitation of immunoglobulin G in human cerebrospinal fluid. *J Lab Clin Med* **76**:816, 1970.

71. J. Savory and M.G. Heintges, Cerebrospinal fluid levels of IgG, IgA, and IgM in neurologic diseases. *Neurology* **23**:953–958, 1973.

72. R.F. Ritchie and J. Graves, Automated analysis of cerebrospinal fluid proteins. *In Advan Automat Anal Technicon International Congress, 1970,* Vol. 1, E.C. Barton et al. (eds.), Thurman Assoc., Miami, Fla., 1971, p. 25.

73. J. Savory, M.G. Heintges, L.M. Killingsworth, and J.M. Potter, Manual and automated determination of immunoglobulins in unconcentrated cerebrospinal fluid. *Clin Chem* **18**:37, 1972.

74. L.M. Killingsworth and J. Savory, Measurement of immunoglobulins in cerebrospinal fluid employing nephelometric immunoprecipitin techniques. *Clin Chem Acta* **43**:279, 1973.

75. Ganrot and Laurell, Measurement of IgG and albumin content of cerebrospinal fluid, and its interpretation, *Clin Chem* **20**:571–573, 1974.

76. J. Savory, G. Buffone, and R. Reich, Kinetics of the IgG anti-IgG reaction as evaluated by conventional and stopped flow nephelometry. *Clin Chem* **20**:1071, 1974.

INDEX